BIOCHEMISTRY AND MOLECULAR BIOLOGY

FOURTH EDITION

BIOCHEMISTRY AND MOLECULAR BIOLOGY

FOURTH EDITION

Todd A. Swanson, M.D., Ph.D.
Resident in Radiation Oncology
William Beaumont Hospital
Royal Oak, Michigan

Sandra I. Kim, M.D., Ph.D.
Resident in Internal Medicine
Beth Israel Deaconess Medical Center
Harvard Medical School
Boston, Massachusetts

Marc J. Glucksman, Ph.D.
Professor of Biochemistry and Molecular Biology
Director of Midwest Proteome Center
Rosalind Franklin University of Medicine and Science
The Chicago Medical School
North Chicago, Illinois

Wolters Kluwer | Lippincott Williams & Wilkins
Health
Philadelphia • Baltimore • New York • London
Buenos Aires • Hong Kong • Sydney • Tokyo

Acquisitions Editor: Nancy Anastasi Duffy
Managing Editor: Stacey L. Sebring
Marketing Manager: Emilie Linkins
Production Editor: Julie Montalbano
Designer: Holly Reid McLaughlin
Compositor: Circle Graphics, Inc.
Printer: Courier Corporation—Westford

First Edition, 1990
Second Edition, 1994
Third Edition, 1999

Library of Congress Cataloging-in-Publication Data
Swanson, Todd A.
  Biochemistry and molecular biology / Todd A. Swanson, Sandra I. Kim, Marc J. Glucksman.
  — 4th ed.
    p. ; cm. — (Board review series)
  Includes index.
  Rev. ed. of: Biochemistry / Dawn B. Marks. 3rd ed. c1999.
  ISBN-13: 978-0-7817-8624-9 (alk. paper) 1.
Biochemistry—Examinations, questions, etc. 2. Molecular biology—Examinations, questions, etc. I. Kim, Sandra. II. Glucksman, Marc J. III. Marks, Dawn B. Biochemistry. IV. Title. V. Series.
  [DNLM: 1. Biochemistry—Examination Questions. 2. Biochemistry—Outlines. 3. Molecular Biology—Examination Questions. 4. Molecular Biology—Outlines. QU 18.2 S972b 2007]
  QP518.3.S93 2007
  572.8'076—dc22
                    2006020979

To Roberta Swanson

For all your help and dedication on this project and all of my endeavors. Having a mother like you, I know I have been truly blessed.

Preface

We have written this book under the advice of many medical students who have taken the USMLE over the past few years. We have been told many times that it is very hard to find a good biochemistry and molecular biology review book that is high yield enough yet has enough depth to be used as a primary study source. Our advice is to find one review book that is short yet thorough and stick with it, so you become familiar and comfortable with that book under the great time pressure you have.

Even if you feel you have mastered biochemistry and molecular biology as an undergrad, it is important to be aware that medical school biochemistry and molecular biology emphasizes a different knowledge base. When biochemistry and molecular biology is tested on USMLE Steps 1 and 2, it is medical biochemistry and molecular biology that is tested (i.e., why is so-and-so enzyme important in disease and medications, what are knockout mice, how is this enzyme regulated, etc.), rather than strictly basic science biochemistry and molecular biology (i.e., the third enzyme of the Krebs cycle converts what to what, calculate the ΔG, etc.).

This review book focuses on medical biochemistry and molecular biology facts that will be tested on the newly formatted USMLE and will be asked in your medical class group sessions or course exams. We have designed the chapters so that it is easier and faster to look up specific topics you do not understand well. Clinical correlations are included to draw your focus to the function and regulation of genes and proteins that are most relevant to disease or medications. We also include more than 500 questions with explanations both at the end of each chapter and in a comprehensive examination.

In addition, BRS Biochemistry and Molecular Biology Flash Cards are available for use with this book. We welcome your suggestions for improvement, either for the review book or flash cards, so please e-mail us via LWW.com.

Todd Swanson
Sandra Kim
Marc Glucksman

Acknowledgments

We (T.A.S. and S.I.K.) would like to acknowledge, first and foremost, the support and encouragement of Arthur Schneider, M.D. His help has been instrumental in paving the way for us to become medical educators.

M.J.G. would like to thank his family and colleagues for suggestions during this endeavor in medical education. This tome could not have been accomplished without the thousands of students taught in classes and mentored over the last 20 years at three of the finest medical schools. For asking for my participation, I would also like to especially thank two of my recent and most brilliant students . . . my coauthors.

We also would like to acknowledge the help of Michael Myers, M.D. As a medical student, he contributed significantly to the USMLE-style questions found in this book. He has also been a steadfast contributor to our accompanying BRS Biochemistry and Molecular Biology Flash Cards.

Last, but not least, we would like to thank the editors at various levels at Lippincott Williams & Wilkins, including Nancy Duffy, Acquisitions Editor; Stacey Sebring, Managing Editor; and Julie Montalbano, Production Editor. We would also like to thank Dvora Konstant for her fine developmental editing of the book.

Contents

Biomolecules:
Life's Building Blocks

I. Brief Review of Organic Chemistry

- Biochemical reactions involve the functional groups of molecules.

A. **Identification of carbon atoms** (Figure 1-1)

   - Carbon atoms are either **numbered** or given **Greek letters**.

B. **Functional groups in biochemistry**

   - Types of functional groups include: alcohols, aldehydes, ketones, carboxyl groups, anhydrides, sulfhydryl groups, amines, esters, and amides. All of these are important components of biochemical compounds (Figure 1-2).

C. **Biochemical reactions**

   1. Reactions are classified according to the functional groups that react (e.g., esterifications, hydroxylations, carboxylations, and decarboxylations).
   2. Oxidations of sulfhydryl groups to disulfides, of alcohols to aldehydes and ketones, and of aldehydes to carboxylic acids frequently occur.
      a. Many of these oxidations are reversed by **reductions.**
      b. In **oxidation** reactions, electrons are lost.
      c. In **reduction** reactions, electrons are gained.

> cc *1.1*   **Foodstuffs are oxidized** as electrons are released and passed through the electron transport chain. Adenosine triphosphate (**ATP**) is generated and supplies the energy to drive various functions of the body.

II. Acids, Bases, and Buffers

A. **Water**

   1. Water (H_2O) is the **solvent of life.** It dissociates into hydrogen ions and (H^+) and hydroxide ions (OH^-).

   $$H_2O \leftrightharpoons H^+ + OH^-$$

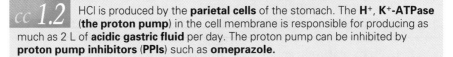

Figure 1-1   Identification of carbon atoms in an organic compound. Carbons are numbered starting from the most oxidized carbon-containing group, or they are assigned Greek letters, with the carbon next to the most oxidized group designated as the α-carbon. This compound is 3-hydroxybutyrate or β-hydroxybutyrate. It is a ketone body.

with an equilibrium constant of

$$K = [H^+][OH^-]/[H_2O]$$

2. Because the extent of dissociation is not appreciable, H_2O remains constant at 55.5 M, and the ion product of H_2O is

$$K_w = [H^+][OH^-] = 1 \times 10^{-14}$$

3. The pH of a solution is the negative $\log_{10}$ of its hydrogen ion concentration $[H^+]$:

$$pH = -\log_{10}[H^+]$$

- For pure water, it's

$$[H^+] = [OH^-] = 1 \times 10^{-7}$$

Therefore, **the pH of pure water is 7**, also referred to as **neutral pH.**

B. **Acids and bases**

- Acids are compounds that donate protons, and bases are compounds that accept protons.

1. *Acids dissociate*
    a. **Strong acids,** such as hydrochloric acid (HCl), dissociate completely.

> cc *1.2*   HCl is produced by the **parietal cells** of the stomach. The **H^+, K^+-ATPase (the proton pump)** in the cell membrane is responsible for producing as much as 2 L of **acidic gastric fluid** per day. The proton pump can be inhibited by **proton pump inhibitors (PPIs)** such as **omeprazole.**

    b. **Weak acids,** such as acetic acid, dissociate only to a limited extent:

$$HA \leftrightharpoons H^+ + A^-$$

    where HA is the acid, and A^- is its conjugate base.
    c. The **dissociation constant** for a weak acid is

$$K = [H^+][A^-]/[HA]$$

2. The **Henderson-Hasselbalch equation** was derived from the equation for the dissociation constant:

$$pH = pK + \log_{10}[A^-]/[HA]$$

where pK is the negative $\log_{10}$ of K, the dissociation constant.

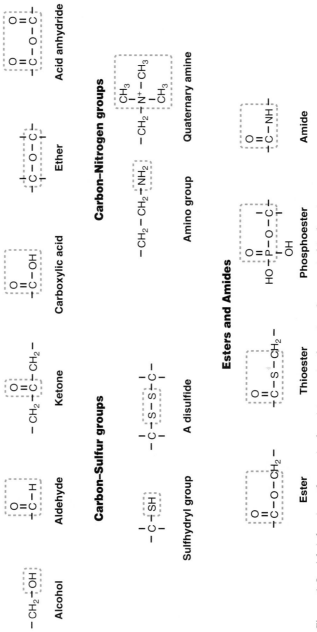

Figure 1-2 A brief review of organic chemistry: major functional groups in biochemistry.

3. The **major acids** produced by the body include **phosphoric acid, sulfuric acid, lactic acid, hydrochloric acid**, and the ketone bodies, acetoacetic acid and β-hydroxybutyric acid. CO_2 is also produced, which combines with H_2O to form **carbonic acid** in a reaction catalyzed by carbonic anhydrase:

$$CO_2 + H_2O \leftrightarrows H_2CO_3 \leftrightarrows H^+ + HCO_3^-$$

> *cc* **1.3**   The **carbonic anhydrase inhibitor, acetazolamide,** blocks the above reaction and is used for the **treatment of glaucoma** as well as altitude sickness.

C. **Buffers**

1. Buffers consist of **solutions of acid-base conjugate pairs,** such as acetic acid and acetate.
    a. Near its pK, a buffer maintains the pH of a solution, resisting changes due to addition of acids or bases (Figure 1-3). For a weak acid, the pK is often designated pK_a.
    b. At the pK_a, $[A^-]$ and $[HA]$ are equal, and the buffer has its maximal capacity.
2. Buffering mechanisms in the body
    • The **normal pH range** of arterial blood is **7.37 to 7.43.**
    a. The major buffers of blood are **bicarbonate** (HCO_3^-/H_2CO_3) and **hemoglobin** (Hb/HHb).
    b. These buffers act in conjunction with mechanisms in the kidneys for excreting protons and mechanisms in the lungs for exhaling CO_2 to maintain the pH within the normal range.

> *cc* **1.4**   Metabolic acidosis can result from accumulation of metabolic acids (lactic acid or the ketone bodies, β-hydroxybutyric acid, and acetoacetic acid) or ingestion of acids or compounds that are metabolized to acids (e.g., methanol, ethylene glycol).

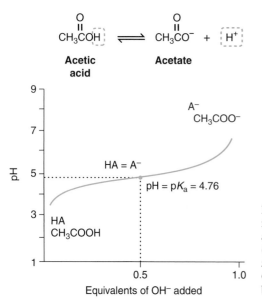

Figure 1-3 The titration curve of acetic acid. The molecular species that predominate at low (acetic acid) and high pH (acetate) are shown. At low pH (high $[H^+]$), the molecule is protonated and has zero charge. As alkali is added, $[H^+]$ decreases (H^+ + $OH^- \rightarrow H_2O$), acetic acid dissociates, and the carboxyl group becomes negatively charged.

> **cc 1.5** **Metabolic alkalosis** is due to increased HCO_3^-, which is accompanied by an increased pH. Acid-base disturbances lead to compensatory responses that attempt to restore normal pH. For example, a metabolic acidosis causes hyperventilation and the release of CO_2, which tends to lower the pH. During metabolic acidosis, the kidneys excrete NH_4^+, which contains H^+ buffered by ammonia:
>
> $$H^+ + NH_3 \leftrightarrows NH_4^+$$

III. Carbohydrate Structure

A. Monosaccharides

1. *Nomenclature*
   a. The simplest monosaccharides have the formula $(CH_2O)_n$. Those with three carbons are called **trioses**; four, **tetroses**; five, **pentoses**; and six, **hexoses.**
   b. They are called **aldoses** or **ketoses,** depending on whether their most oxidized functional group is an aldehyde or a ketone (Figure 1-4).
2. *D and L sugars*
   a. The configuration of the asymmetric carbon atom farthest from the aldehyde or ketone group determines whether a monosaccharide belongs to the D or L series. In the D form, the hydroxyl group is on the right; in the L form, it is on the left (see Figure 1-4).
   b. An asymmetric carbon atom has four different chemical groups attached to it.
   c. **Sugars of the D series,** which are related to D-glyceraldehyde, are the most common in nature (Figure 1-5).
3. *Stereoisomers, enantiomers, and epimers*
   a. **Stereoisomers** have the same chemical formula but differ in the position of the hydroxyl groups on one or more of their asymmetric carbons (see Figure 1-5).
   b. **Enantiomers** are stereoisomers that are mirror images of each other (see Figure 1-4).

> **cc 1.6** The antiepileptic drug **mephenytoin** is **hydroxylated in the S-enantiomer,** which is normally eliminated within hours. The R-enantiomer accumulates, requiring days or weeks for elimination.

   c. **Epimers** are stereoisomers that differ in the position of the hydroxyl group at only one asymmetric carbon. For example, D-glucose and D-galactose are epimers that differ at carbon 4 (see Figure 1-5).

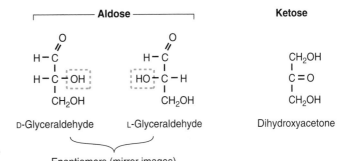

Figure 1-4 Examples of trioses, the smallest monosaccharides.

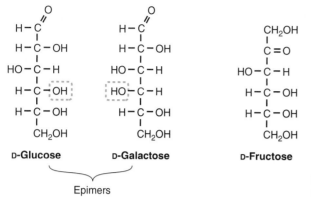

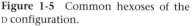

Figure 1-5 Common hexoses of the D configuration.

4. *Ring structures of carbohydrates*

    a. Although **monosaccharides** are often drawn as straight chains (Fischer projections), they exist mainly as ring structures in which the aldehyde or ketone group has reacted with a hydroxyl group in the same molecule (Figure 1-6).

    b. **Furanose** and **pyranose** rings contain five and six members, respectively, and are usually drawn as Haworth projections (see Figure 1-6).

    c. The **hydroxyl group on the anomeric carbon** may be in the α or β configuration.

        (1) In the α **configuration**, the hydroxyl group on the anomeric carbon is on the right in the Fischer projection and below the plane of the ring in the Haworth projection.

        (2) In the β **configuration**, it is on the left in the Fischer projection and above the plane in the Haworth projection (Figure 1-7).

    d. In solution, **mutarotation occurs.** The α and β forms equilibrate via the straight-chain aldehyde form (see Figure 1-7).

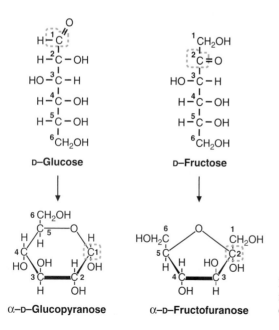

Figure 1-6 Furanose and pyranose rings formed by glucose and fructose. The anomeric carbons are surrounded by *dashed lines*.

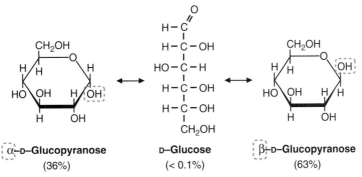

Figure 1-7   Mutarotation of glucose in solution. The percentage of each form is indicated.

B. Glycosides

    1. *Formation of glycosides*

        a. Glycosidic bonds form when the **hydroxyl** group on the anomeric carbon of a monosaccharide reacts with an –OH or –NH group of another compound.

> *CC 1.7*   The **glycoside digitalis** and its derivatives are of clinical significance because they **inhibit the Na⁺-K⁺ ATPase** on cell membranes. Such drugs are used in the treatment of **congestive heart failure.**

        b. **α-Glycosides** or **β-glycosides** are produced depending on the position of the atom attached to the anomeric carbon of the sugar.

    2. *O-Glycosides*

        a. **Monosaccharides** can be linked via *O*-glycosidic bonds to another monosaccharide, forming *O*-glycosides.

        b. **Disaccharides** contain two monosaccharides. Sucrose, lactose, and maltose are common disaccharides (Figure 1-8).

        c. **Oligosaccharides** contain up to approximately 12 monosaccharides.

        d. **Polysaccharides** contain more than 12 monosaccharides; for example, glycogen, starch, and glycosaminoglycans.

    3. *N-Glycosides*

        • Monosaccharides can be linked via *N*-glycosidic bonds to compounds that are not carbohydrates. Nucleotides contain *N*-glycosidic bonds.

C. Derivatives of carbohydrates

    1. **Phosphate groups** can be attached to carbohydrates.

        a. Glucose and fructose can be phosphorylated on carbons 1 and 6.

        b. Phosphate groups can link sugars to nucleotides, as in UDP-glucose.

    2. **Amino groups,** which are often acetylated, can be linked to sugars (e.g., glucosamine and galactosamine).

    3. **Sulfate groups** are often found on sugars (e.g., chondroitin sulfate and other glycosaminoglycans) (Figure 1-9).

D. Oxidation of carbohydrates

    1. *Oxidized forms*

        a. The anomeric carbon of an aldose (C1) can be oxidized to an acid.

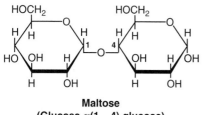

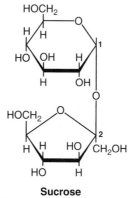

Maltose
(Glucose-α(1→4)-glucose)

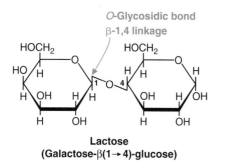

Lactose
(Galactose-β(1→4)-glucose)

Sucrose
(Glucose-α(1→2)-fructose)

Figure 1-8 The most common disaccharides.

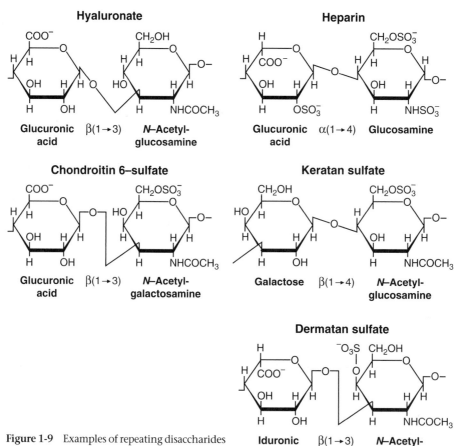

Figure 1-9 Examples of repeating disaccharides of glycosaminoglycans.

- Glucose forms **gluconic acid** (gluconate). **6-Phosphogluconate** is an inter-mediate in the pentose phosphate pathway.

> **cc 1.8** The oxidation of glucose by **glucose oxidase** (a highly specific test for glucose) is used by clinical and other laboratories to measure the amount of **glucose in urine** using a **dipstick.**

  b. **Carbon 6 of a hexose** can be oxidized to a uronic acid.
   (1) Uronic acids are found in glycosaminoglycans of proteoglycans (see Figure 1-9).
   (2) Glucose forms **glucuronic acid.** Conjugation with glucuronic acid makes lipid compounds more water soluble (e.g., bilirubin diglucuronide).

> **cc 1.9** Infants have a **decreased ability to conjugate glucuronic acid** onto drugs such as **chloramphenicol.** Administration of this antibiotic dur-ing the neonatal period can result in elevated plasma levels of the drug and a fetal shock-like syndrome referred to as **Gray baby syndrome.**

2. *Test for reducing sugars*
   - Reducing sugars contain a free anomeric carbon that can be oxidized.
   a. When the anomeric carbon is oxidized, another compound is reduced. If the reduced product of this reaction is colored, the intensity of the color can be used to determine the amount of the reducing sugar that has been oxidized.
   b. This reaction is the basis of the reducing-sugar test, which is used by clinical laboratories. The test is not specific. Aldoses such as glucose give a positive test result. Ketoses such as fructose are also reducing sugars because they form aldoses under test conditions.

> **cc 1.10** Because dipsticks only detect glucose, many clinical laboratories use a chemical test for reducing sugars, a modified **Benedict's Test for Reducing Sugars,** which also will detect the presence of **sucrose, galactose,** and **fructose.** Most newborn and **infant urine is routinely screened** for reducing sugars to detect **in-born errors in metabolism.**

E. Reduction of carbohydrates

   1. The aldehyde or ketone group of a sugar can be reduced to a hydroxyl group, forming a **polyol** (polyalcohol).
   2. Glucose is reduced to **sorbitol,** and galactose to **galactitol.**

> **cc 1.11** **Sorbitol** does not readily diffuse out of cells. As it accumulates in cells, it causes **osmotic damage** to cells of the nervous system, resulting in **cataracts** and **neuropathy.**

F. Glycosylation of proteins

   - Addition of sugar moieties to proteins can alter proteins in many ways including modifying their function, protect them from proteolysis, and direct their intra-cellular traffic, as well as direct cellular movement.

> **cc 1.12** Patients with **leukocyte adhesion deficiency (LAD) II** have a congenital **deficiency in the ability to glycosylate** ligands for cell surface **selectins,** which mediate immune cell migration. Such patients are prone to **recurrent life-threatening infections.**

IV. Proteoglycans, Glycoproteins, and Glycolipids

A. Proteoglycans are found in the extracellular matrix or ground substance of connective tissue, synovial fluid of joints, vitreous humor of the eye, secretions of mucus-producing cells, and cartilage.

1. Proteoglycans consist of a core protein with long unbranched polysaccharide chains (**glycosaminoglycans**) attached. The overall structure resembles a bottle brush (Figure 1-10).
2. These chains are composed of **repeating disaccharide units**, which usually contain a **uronic acid** and a **hexosamine** (see Figure 1-9). The uronic acid is generally D-glucuronic or L-iduronic acid.

> cc *1.13* **Heparin is a glycosaminoglycan,** which is an important **anticoagulant** found in the granules of mast cells. It can be used during the treatment of **myocardial infarction** as well as for the **prevention of deep venous thrombosis** during hospitalizations.

3. The amino group of the hexosamine is usually **acetylated**, and **sulfate** groups are often present on carbons 4 and 6.
4. A xylose and two galactose residues connect the chain of repeating disaccharides to the core protein.

B. Glycoproteins serve as enzymes, hormones, antibodies, and structural proteins. They are found in extracellular fluids and in lysosomes and are attached to the cell membrane. They are involved in cell–cell interactions.

1. The **carbohydrate** portion of glycoproteins differs from that of proteoglycans in that it is **shorter** and often **branched** (Figure 1-11).
   a. Glycoproteins contain mannose, L-fucose, and N-acetylneuraminic acid (NANA) in addition to glucose, galactose, and their amino derivatives. NANA is a member of the class of sialic acids.

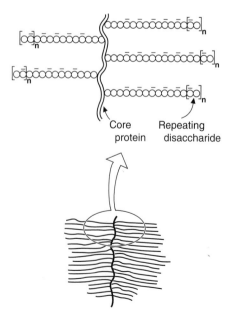

Core protein   Repeating disaccharide

Figure 1-10 "Bottle brush" structure of a proteoglycan with a magnified segment.

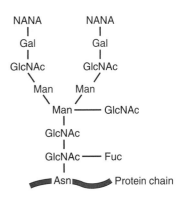

Figure 1-11   Example of the carbohydrate moiety of a glycoprotein. Note that, in this case, the carbohydrate is attached to an asparagine (*N*-linked). NANA = *N*-acetylneuraminic acid, Gal = galactose, GlcNAc = *N*-acetylglucosamine, Man = mannose, Fuc = fucose.

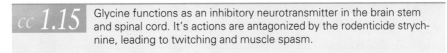

cc **1.14**   The **influenza virus** infects cells by binding its viral hemagglutinin to **sialic acid** on the surface of epithelial cells.

    b. The antigenic determinants of the ABO and Lewis blood group substances are sugars at the ends of these carbohydrate branches.

  2. The carbohydrates are attached to the protein via the hydroxyl groups of **serine and threonine** residues or the amide N of **asparagine.**

C. Glycolipids

  1. Glycolipids (or sphingolipids) are derived from the lipid ceramide. This class of compounds includes cerebrosides and gangliosides.

    a. Cerebrosides are synthesized from ceramide and UDP-sugars.

    b. Gangliosides have NANA residues (derived from CMP-NANA) branching from the linear oligosaccharide chain.

  2. Glycolipids are found in the cell membrane with the carbohydrate portion extending into the extracellular space.

V. Amino Acids

A. Structures of the amino acids (Figure 1-12)

  1. Most amino acids contain a **carboxyl group**, an **amino group**, and a **side chain** (R group), all attached to the α-carbon.

    Exceptions are:

    a. Glycine, which does not have a side chain. Its α-carbon contains two hydrogens.

cc **1.15**   Glycine functions as an inhibitory neurotransmitter in the brain stem and spinal cord. It's actions are antagonized by the rodenticide strychnine, leading to twitching and muscle spasm.

    b. Proline, in which the nitrogen is part of a ring, and is an **imino acid.**

  2. All of the 20 amino acids, except glycine, are of the L configuration. Because glycine does not contain an asymmetric carbon atom, it is not optically active, and thus, it is neither D nor L.

  3. The **classification** of amino acids is based on the chemistry of their side chains.

    a. Hydrophobic amino acids have side chains that contain **aliphatic** groups (valine, leucine, and isoleucine) or **aromatic groups** (phenylalanine, tyrosine, and tryptophan) that can form hydrophobic interactions.

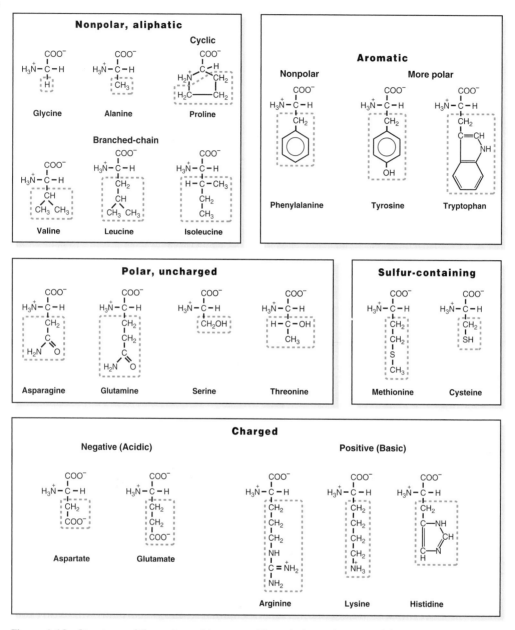

Figure 1-12 Structures of the amino acids, grouped by polarity and structural features.

- **Tyrosine** has a phenolic group that carries a negative charge above its pK_a (≈ 10.5), so it is not hydrophobic in this pH range.
  b. **Hydroxyl groups** found on serine and threonine can form hydrogen bonds.
  c. **Sulfur** is present in cysteine and methionine.
  - The **oxidation** of the **sulfhydryl groups** of two cysteines can form a **disulfide bond**, producing cystine.
  d. **Ionizable groups** are present on the side chains of seven amino acids. They can **carry a charge**, depending on the pH. When charged, they can form **electrostatic interactions**.

e. Amides are present on the side chains of asparagine and glutamine.
f. The side chain of **proline forms a ring** with the nitrogen attached to the α-carbon.

B. **Charges on amino acids** (Figure 1-13)
1. *Charges on α-amino and α-carboxyl groups*
   - At physiologic pH, the **α-amino group** is protonated ($pK_a \approx 9$) and carries a **positive charge**, and the **carboxyl group** is dissociated ($pK_a \approx 2$) and carries a **negative charge**.
2. *Charges on side chains*
   a. **Positive charges** are present on the side chains of the basic amino acids **arginine, lysine,** and **histidine** at pH 7.
   b. **Negative charges** are present on the side chains of the acidic amino acids **aspartate and glutamate** at pH 7.

> *cc 1.16* Glutamate is the amino acid in the highest concentration in the brain and functions as a neurotransmitter in the brain and spinal cord. Memantine is an anti-glutamatergic drug used for treatment in Alzheimer's disease. Glutamate antagonism is implicated in schizophrenia, where drugs of abuse, like ketamine and phencyclidine, affect glutamate binding to its receptor.

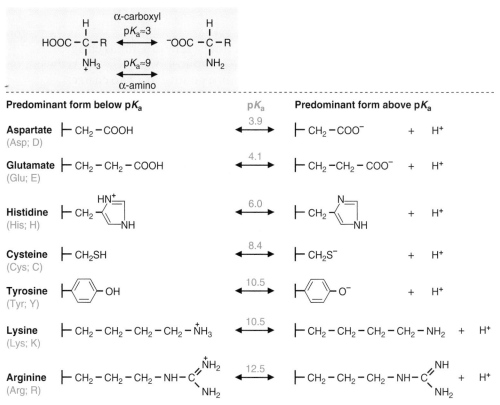

Figure 1-13 Side chains that are ionizable. For each amino acid, the species that predominates at a pH below the pK_a is shown on the left; the species that predominates at a pH above the pK_a is shown on the right. Note that the charge changes from 0 to– or from + to 0. At the pK_a, equal amounts of both species are present.

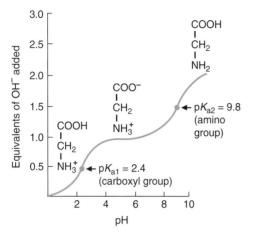

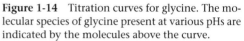

Figure 1-14 Titration curves for glycine. The molecular species of glycine present at various pHs are indicated by the molecules above the curve.

c. The isoelectric point (pI) is the pH at which the number of positive charges equals the number of negative charges.

C. Titration of amino acids

- Ionizable groups on amino acids carry protons at low pH (high [H⁺]) that dissociate as the pH increases.
1. For an amino acid that does not have an ionizable side chain, two pKₐs are observed during titration (Figure 1-14).
   a. The first (**pKₐ₁**) corresponds to the **α-carboxyl group** (pKₐ₁ ≈ 2). As the proton dissociates, the carboxyl group goes from a zero to a minus charge.
   b. The second (**pKₐ₂**) corresponds to the **α-amino group** (pKₐ₂ ≈ 9). As the proton dissociates, the amino group goes from a positive to a zero charge.
2. For an amino acid with an ionizable side chain, **three pKₐs** are observed during titration (Figure 1-15).
   a. The α-carboxyl and α-amino groups have pKₐs of about 2 and 9, respectively.
   b. The **third pKₐ** varies with the amino acid and depends on the pKₐ of the side chain (see Figure 1-15).

D. Peptide bonds

- Peptide bonds covalently join the α-carboxyl group of each amino acid to the α-amino group of the next amino acid in the protein chain (Figure 1-16).
1. *Characteristics*
   a. The **atoms** involved in the peptide bond form a **rigid, planar unit.**
   b. Because of its **partial double-bond character**, the planar peptide bond itself has no freedom of rotation.
   c. However, the bonds involving the **α-carbon** can **rotate freely.**
2. Peptide bonds are extremely stable. Cleavage generally involves the hydrolytic action of proteolytic enzymes.

VI. Lipids

A. Fatty acids exist "free" or esterified to glycerol (Figure 1-17).

1. In humans, fatty acids usually have an even number of carbon atoms, are 16 to 20 carbon atoms in length, and may be saturated or unsaturated (containing dou-

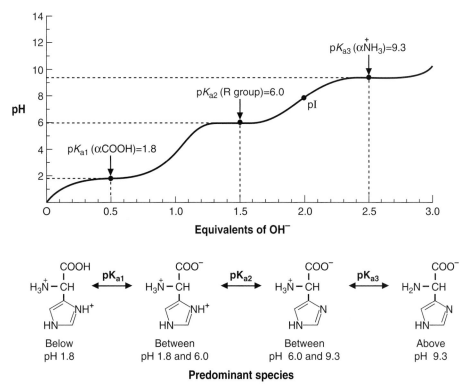

Predominant species

Figure 1-15 Titration curves for histidine. For histidine, pK_{a2} is the dissociation constant of the imidazole (side chain) group.

ble bonds). They are described by the number of carbons and the positions of the double bonds (e.g., arachidonic acid, which has 20 carbons and 4 double bonds, is $20:4,\Delta^{5,8,11,14}$).

2. Polyunsaturated fatty acids are often classified according to the position of the first double bond from the ω-end (the carbon furthest from the carboxyl group; e.g., ω-3 or ω-6).

B. **Monoacylglycerols (monoglycerides), diacylglycerols (diglycerides), and triacylglycerols (triglycerides)** contain one, two, and three fatty acids esterified to glycerol, respectively.

C. **Phosphoglycerides** contain fatty acids esterified to positions 1 and 2 of the glycerol moiety and a phosphoryl group at position 3 (e.g., phosphocholine).

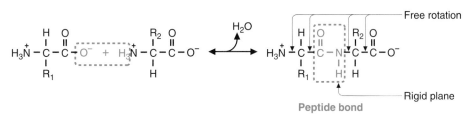

Figure 1-16 The peptide bond.

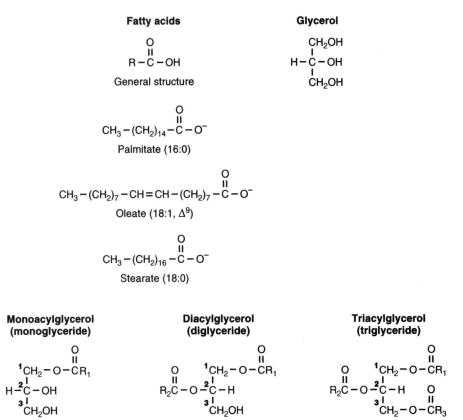

Figure 1-17 The structures of fatty acids, glycerol, and the acylglycerols. *R* indicates a linear aliphatic chain. Fatty acids are identified by the number of carbons and the number of double bonds and their positions (e.g., 18:1, Δ^9).

D. **Sphingolipids** contain ceramide with a variety of groups attached.

1. Sphingomyelin contains phosphocholine.
2. Cerebrosides contain a sugar residue.
3. Gangliosides contain a number of sugar residues.

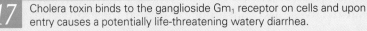

cc 1.17 Cholera toxin binds to the ganglioside Gm_1 receptor on cells and upon entry causes a potentially life-threatening watery diarrhea.

E. **Cholesterol** contains four rings and an aliphatic side chain.

• Bile salts and steroid hormones are derived from cholesterol.

F. **Prostaglandins and leukotrienes** are derived from polyunsaturated fatty acids such as arachidonic acid.

G. **The fat-soluble vitamins** include vitamins A, D, E, and K.

VII. Membranes

A. Membrane structure

1. **Membranes** are composed mainly of lipids and proteins (Figure 1-18).

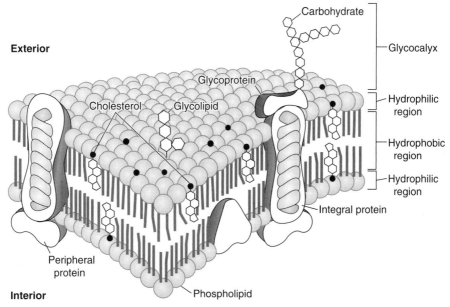

Figure 1-18   The structure of the cell membrane.

2. Phosphoglycerides are the major membrane lipids, but sphingolipids and cholesterol are also present.
   • **Phospholipids** form a bilayer, with their hydrophilic head groups interacting with water on both the extracellular and intracellular surfaces and their hydrophobic fatty acyl chains in the central portion of the membrane.
3. Peripheral proteins are attached at the periphery of the membrane; integral proteins span from one side of the membrane to the other.
4. Carbohydrates are attached to proteins and lipids on the exterior side of the cell membrane. They extend into the extracellular space.
5. Lipids and proteins can diffuse laterally within the plane of the membrane. Therefore, the membrane is termed "fluid mosaic."

> *cc 1.18*   Patients with spur cell anemia have an increased cholesterol content (>40%) in the membranes of their erythrocytes, resulting in decreased membrane fluidity. Membrane fluidity is required for proper movement of erythrocytes through capillaries of the spleen. Thus, erythrocytes from these patients are destroyed in the spleen.

B.   **Membrane function**

1. Membranes serve as **barriers** that separate the contents of a cell from the external environment or the contents of individual organelles from the remainder of the cell.
2. The **proteins** in the cell membrane have many functions.
   a. Some are involved in the **transport** of substances across the membrane.

> *cc 1.19*   The **cystic fibrosis transmembrane regulator** (CFTR) is a chloride ion channel found on cell membranes. Mutation in this protein (the most common of which is the loss of a phenylalanine residue at position 508, known as the ΔF_{508} mutation) results in cystic fibrosis (CF). CF is the most common lethal genetic disease in Caucasians, which results in viscous secretions of the respiratory tract with recurrent life-threatening pulmonary infections.

    b. Some are **enzymes** that catalyze biochemical reactions.

    c. Those on the exterior surface can function as **receptors** that bind external ligands such as hormones or growth factors.

    d. Others are **mediators** that aid the ligand–receptor complex in triggering a sequence of events (e.g., G proteins) known as **signal transduction;** as a consequence, **second messengers** (e.g., cyclic adenosine monophosphate [cAMP]) that alter metabolism are produced inside the cell. Therefore, an external agent, such as a hormone, can elicit effects intracellularly without entering the cell.

VIII. Nucleotides

A. **Nucleotide structure**

    1. Heterocyclic, basic compounds composed of purine and pyrimidines (Figure 1-19)

    2. Derivatives of nucleotides that contain sugars linked to a nitrogenous base are termed **nucleosides.**

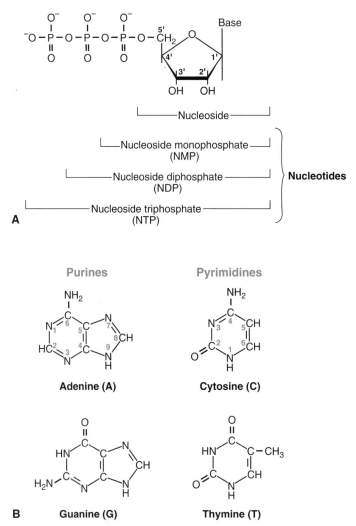

Figure 1-19 Nucleotide and nucleoside. **(A)** Generalized structure. **(B)** Nitrogenous bases.

    a. Ribonucleosides contain the purine or pyrimidine base linked through a **β-*N*-glycosidic bond** to either the **N-1 of pyrimidines** or the **N-9 of a purine** to the sugar **D-ribose.**

    b. Deoxyribonucleotides have a similar structure, but instead, the sugar linked to the base is a **2-deoxy-D-ribose.**

    c. Nucleotides are nucleosides with **phosphoryl groups** esterified to a **hydroxyl group of the sugar.** These can contain one (mononucleotides), two (dinucleotides), and three (trinucleotides) phosphodiester bonds, adding additional high-energy phosphate bonds.

    d. Polynucleotides result from polymerization of dinucleotides through a **3′ to 5′ phosphodiesterase** bond between the phosphate of one monomer to the 3′OH of the pentose sugar.

B. Nucleotide function

    1. Serves as energy stores (i.e., ATP).

    2. Forms portions of several coenzymes (i.e., nicotinamide adenine dinucleotide [NAD$^+$]).

    3. Serves as signaling intermediates (i.e., cAMP, cyclic guanosine monophosphate [cGMP]).

    4. Regulators of enzymatic functions serving as allosteric regulators.

    5. Conveys genetic information (DNA and RNA).

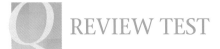

REVIEW TEST

*Directions: Each of the numbered questions or incomplete statements in this section is followed by answers or by completions of the statement. Select the **one** lettered answer or completion that is **best** in each case.*

1. What functional groups are present in the following molecule?

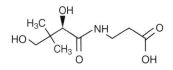

(A) Ketone, alcohol, amide, aldehyde
(B) Esther, ketone, alcohol, amide
(C) Carboxylic acid, amide, alcohol
(D) Alcohol, amide, carboxylic acid
(E) Thioester, quaternary amine, acid anhydride

2. The conversion of β-hydroxybutyrate to acetoacetate occurs by what type of reaction?

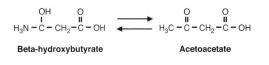

Beta-hydroxybutyrate   **Acetoacetate**

(A) Oxidation
(B) Reduction
(C) Dehydration
(D) Dehydroxylation
(E) Esterification

3. If the pK_a of a weak acid is 5.4, at physiologic pH (7.4), the acid would be:

(A) almost completely protonated.
(B) almost completely unprotonated.
(C) approximately 90% protonated.
(D) approximately 90% unprotonated.
(E) approximately 50% protonated.

4. Which of the values below is nearest to the concentration of hydrogen ion in blood?

(A) 4 M
(B) 7 M
(C) 6 mM
(D) 0.00000004 M
(E) 1 M

5. A solution contains 2×10^{-3} moles per liter of a weak acid (pK = 3.5) and 2×10^{-3} moles per liter of its conjugate base. Its pH is what?

(A) 4.1
(B) 3.9
(C) 3.5
(D) 3.1
(E) 2.7

6. The sugar shown below:

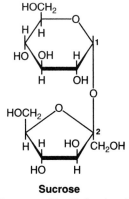

Sucrose
(Glucose-α(1→2)-fructose)

(A) contains a β-1,4-glycosidic bond.
(B) is cleaved by lactase.
(C) undergoes mutarotation.
(D) contains a pentose sugar.
(E) is sucrose (table sugar).

7. The enzyme that interconverts UDP-galactose and UDP-glucose is called an epimerase. This name is appropriate because glucose and galactose are epimers, which means that they are:

(A) mirror images of each other.
(B) ketoses rather than aldolases.
(C) hexoses of the L configuration.
(D) monosaccharides that differ only in the position of one hydroxyl group.
(E) disaccharides that contain a β-1, 4-glycosidic bond.

8. In sickle cell anemia, the hemoglobin molecule (HbS) is abnormal. If the β chains of normal hemoglobin (HbA) and HbS have the N-terminal sequences shown below and the chains are otherwise the same, which of the following statements is correct?

HbA: Val-His-Leu-Thr-Pro-Glu-Glu-Lys-Ser-Ala-Val-Thr. . .

HbS: Val-His-Leu-Thr-Pro-Val-Glu-Lys-Ser-Ala-Val-Thr. . .

(A) HbS contains one more hydrophobic amino acid than HbA.
(B) HbS contains one more negative charge than HbA.
(C) Neither HbS nor HbA contains an amino acid that has a side chain with a pK_a of 6.
(D) The entire sequences shown for both HbA and HbS can form α-helices.
(E) HbA and HbS differ by more than one amino acid.

9. Which one of the following characteristics of phospholipids is correct?

(A) They always contain choline and glycerol.
(B) They are an important source of energy during fasting.
(C) They are a major component of membranes.
(D) They are not charged in the body.
(E) They are not soluble in water.

10. Adenosine triphosphate (ATP) is the major energy currency within the cell. Which of the following best describes the type of compound ATP is?

(A) Phospholipid
(B) Imino acid
(C) Nucleotide
(D) Triacylglycerol
(E) Glycoprotein

11. A 67-year-old man suffers from congestive heart failure. He is taking digoxin, which helps the heart to beat more strongly and regularly. Digoxin is an ester that contains a sugar component (glycol) and a non-sugar (aglycone) component attached via oxygen. Digoxin would be best classified as a:

(A) Glycoprotein
(B) Glycoside
(C) Oligosaccharide
(D) Glucosteroid
(E) Thioester

12. A 57-year-old man with a long history of alcohol abuse comes to the emergency room with symptoms of confusion and an enlarged liver on examination. The patient also has a flapping tremor at the wrist (asterixis). He is diagnosed with hepatic encephalopathy, which can be treated with a diet of branched-chain amino acids. Which of the following sets of amino acids would you suggest?

(A) Tryptophan, phenylalanine, tyrosine
(B) Aspartate, glutamate, asparagine
(C) Valine, leucine, isoleucine
(D) Glycine, alanine, serine
(E) Methionine, proline, cysteine

13. A 28-year-old man complains of a rash on his sun-exposed skin, diarrhea, and loss of balance. His urinalysis results are significant for an increase in neutral amino acids. The patient is diagnosed with Hartnup's disease, a defective transport of neutral amino acids in the kidney. Which of the following amino acids would have been found in the urine sample?

(A) Lysine
(B) Phenylalanine
(C) Arginine
(D) Histidine
(E) Glutamate

14. A teenager presents to the emergency room 2 hours after an overdose of salicylic acid (aspirin). The ER physician administers sodium bicarbonate to increase systemic pH. Salicylate anions become trapped within the renal tubule, preventing back-diffusion across the renal epithelium into the patient's systemic circulation. What will be the ratio of aspirin secreted if the renal dialysate has a pH of 6.0 (salicylic acid pKa ≈ 3.0)?

(A) 10,000:1
(B) 1000:1

(C) 100:1

(D) 1:100

(E) 1:1000

15. A young infant, who was nourished with a synthetic formula, had a sugar in the blood and urine. This compound gave a positive reducing-sugar test but was negative when measured with glucose oxidase. Treatment of blood and urine with acid (which cleaves glycosidic bonds) did not increase the amount of reducing sugar measured. Which of the following compounds is most likely to be present in this infant's blood and urine?

(A) Glucose

(B) Fructose

(C) Sorbitol

(D) Maltose

(E) Lactose

16. A medical student is assigned to a patient in the intensive care unit. A review of the patient's medications shows that he is given a proton pump inhibitor (PPI). This class of drugs inhibits the production of which of the following major acids produced by the body?

(A) Phosphoric acid

(B) Sulfuric acid

(C) Lactic acid

(D) β-Hydroxybutyric acid

(E) Hydrochloric acid

17. A 76-year-old woman who is bed bound in a nursing home begins to develop swelling of her left leg. She is evaluated with venous Doppler ultrasound and is found to have a deep vein thrombosis. She is immediately started on heparin to further prevent the clot from enlarging. Heparin is an example of a:

(A) sphingolipid.

(B) cerebroside.

(C) ganglioside.

(D) glycosaminoglycan.

(E) prostaglandin.

18. A 46-year-old longshoreman is brought to the emergency room with muscle twitching, spasms, and difficulty swallowing. Apparently, the cargo container he was unloading from Indonesia contained the rodenticide strychnine. Strychnine interferes with one of the functions of which of the following nonpolar, aliphatic amino acids?

(A) Tyrosine

(B) Asparagine

(C) Glycine

(D) Glutamate

(E) Lysine

19. A 43-year-old, alcoholic male has been taking the drug cimetidine for gastric reflux. His primary care physician warns that this is not a good idea given his poor liver function, and therefore, his decreased ability to metabolize the drug by glucuronidation. Glucuronidation involves the addition of a glucose molecule that has been changed by which of the following mechanisms to form gluconic acid?

(A) Oxidation

(B) Sulfonation

(C) Reduction

(D) Phosphorylation

(E) Mutarotation

20. A newborn girl is delivered after her mother had an uncomplicated 9-month pregnancy. The family is concerned because their 10-year-old son has been diagnosed with cystic fibrosis and has already developed several severe pulmonary infections requiring hospitalization. They request that their pediatrician order a sodium chloride sweat test to determine if their newborn daughter has the disease. The disease is due to a defect in which of the following?

(A) A peripheral membrane protein

(B) A transmembrane protein

(C) Increased cholesterol content of the lipid bilayers

(D) An enzyme

(E) The ability to glycosylate ligands for selectins

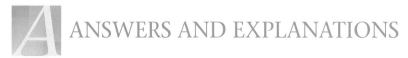

ANSWERS AND EXPLANATIONS

1–D. The molecule shown is vitamin B_5, pantothenic acid, which contains a primary and secondary alcohol, an amide, and a carboxylic acid group. This vitamin is a component of coenzyme A, which is involved in the synthesis of cholesterol.

2–A. An alcohol is oxidized to a ketone when β-hydroxybutyrate is converted to acetoacetate. These compounds are ketone bodies.

3–B. Because pK_a – pH – log (protonated/unprotonated) = 1/100, ~99% or almost all of the acid would be in the unprotonated form. At pH 5.4, the acid is 50% unprotonated; at pH 6.4, the acid is 90% unprotonated; at pH 7.4, the acid is 99% unprotonated.

4–D. The Law of Mass Action applied to the dissociation of water $-\log [H^+]$ 4×10^8 = pH 7.4.

5–C. The pH and pK are related as follows: pH = pK + log([A⁻]/[HA]). Thus, when the concentrations of a weak acid and its base are equal, the pH equals the pK.

6–E. This sugar is sucrose. It contains glucose and fructose (two hexoses) joined by their anomeric carbons; thus, it is not a reducing sugar and does not mutarotate.

7–D. Glucose and galactose are not mirror images (enantiomers). These two monosaccharides differ only in that they contain hydroxyl groups on different sides of carbon 4 (i.e., they are epimers). They are aldoses, not ketoses. They are hexoses (containing six carbons) in the D configuration.

8–A. The glutamate at position 6 in HbA is replaced by valine in HbS. Therefore, HbS has one more hydrophobic amino acid and one less negative charge than HbA. Both HbA and HbS contain histidine, which has a side chain with a pK_a of 6. Both sequences contain proline, which is cyclic and interrupts formation of an α-helix.

9–C. Phospholipids are important components of membranes but are also found in blood lipoproteins and in lung surfactant. They are amphipathic molecules that are not involved in storing energy but in interfacing between body lipids and their aqueous environment. They are soluble in water because they contain a phosphate residue that is negatively charged, and they often contain choline, ethanolamine, or serine residues that have a positive charge at physiologic pH. (A serine residue will contain both a negative charge and a positive charge.)

10–C. Adenosine triphosphate is a nucleotide. Nucleotides are composed of a sugar linked to a nitrogenous ring, either a purine or pyrimidine. Nucleotides have many cellular functions including energy storage and signal transduction and as allosteric regulators and the building blocks of genetic information. Phospholipids are membrane components, whereas proline is an example of an imino acid. Triacylglycerols contain 3 fatty acids esterified to glycerol. Glycoproteins have numerous functions within the cell and are composed of glycosylated polypeptides.

11–B. Digoxin is a medication that can improve the contraction of the heart. It is a drug that has been around for centuries and is made from the foxglove plant. As stated in the question stem, the definition of a glycoside is an ester containing a sugar component (glycol) and a nonsugar (aglycone) component attached via oxygen or nitrogen bond; hydrolysis of a glycoside yields one or more sugars.

12–C. The branched-chain amino acids (BCAAs) comprise the three essential amino acids L-leucine, L-isoleucine, and L-valine. These amino acids are found in proteins of all life forms. Dietary sources of the branched-chain amino acids are principally derived from animal and vegetable proteins.

13–B. Phenylalanine is the only answer choice that that does not have an ionizable side chain. The symptoms of dermatitis (rash), diarrhea, and dementia are the "3 Ds" of pellagra. Pellagra is a congregate of symptoms resulting from vitamin B_3 (niacin) deficiency of which tryptophan is a precursor.

14–B. Manipulating the Henderson-Hasselbalch equation to $pK_a - pH = \log$ (ionized/ nonionized) results in $10^3 =$ ionized/nonionized $= 1000$.

15–B. Fructose gives a positive result in a reducing-sugar test and a negative result in a glucose oxidase test. It is a monosaccharide and, thus, is not cleaved by acid. Glucose gives a positive test result with the enzyme glucose oxidase. Sorbitol has no aldehyde or ketone group and, thus, cannot be oxidized in the reducing-sugar test. Maltose and lactose are disaccharides that undergo acid hydrolysis, which doubles the amount of reducing sugar.

16–E. The proton pump inhibitors, such as omeprazole, inhibit the H^+, K^+-ATPase, which is responsible for the production of hydrochloric acid by the gastric parietal cells. Many patients are given these medications in the hospital to prevent the development of gastric ulcers. Phosphoric acid and sulfuric acid are important acids that are byproducts of normal metabolism. Lactic acid is yet another product of metabolism, primarily anaerobic glycolysis. β-Hydroxybutyric acid is a ketone that results from lipid metabolism.

17–D. Heparin is a glycosaminoglycan, a long repeating chain of disaccharide units. The sugar residues of heparin are sulfonated. Cerebrosides and gangliosides are both examples of sphingolipids derived from the lipid ceramide. Prostaglandins are derived from the polyunsaturated fatty acid, arachidonic acid.

18–C. Strychnine interferes with neurotransmission by the amino acid glycine. Glycine is actually the only nonpolar amino acid listed. Tyrosine is a polar aromatic amino acid. Asparagine and glutamine are polar, uncharged amino acids. And lastly, lysine is a charged amino acid.

19–C. Glucuronidation makes the drug more water soluble and, therefore, secretable by the kidneys by the addition of glucose molecules that have been oxidized to form gluconic acid. Sulfonated sugars are found in glycosaminoglycans. Reduction of glucose forms sorbitol, whereas phosphorylation of glucose traps glucose within the cell and commits it to metabolism. Mutarotation occurs when α glucose becomes β glucose, a process that requires passage through a straight-chain aldehyde.

20–B. The protein involved in this disease is the cystic fibrosis transmembrane conductance regulator (CFTR) gene and over 90% have a particular mutation known as the Δ508. It is one of the most common lethal genetic disorders in white populations, with death due to respiratory failure secondary to repeat pulmonary infections and buildup of thick, tenacious mucous in the respiratory passages. There are numerous diseases associated with defects in enzymes, particularly those of key metabolic enzymes. Increased cholesterol content of lipid bilayer can result in spur cell anemia. Defects in the ability to glycosylate ligands for selectins are found in leukocyte adhesion deficiency II.

chapter 2

Protein Structure/Function

I. General Aspects of Protein Structure (Figure 2-1)

A. **The linear sequence of amino acid residues** in a polypeptide chain determines the three-dimensional configuration of a protein.

B. **The structure of a protein** determines its function.

1. The **primary structure** is the sequence of amino acids along the polypeptide chain.
   a. By convention, the **sequence** is written from left to right, starting with the **N-terminal** amino acid and ending with its C-terminal amino acid.
   b. Because there are no dissociable protons in peptide bonds, the **charges** on a polypeptide chain are due only to the N-terminal amino group, the C-terminal carboxyl group, and the side chains on amino acid residues.
   c. A protein will **migrate** in an **electric field,** depending on the sum of its charges at a given pH (the net charge).
      (1) **Positively charged** proteins are cations and migrate toward the **cathode** (−).
      (2) **Negatively charged** proteins are anions and migrate toward the **anode (+).**
   d. At the **isoelectric pH** (the pI), the net charge is zero, and the protein does not migrate.
2. **Secondary structure** includes various types of local conformations in which the atoms of the side chains are not involved.
   a. An **α-helix** is generated when each carbonyl of a peptide bond forms a **hydrogen bond** with the −NH of a peptide bond four amino acid residues further along the chain (Figure 2-1).
   b. The side chains of the amino acid residues extend outward from the central axis of the rod-like structure. This allows the formation of high tensile strength fibrillary proteins.

> *cc* **2.1** **Marfan syndrome** results from mutations in the gene for the highly α-helical fibrillary protein *fibrillin,* which is a major component of microfibrils found in the extracellular matrix. Patients have defective connective tissue, particularly in the ligaments and aorta. They present with **excessively long extremities and fingers, arachnodactyly,** and a predisposition to **dissecting aortic aneurysms** and valvular disease.

   c. The α-helix is disrupted by proline residues, in which the ring imposes geometric constraints, and by regions in which numerous amino acid residues have charged groups or large, bulky side chains (Figure 2-2).

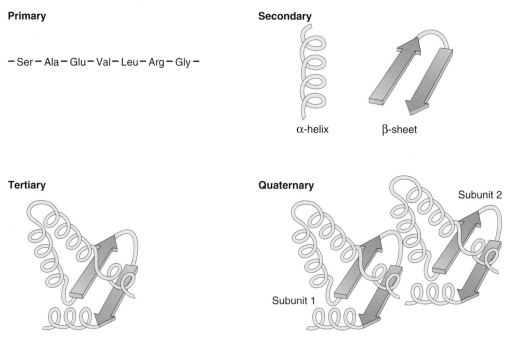

Primary

− Ser − Ala − Glu − Val − Leu − Arg − Gly −

Secondary

α-helix   β-sheet

Tertiary

Quaternary

Subunit 2

Subunit 1

Figure 2-1   Schematic diagram of the primary, secondary, tertiary, and quaternary structure of a protein.

3. **β-Sheets** are formed by **hydrogen bonds** between two extended polypeptide chains or between two regions of a single chain that folds back on itself (Figure 2-3).
   a. These **interactions** are between the **carbonyl** of one peptide bond and the –NH of another.
   b. The chains may run in the same direction (parallel) or in opposite directions (anti-parallel).

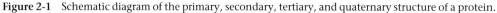

> *cc* **2.2** Prion diseases, like **Creutzfeldt-Jakob disease (CJD),** result from the transmission of a proteinaceous agent that is capable of **altering the normal α-helical arrangement** of the prion protein and replacing them with **β-pleated sheets** like the pathogenic form. The resulting misfolded protein is resistant to degradation, with death of the affected neurons. Patients suffer pronounced involuntary jerking movements (**startle myoclonus**) and rapidly **deteriorating dementia.**

   c. **Supersecondary structures**
   (1) Certain motifs involving a combination of α-helices and β-sheets are frequently found and include the **helix-turn-helix, leucine zipper,** and **zinc finger.** These motifs are often found in **transcription** factors as they help mediate **binding of proteins to DNA.**

> *cc* **2.3** The family of transcriptions factors known as **homeobox proteins** contain **helix-turn-helix** motifs. They play a significant role in pattern development during development of the limbs and other body parts. Disruption of **protein-DNA** results in congenital malformations.

   (2) Other types of **helices** or **loops** and **turns** can occur that differ from one protein to another (random coils).

C. **The tertiary structure of a protein** refers to its overall three-dimensional **conformation.** It is produced by interactions between disparate amino acid residues that may

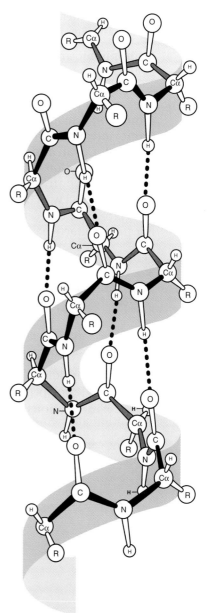

Figure 2-2 An α-helix. The enlarged segment shows the hydrogen bonding that occurs between the carbonyl (C = O) of one peptide bond and the –NH of another peptide bond that is four amino acid residues further along the chain.

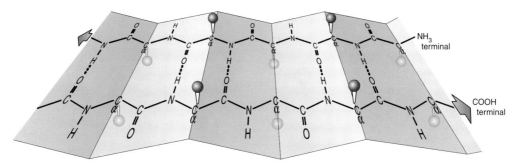

Figure 2-3 The structure of an antiparallel β-sheet. The orientation is indicated by *arrows*.

be located at a considerable distance from each other in the primary sequence of the polypeptide chain (Figure 2-4).

1. **Hydrophobic amino acid residues** tend to reside and cluster in the **interior** of globular proteins, where they exclude water, while **hydrophilic** residues are usually found on the **surface,** where they interact with water.
2. The types of interactions between amino acid residues that produce the **three-dimensional shape** of a protein include hydrophobic interactions, **electrostatic (ionic)** interactions, **hydrogen bonds,** and van der Waals, all of which are **noncovalent. Covalent disulfide bonds** also occur.
3. All the information required for proteins to correctly assume their tertiary structure is defined by their primary sequence. Sometimes molecules known as "chaperones" interact with the polypeptide **to help find the correct tertiary structure.** Such proteins either catalyze the rate of folding or protect the protein from forming "nonproductive" intramolecular tangles during the folding process.

> *cc* **2.4**   **Heat shock proteins** (hsps) are a group of **chaperones.** Mutations in such proteins sometimes lead to human disease. Some patients with **Charcot-Marie-Tooth disease (CMT),** one of the most common inherited **neuromuscular diseases,** have been found to have mutations in hsps.

D.   **Quaternary structure** refers to the spatial arrangement of subunits in a protein containing more than one polypeptide chain (see Figure 2-1).

   • The subunits are joined together by the same types of **noncovalent interactions** within a single polypeptide to form its tertiary structure.

E.   **Denaturation and renaturation**

1. Proteins can be **denatured** by agents such as **heat** and **urea** that unfold polypeptide chains without causing hydrolysis of peptide bonds.

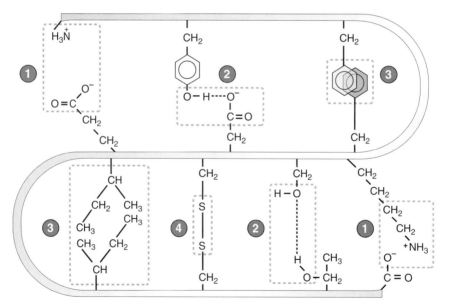

Figure 2-4   Interactions between amino acid residues in a polypeptide chain. (1) Electrostatic interactions; (2) hydrogen bonds; (3) hydrophobic interactions; and (4) a disulfide bond.

2. If a denatured protein returns to its native state after the denaturing agent is removed, the process is called **renaturation.**

F. Protein misfolding

1. Misfolded proteins can result spontaneously from **mutations in the gene encoding the protein.**

> *cc 2.5* Mutations in patients with **alpha-antitrypsin (AAT) deficiency** result in a misfolded protein that gets trapped within the cell. Patients with decreased levels of this protease inhibitor manifest with **cirrhosis** and **emphysema.**

> *cc 2.6* **Huntington's disease** results from the expansion of a region of **polyglutamine repeats** within the *huntington* **protein.** The protein aggregates and forms intranuclear inclusions, resulting in neuronal cell death. Patients present with **progressive movement disorders and dementia.**

2. Misfolded proteins can aggregate to form insoluble β-pleated fibrils, or amyloid. These fibrils accumulate in tissue, often resulting in worsening pathology as the amyloid accumulates. See Table 2-1 for some clinically relevant **amyloidopathies.**

G. Post-translational modifications of proteins occur after the protein has been synthesized on the ribosome. A given protein can have many combinations of modifications.

TABLE 2-1	*Amyloidosis and Human Disease*		
	Amyloid Protein Component	**Associated Disease**	**Notes**
cc 2.7	Beta amyloid	Alzheimer's disease	The most common cause of **progressive dementia.**
cc 2.8	β_2-microglobulin	Hemodialysis-associated amyloidosis	Deposition of amyloid in bone joints results in arthritis and cartilage and bone destruction.
cc 2.9	Calcitonin	Medullary carcinoma of the thyroid	Deposition of **amyloid around the C-cells of the thyroid,** the source of the calcitonin.
cc 2.10	Immunoglobulin light chain	Multiple myeloma	Patients have renal (**myeloma kidney**) and **heart failure** due to accumulation of protein in these tissues.
cc 2.11	Islet amyloid protein	Type 2 diabetes mellitus	Deposition of the islet amyloid protein, normally secreted with insulin, may contribute to further **islet dysfunction.**
cc 2.12	Transthyretin	Familial amyloidotic neuropathies	Deposition of amyloid in neurons with axonal degeneration.

1. **Post-translation modifications** include: phosphorylation, glycosylation, ADP-ribosylation, hydroxylation, and acetylation.
2. Such modifications alter the charge on proteins and the interactions between amino acid residues, **altering the three-dimensional configuration** and, thus, the function of the protein.
3. See Table 2-2 for medically relevant post-translation modifications.

TABLE 2-2	*Various Post-Translation Modifications*		
	Modification	**Protein Target**	**Clinical Consequence**
cc 2.13	Acetylation	Histones	Involved in the regulation of protein-DNA interactions as histone proteins are often acetylated.
cc 2.14	Acylation	RAS (p21)	RAS is anchored to the inner cytoplasmic membrane by **farnesyl (a fatty acyl moiety).** Inhibitors of this modification are being developed to **suppress the oncogenicity of RAS.**
cc 2.15	ADP-Ribosylation	Rho (a small GTP protein)	*Clostridium botulinum* toxin is an enzyme that **ADP-ribosylates Rho** leading to **inhibition of the release of acetylcholine** and a subsequent **flaccid paralysis.**
cc 2.16	Carboxylation	Clotting factors	Carboxylation of **factors VII, IX, X, fibrinogen, and proteins C and S** are required for coagulation. This process is inhibited by the drug **warfarin.**
cc 2.17	Disulfide bond formation	Antibodies	Antibodies are complex immune molecules whose function requires numerous intra- as well as intermolecular disulfide bonds.
cc 2.18	Glycation	Hemoglobin	**Nonenzymatic addition of sugar** to proteins contributes to disease complications. **Glycated hemoglobin, HBA$_{1c}$,** is normally 6% of the total hemoglobin but increases when red blood cells are exposed to high levels of blood glucose and is a measure of **long-term glucose control** in diabetic patients.
cc 2.19	Glycosylation	Red blood cell proteins	Different **sugars added to red blood cell proteins** determine an individual's **blood type. Transfusions** of blood products and successful **transplantation** require correct blood type matching.

TABLE 2-2	*Various Post-Translation Modifications (continued)*		
	Modification	**Protein Target**	**Clinical Consequence**
cc **2.20**	Glycosyl phosphatidyl inositol (GPI)	Complement regulatory proteins	Patients with **paroxysmal nocturnal hemoglobin** (PNH) lack the ability to form **GPI linkage.** Such patients cannot produce cell surface complement regulatory proteins, causing **red blood cell destruction** and subsequent **anemia.**
	Hydroxylation	Collagen	See text.
cc **2.21**	Phosphorylation	Growth factor receptors	**Phosphorylation of proteins usually results in growth-promoting signals.** A number of newly developed anti-cancer drugs seek to prevent phosphorylation.
	Ubiquitination	Proteins targeted for degradation	Improper ubiquitination and degradation of various proteins can lead to abnormalities in protein folding. Aberrant protein folding can lead to diseases such as Alzheimer disease.

H. Protein degradation

1. Proteins from the intracellular environment may be targeted for degradation by the **ubiquitin–proteasomal pathway** (Figure 2-5).
    a. **Ubiquitin,** a small globular protein, is covalently attached to the target protein to be degraded.
    b. **Further** ubiquitination of the target protein results in **polyubiquitination.**
    c. Polyubiquitinated "tagged" proteins are then recognized by a large multiprotein proteolytic complex, known as the **proteasome.**

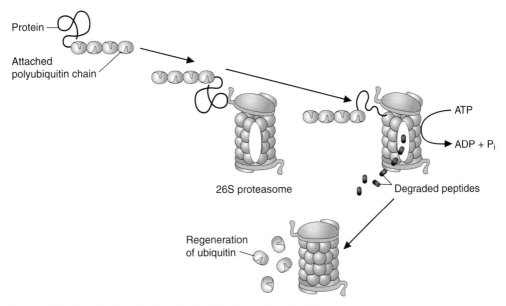

Figure 2-5 Protein degradation of ubiquitinated proteins by the proteasome.

   d. The **proteasome** degrades proteins into small peptides, which are then further degraded into amino acid precursors or presented on the surface of cells as small peptides for immune recognition.

> *cc 2.22* The novel anti-cancer drug **bortezomib (Velcade)** is used for the treatment of **multiple myeloma** and **inhibits the proteasome.** It is believed that cancer cells are more dependent on proteasomal degradation than normal cells for proliferation, metastasis, and survival.

  2. Alternatively, some proteins are degraded in a **PEST sequence**–dependent manner.
    • Proteins that have **PEST** sequences in their N terminus (proline [P], glutamate [E], serine [S], and threonine [T]) are targeted for rapid degradation after synthesis by nonspecific proteases.

  3. Proteins from the extracellular environment are degraded within lysosome.
    a. Material enters the cell by endocytosis.
    b. The endocytic vesicle fuses with the lysosome to form the phagolysosome.
    c. The proteolytic enzymes within the lysosome digest the endocytosed material into peptides.
    d. These peptides can then be completely degraded or, in some cases, be presented to cells of the immune system.

> *cc 2.23* Patients with **Chédiak-Higashi syndrome** have a defect in the ability to **transfer enzymes from lysosomes to phagocytic vesicles.** They have **recurrent infections** due to a lack of microbial killing, anemia, and thrombocytopenia.

II.   Examples of Medically Important Proteins

A. Hemoglobin (Figure 2-6) is a globular oxygen transport protein necessary for human life, whose biochemistry is well studied.

  1. *Structure of hemoglobin*
    • Adult hemoglobin (HbA) consists of **four polypeptide chains** (two α and two β chains), each containing a molecule of **heme.**
    a. The α **and** β **chains** of HbA are **similar** in three-dimensional configuration to each other and to the single chain of muscle myoglobin, although their amino acid sequences differ.

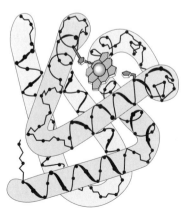

Figure 2-6 The structure of the β chain of hemoglobin. Cylindrical regions contain α-helices. The planar structure near the top center of the polypeptide chain is heme. (From: Enzyme Structure and Mechanism by Fersht © 1977 by W. H. Freeman and Company. Used with permission.)

> *cc* **2.24** Many types of **mutations** produce alterations in the structure of hemo-globin. One common mutation results in **sickle cell anemia,** in which the β chain of hemoglobin contains a **valine rather than a glutamate at position 6.** Thus, in the mutant hemoglobin (HbS), a hydrophobic amino acid replaces an amino acid with a negative charge. This change allows **deoxygenated molecules of HbS to polymerize.** Red blood cells that contain large complexes of HbS molecules can as-sume a sickle shape. These cells undergo **hemolysis,** and an **anemia** results. Painful **vaso-occlusive crises** also occur, and **end-organ damage** may result.

  b. Eight α-helices occur in each chain.
  c. **Heme,** a complex of a **porphyrin ring** and a **ferrous (Fe²⁺)** ion, fits into a crevice in each globin chain and interacts with two histidine residues.

2. *Function of hemoglobin*
  a. The oxygen saturation curve for hemoglobin is sigmoidal (Figure 2-7).
    (1) **The iron of each heme** binds **one O_2** molecule, for a total of four O_2 mol-ecules per HbA molecule. HbA changes from the taut or tense **(T) form** to the relaxed **(R) form** when oxygen binds.
    (2) Binding of O_2 to one heme group in hemoglobin increases the affinity for O_2 of its other heme groups. This allosteric effect produces the sigmoidal oxygen saturation curve.

> *cc* **2.25** **Hemoglobin has approximately 250× the affinity for carbon monoxide** than oxygen. Prolonged and/or heavy exposure to carbon monoxide results in a disorientation, headache, and **potentially fatal asphyxiation.** Patients may have "**cherry-red mucous membranes**" due to the accumulation **of carboxyhemoglobin.**

  b. The binding of **protons** to HbA stimulates the release of O_2, a manifestation of the **Bohr effect** (see Figure 2-7).
    (1) Thus, O_2 is readily released in the tissues where [H⁺] is high due to the pro-duction of CO_2 by metabolic processes:

$$CO_2 + H_2O \leftrightarrows H_2CO_3 \leftrightarrows H^+ + HCO_3^-$$
Tissues $H^+ + HbAO_2 \leftrightarrows HHbA + O_2$ **Lungs**

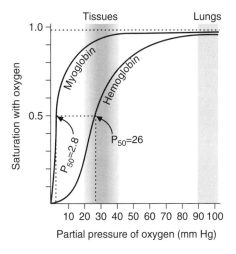

Figure 2-7 Oxygen saturation curves for myoglobin and adult hemoglobin (HbA). Myoglobin has a hyper-bolic saturation curve. HbA has a sigmoidal curve. The HbA curve shifts to the right at lower pH, with higher concentrations of 2,3-biphosphoglycerate (BPG), or as CO_2 binds to HbA in the tissues. Under these conditions, O_2 is released more readily. P_{50} is the partial pressure of O_2 at which half-saturation with O_2 occurs.

(2) These reactions are reversed in the lung. O_2 binds to HbA, and CO_2 is exhaled.
  c. Covalent binding of CO_2 to HbA in the tissues also causes O_2 release.
  d. Binding of **2,3-bisphosphoglycerate (BPG)** (formerly known as 2,3-diphosphoglycerate [DPG]), a side product of glycolysis in red blood cells, decreases the affinity of HbA for O_2. Consequently, O_2 is more readily released in tissues when BPG is bound to HbA.

B. **Collagen** refers to a group of very similar structural proteins that are found in the **extracellular matrix**, the **vitreous humor** of the eye, and in **bone and cartilage**. There are numerous other structural proteins important in human disease; for other select examples, see Table 2-3.

  1. *Structure of collagen*
     a. Collagen consists of three chains that intertwine to form a triple helix (Figure 2-8).

> *cc 2.30* **Osteogenesis imperfecta** is a group of related disorders in the **synthesis of type I collagen.** Such defects have a wide spectrum of clinical consequence, although they all share bone fragility (with a predisposition to **multiple childhood fractures**), hearing loss, and a **distinctive blue sclera.**

  b. Collagen contains approximately 1000 amino acids, one third of which are **glycine.** The sequence Gly-X-Y frequently occurs, in which X is often **proline** and Y is **hydroxyproline** or **hydroxylysine**.
  2. *Synthesis of collagen*
     a. The polypeptide chains of **preprocollagen** are synthesized on the **rough endoplasmic reticulum**, and the signal (pre) sequence is cleaved.

TABLE 2-3	*Structural Proteins and Disease*		
	Protein	**Disease**	**Disease Characteristics**
cc 2.26	Spectrin	Hereditary spherocytosis	**Hereditary anemia and** splenomegaly; treatment sometimes involves **splenectomy.**
cc 2.27	Dystrophin	Muscular dystrophy	**Progressive motor weakness,** eventual respiratory failure, and cardiac decompensation. **X-linked inheritance.**
cc 2.28	β-myosin heavy chain	Familial hypertrophic cardiomyopathy	Enlargement of the heart with outlet obstruction. **Most common cause of sudden, otherwise unexplainable death in young athletes.**
cc 2.29	Collagen (α5 chain of type IV collagen)	Alport syndrome	**X-linked syndrome** characterized by **renal failure, nerve deafness,** and **cataracts.**

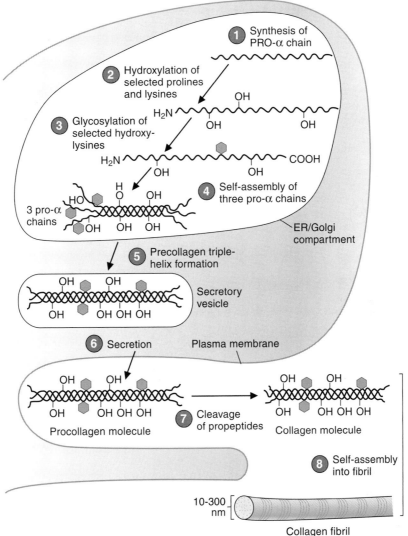

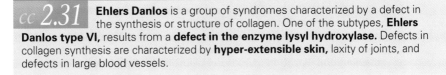

Figure 2-8 Steps in the formation of mature collagen fibrils.

b. **Proline** and **lysine** residues are **hydroxylated** by a reaction that requires O_2 and **vitamin C**.

> *cc* **2.31** **Ehlers Danlos** is a group of syndromes characterized by a defect in the synthesis or structure of collagen. One of the subtypes, **Ehlers Danlos type VI,** results from a **defect in the enzyme lysyl hydroxylase.** Defects in collagen synthesis are characterized by **hyper-extensible skin,** laxity of joints, and defects in large blood vessels.

c. **Galactose** and **glucose** are added to hydroxylysine residues.
d. The **triple helix** forms, procollagen is secreted from the cell, and cleaved to form collagen.
e. **Cross-links** are produced. The side chains of lysine and hydroxylysine residues are oxidized to form aldehydes, which can undergo aldol condensation or form Schiff bases with the amino groups of lysine residues.

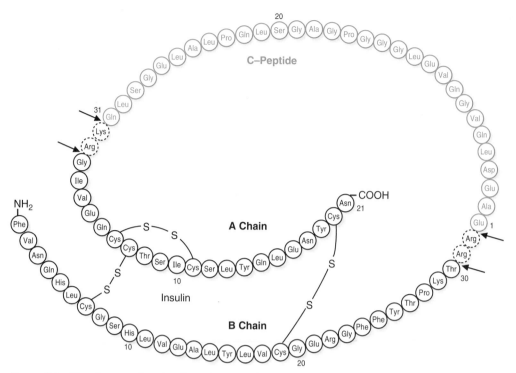

Figure 2-9 The cleavage of proinsulin to form insulin. Cleavage occurs at the arrows, which release the C-peptide. The A and B chains of insulin are joined by disulfide bonds. (From Murray RK, et al. *Harper's Biochemistry,* 23rd ed. Stamford, CT: Appleton & Lange, 1993:500.)

C. Insulin

1. *Structure of insulin* (see Figure 2-8)
   - Insulin is a polypeptide hormone that is produced by the **β cells** of the **pancreas.** The mature form has 51 amino acids in **two polypeptide chains (A and B),** which are linked by two **disulfide bridges.**
2. *Synthesis of insulin* (Figure 2-9)
   a. **Preproinsulin,** consisting of the A and B chains joined by a C-peptide, is synthesized on the rough endoplasmic reticulum and the pre- (signal) sequence is removed to form proinsulin.
   b. In secretory granules, **proinsulin** is cleaved, and the **C-peptide** is released. The remainder of the molecule forms the active hormone.

> *cc* **2.32** **C-peptide levels are used to differentiate the causes of high insulin in patients.** In cases of low blood glucose due to increased levels of circulating insulin via endogenous production, as in **tumors of pancreatic β cells,** serum levels of **C-peptide will also be elevated.** However, in cases of **surreptitious insulin administration** (purposeful injection of insulin), **C-peptide is not elevated,** as commercial insulin preparations have purified away this contaminate.

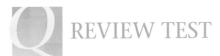

Directions: *Each of the numbered questions or incomplete statements in this section is followed by answers or by completions of the statement. Select the **one** lettered answer or completion that is **best** in each case.*

1. Proteins are effective buffers because they contain:

(A) a large number of amino acids.
(B) amino acid residues with different pK_as.
(C) N-terminal and C-terminal residues that can donate and accept protons.
(D) peptide bonds that readily hydrolyze, consuming hydrogen and hydroxyl ions.
(E) a large number of hydrogen bonds in α-helices.

2. At physiologic pH (7.4), the hexapeptide (Asp-Ala-Ser-Glu-Val-Arg) will contain a net charge of:

(A) −2.
(B) −1.
(C) 0.
(D) +1.
(E) +2.

3. The formation of a disulfide bond is an example of what type of protein structure?

(A) Primary
(B) Secondary
(C) Super secondary
(D) Tertiary
(E) Quaternary

4. Which one of the following conditions causes hemoglobin to release oxygen more readily?

(A) Metabolic alkalosis
(B) Increased production of 2,3-bisphosphoglycerate (BPG)
(C) Hyperventilation, leading to decreased levels of CO_2 in the blood
(D) Replacement of the β subunits with γ subunits
(E) High concentrations of carbon monoxide

5. What molecular property do the following elements of life as we know it share: boiling an egg, allostery in oxygen binding or effectors binding to enzymes, a hair permanent, and cleaning clothes in the washer?

(A) Microelectrophoretic properties of proteins
(B) Ionization of tyrosine side chains at pH 11
(C) Post-translational chemical modification of proteins
(D) Changes in secondary and tertiary structure of proteins
(E) Proteolysis of peptide bonds

6. Proteins can often unfold under conditions of high salt or extremes of pH. Which of the following interactions is likely to be disrupted at pH 4.0?

(A) A hydrogen bond between the carboxyl and amino termini
(B) A disulfide (cystine) linkage
(C) A salt bridge (electrostatic interaction) between Arg and Asp
(D) A hydrogen bond between the hydroxyl group of a Tyr side chain and a backbone carbonyl oxygen
(E) A hydrogen bond between the side chain hydroxyl of Ser and the imidazole group of His

7. Type I collagen:

(A) forms fibrils through intermolecular cross-links.
(B) is assembled into triple helices in the extracellular space.
(C) is a homotrimer.
(D) is characterized by repeating RGD sequences.
(E) contains hydroxyserine residues.

8. Which of the following binds to the hemoglobin molecule at the same site as O_2?

(A) CO_2
(B) H^+
(C) 2,3 bisphosphoglycerate (BPG)

(D) CO
(E) ATP

9. Which of the following characteristics contributes to a tight protein–protein interface (Kd ~ 0.1 nM)?

(A) A small surface area between molecules at the interface
(B) Amino acids, such as Met, Ser, and Thr, at the interface
(C) Salt molecules within each molecule, not between molecules at the interface
(D) Hydrophobic interactions at the interface
(E) A β-sheet structure between molecules at the interface

10. In the figure below, four bonds are indicated by numbers. Choose the correct structure.

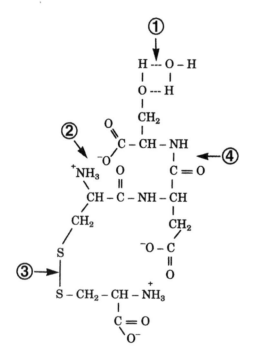

(A) (1) Electrostatic interaction; (2) hydrogen bond; (3) disulfide bond; (4) peptide bond
(B) (1) Hydrogen bond; (2) peptide bond; (3) disulfide bond; (4) electrostatic interaction

(C) (1) Hydrogen bond; (2) disulfide bond; (3) electrostatic interaction; (4) peptide bond
(D) (1) Hydrogen bond; (2) electrostatic interaction; (3) disulfide bond; (4) peptide bond
(E) (1) Hydrogen bond; (2) electrostatic interaction; (3) peptide bond; (4) disulfide bond

11. A young female presents to the physician's office for a sports physical before participation in volleyball. She appears to have a perfect habitus for the sport because she is much taller than her peers and has exceptionally long arms and fingers. Upon auscultation of her heart, there is a midsystolic click associated with a murmur of mitral valve prolapse. The physician suspects she may have Marfan's syndrome, which is a defect in which of the following proteins?

(A) Myosin heavy chain
(B) Spectrin
(C) Ankyrin
(D) Fibrillin
(E) Collagen

12. A 65-year-old man with a history of type 2 diabetes is complaining of blurred vision and numbness in his toes. Lab results were significant for an increased BUN and creatinine, indicative of renal failure. Lab work also revealed an HbA$_{1C}$ of 9.0. One of the mechanisms for the damage responsible for the man's symptoms is the nonenzymatic covalent bonds formed between glucose and structural proteins. This reaction would best be classified as:

(A) acylation.
(B) carboxylation.
(C) glycation.
(D) hydroxylation.
(E) esterification.

13. A 47-year-old woman passes out at work and is brought to the emergency room. Her blood sugar is 24 mg/dL (normal > 70 mg/dL). She is also tested for C-peptide, which is much higher than

normal. What is a possible cause of this woman's state?

(A) Anorexia
(B) High-protein diet
(C) Exogenous administration of insulin
(D) Insulin-secreting islet cell tumor
(E) High-glucose diet

14. A social worker refers a 2-year-old child to the physician because of suspected child abuse. On physical examination, the child has blue sclerae and diminished hearing in both ears, and radiographs of the child's extremities show recent and healing long bone fractures. The child is diagnosed with osteogenesis imperfecta. This disorder is a defect in the synthesis of which of the following proteins?

(A) Transthyretin
(B) Calcitonin
(C) Spectrin
(D) β-Mysosin heavy chain
(E) Collagen

15. In 1795, the British navy began to dispense limes during long sea voyages (hence the name "limeys" for British sailors), a measure that was largely successful in preventing scurvy. Scurvy is a condition characterized by general weakness, anemia, gum disease (gingivitis), and skin hemorrhages resulting from a lack of ascorbic acid (vitamin C) in the diet. Ascorbic acid plays a crucial role in which of the following processes in collagen synthesis?

(A) Transcription
(B) Glycosylation
(C) Hydroxylation
(D) Covalent cross-linkage
(E) C-peptide cleavage

16. An 18-year-old boy works in the circus as a contortionist due to his hypermobile joints that allow for abnormal flexibility. He also has increased elasticity of his skin and bruises easily. This is a typical presentation of Ehlers-Danlos syndrome, resulting from a defect in collagen. Ehlers-Danlos type VI results in a lysyl oxidase deficiency. Which of the following processes will therefore be impaired?

(A) Transcription
(B) Glycosylation
(C) Hydroxylation
(D) Covalent cross-linkage
(E) Secretion into the extracellular space

17. A 24-year-old bride prepares for her wedding day. After her manicure and pedicure, her hairdresser uses rollers to create a new style for her hair. To create a "permanent wave," the stylist then applies thioglycollate to break apart the –S–S– bonds in cystine units, reducing them to –SH groups. Which level of protein structure is most greatly affected by this treatment?

(A) Primary structure
(B) Secondary structure
(C) Supersecondary structure
(D) Tertiary structure
(E) Quaternary structure

18. A 59-year-old man presents with nephrotic syndrome. Immunoelectrophoresis detects a monoclonal IgG lambda in his serum and free lambda light chains in his urine. A renal biopsy shows amyloidosis. Although several different proteins are precursors to amyloid deposition, all amyloid fibrils share an identical secondary structure, which is which of the following structures?

(A) α-Helix
(B) β-Pleated sheet
(C) Triple helix
(D) Helix-turn-helix
(E) Leucine zipper

19. The above patient with multiple myeloma has failed numerous treatments, and yet his disease has advanced. He sees his oncologist who wants to start him on the drug bortezomib, which works by inhibiting the proteosome. Which intracellular proteins will not be degraded as a result of this drug?

(A) Proteins with PEST sequences
(B) Amyloid proteins
(C) Polyubiquitinated proteins
(D) Immunoglobulin light chains
(E) Tense proteins

20. A 16-year-old, African-American female comes to the emergency room with complaints of painful muscle cramps. She states that she has sickle cell anemia and that she ran out of her pain medication. A complete blood count and smear rapidly confirm the diagnosis, and she is started on intravenous fluids and pain medications. The molecular defect underlying her disease is which of the following?

(A) A valine rather than a glutamine at position 6 of the β-globin protein

(B) A glutamine rather than a valine at position 6 of the β-globin protein

(C) A valine rather than a glutamine at position 6 of the α-globin protein

(D) A glutamine rather than a valine at position 6 of the α-globin protein

(E) Expansion of a polyglutamine repeat within β-globin gene

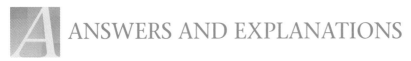

1–B. The side chains of the amino acid residues in proteins contain functional groups with different pK_as. Therefore, they can donate and accept protons at various pH values and act as buffers over a broad pH spectrum. There is only one N-terminal amino group ($pK_a \approx 9$) and one C-terminal carboxyl group ($pK_a \approx 3$) per polypeptide chain. Peptide bonds are not readily hydrolyzed, and such hydrolysis would not provide buffering action. Hydrogen bonds have no buffering capacity.

2–B. The N-terminal aspartate (Asp) contains a positive charge on its N-terminal amino group and a negative charge on the carboxyl group of its side chain. Glutamate (Glu) contains a negative charge on the carboxyl group of its side chain. The C-terminal arginine (Arg) contains a negative charge on its C-terminal carboxyl group and a positive charge on its side chain. Thus, the overall charges are $^+2$ and $^-3$, which gives a net charge of $^-1$.

3–C. The disulfide bond, as well as the noncovalent electrostatic, hydrophobic, and hydrogen bonds, stabilize the tertiary structure. Both the secondary and quaternary structures rely only on covalent bonds for stabilization.

4–B. Increased $[H^+]$, BPG, and CO_2 decrease the affinity of HbA for O_2. Fetal hemoglobin (HbF = $\alpha_2\gamma_2$) has a greater affinity for O_2 than HbA ($\alpha_2\beta_2$). Increased BPG would cause O_2 to be more readily released. High carbon monoxide levels would actually make hemoglobin less likely to release oxygen.

5–D. All of these actions are caused by conformational changes in the three-dimensional structure of proteins. Whereas the other choices do occur in specific circumstances, the most important general properties of protein function lie in their structure.

6–C. An extreme of pH implies that interactions between charged amino acids are responsible for the disruption of function. Thus, disulfides and hydrogen bonds are not the correct answer (the pK_a of His is ~7). At pH 4, the charge of Asp is neutralized, which would block an electrostatic interaction.

7–A. Collagen is cross-linked to form fibrils, is assembled in the Golgi/ER intracellularly, is intertwined as a triple helix (a homotrimer), has an Gly-X-Y repeat (RGD sequences), and has hydroxyproline and hydroxylysine.

8–D. The iron of each heme binds one O_2. CO binds to the same site with ~250× greater affinity than O_2. CO_2 binds to uncharged α-amino groups (A), and H^+ dissociates from a histidine and does not bind to heme (B). Both CO_2 and H^+ are transported to the lungs. BPG binds to the interface formed by two β chains (C), and ATP (E) does not bind.

9–D. Tight protein–protein interfaces are very hydrophobic, without any "pockets" to maximize the strength of the interaction.

10–D. Bond 1: The hydroxyl group of serine forms hydrogen bonds with water. Bond 2: A positively charged amino group (on a cysteine residue) and a negatively charged carboxyl group (on a serine residue) form an electrostatic interaction. Bond 3: Two cysteine residues are covalently joined by a disulfide bond. Bond 4: In peptides, adjacent amino acids are joined covalently by peptide bonds.

11-D. Marfan's syndrome presents similar to the case described and results from an autosomal dominant mutation in the structural protein fibrillin. Familial hypertrophic cardiomyopathy is associated with defects in myosin heavy chain. Hereditary spherocytosis is associated with mutations in spectrin or secondary defects in ankyrin. Collagen defects are seen in Ehlers Danlos syndrome and vitamin C deficiency.

12–C. Glycation refers to the reaction of the glucose aldehydes group reacting with the amino groups of protein. The increased rate of glycation of collagen during hyperglycemia is implicated in the development of complications of diabetes, such as blindness and renal and vascular disease. Clotting factors are often carboxylated; histones can be acylated. Collagen is a prominent example of a protein that is hydroxylated during its production.

13–D. The pancreas synthesizes proinsulin, which is cleaved in the Golgi apparatus to insulin and C-peptide. If the patient is not eating carbohydrates, there will not be a large enough stimulus to result in a high insulin or corresponding C-peptide level. If she was self-administering pharmaceutical insulin, it would not include C-peptide; thus, her serum C-peptide level would not be elevated. Therefore, answer choice D is the most likely answer.

14–E. Osteogenesis imperfecta results from mutations in the gene for type I collagen. As such, the patients have multiple fractures with minimal trauma. The blue sclerae result from defects in the collagen that is found in the eye. Transthyretin forms the amyloid of familial amyloidotic neuropathies, whereas calcitonin forms the amyloid in medullary carcinoma of the thyroid. Spectrin mutations are found in hereditary spherocytosis, and β-myosin heavy chain mutations are found in familial hypertrophic cardiomyopathy.

15–C. Vitamin C (ascorbic acid) is an important cofactor for the enzymes prolyl hydroxylase and lysyl hydroxylase. The hydroxylation of proline stabilizes the triple helix stricture of collagen. The hydroxyl group of lysine is often glycosylated with glucose and galactose. Cross-linkage of collagen results from the hydroxylation of lysine. C-peptide cleavage occurs in insulin processing.

16–D. The triple helix of collagen spontaneously associates into collagen fibrils where the extracellular enzyme, lysyl oxidase, converts lysine to allysine. The newly formed residue then covalently links to the amino group of lysine on a neighboring collagen molecule, giving the fibril increased tensile strength. Transcription, glycosylation, and secretion of proteins into the extracellular space are all generalized mechanisms of numerous protein syntheses and processing.

17–D. The tertiary structure is stabilized by covalent disulfide bonds as well as hydrophobic interactions, electrostatic interactions, and hydrogen bonds. The primary structure is composed of covalent amide bonds. The secondary, supersecondary, and the quaternary structure are stabilized by noncovalent interactions.

18–B. Regardless of the type of amyloid disease, the pathogenesis is related to the accumulation of β-pleated protein. In the case of multiple myeloma, it is the accumulation of immunoglobulin light chains in the kidney and heart. α-Helix proteins include native fibrillary proteins, of which collagen is one that forms a triple helix. Helix-turn-helix and leucine zippers are supersecondary structures that are often found in transcription factors, like homeobox proteins (helix-turn-helix).

19–C. The proteasome normally degrades proteins that have been polyubiquitinated. As such, these proteins will accumulate, leading to a selective adverse effect on the cancer cells (myeloma cells). Proteins with PEST sequences are rapidly degraded by nonspecific intracellular proteases. Indeed, immunoglobulin light chains are the amyloid proteins in this disease, but the drug does not directly affect these molecules.

20–A. Sickle cell anemia results from a single mutation in the β-globulin protein of hemoglobin, a valine rather than a glutamine at position 6. There are other abnormalities of hemoglobin that affect the α chain as well as the β chain. Expansion of a polyglutamine repeat occurs in the huntington protein, resulting in Huntington's disease, a progressive movement disorder.

Enzymes and Kinetics

I. General Properties of Enzymes

A. Naming enzymes

1. Names most often describe the reaction catalyzed with the suffix "**-ase**" to indicate the protein is an enzyme.
2. Common names of enzymes may have no apparent logical basis (e.g., trypsin). A systematic classification system introduced by the Enzyme Commission divided enzymes into **6 general groups** (Table 3-1).

TABLE 3-1	*Systematic Classification of Enzymes and Clinical Correlates*		
	Enzyme Class	**Reaction**	**Clinically Relevant Example**
cc 3.1	Oxidoreductases	Catalyze oxidation-reduction reactions	The superoxide anion radical (O_2^-) is broken down by **superoxide dismutase** to hydrogen peroxide and oxygen. Superoxide is so damaging that mutations in superoxide dismutase can lead to **amyotrophic lateral sclerosis** (ALS), characterized by motoneuron loss in the spinal cord and brain stem.
cc 3.2	Transferases	Catalyze C-, N-, or P-group transfer reactions	**Phosphorylase kinase** catalyzes 4 ATP + 2 phosphorylase b ↔ 4 ADP + phosphorylase a. Inherited enzyme deficiency is responsible for **one fourth of glycogen storage diseases.** Symptoms include hepatomegaly, growth retardation, cirrhosis, and hypercholesterolemia.
cc 3.3	Hydrolases	Catalyze cleavage of bonds by water (hydrolytic) reactions	**Tissue plasminogen activator** cleaves Arg-Val bond in **plasminogen to form active plasmin.** The recombinant protein is used to treat **ischemic stroke and myocardial infarcts** by its **thrombolytic** ability to dissolve blood clots.

TABLE 3-1	*Systematic Classification of Enzymes and Clinical Correlates (continued)*		
	Enzyme Class	**Reaction**	**Clinically Relevant Example**
cc 3.4	Lyases	Catalyze addition groups to double bonds. Cleavage of C-C, C-S, and certain C-N bonds.	**Guanylate cyclase** catalyzes GTP $\leftrightarrow$ 3′,5′-cyclic GMP + diphosphate. A mutation in the retina form of the enzyme leads to **Leber congenital amaurosis,** representing the most **common genetic cause of congenital visual impairment** in infants and children.
cc 3.5	Isomerases	Catalyze racemization/ isomerization reactions	**DNA topoisomerase II (gyrase)** has nicking-closing activity and also catalyzes super-twisting and hydrolysis of ATP of double-stranded DNA. **Ataxia-telangiectasia (AT)** exhibits cerebellar ataxia, telangiectases, immune disorders, and a predisposition to malignancy with chromosomal breakage. Often, DNA topoisomerase II is markedly reduced.
cc 3.6	Ligases	Catalyze condensation of 2 molecules with bonds between C and O, S, N (and cleavage of ATP, GTP)	**Propionyl-CoA carboxylase (PCCase)** catalyzes ATP + propanoyl-CoA + HCO_3 $\leftrightarrow$ ADP + phosphate + (S)-methylmalonyl-CoA. A mutation in the enzyme causes **propionic acidemia** with vomiting, ketosis, neutropenia, periodic thrombocytopenia, developmental retardation, and intolerance to protein.

ADP = adenosine diphosphate; ATP = adenosine triphosphate; GTP = guanosine triphosphate.

B.   The reactions of the cell would not occur rapidly enough to sustain life if enzyme catalysts were not present. Enzymes **"speed" up reactions** 10^6- to 10^{11}-fold.

cc 3.7   **Catalase:** $2H_2O_2$ to $2H_2O + O_2$ has one of the highest turnover rates for all enzymes: one molecule of catalase can convert 6 million molecules of hydrogen peroxide to water and oxygen per second. **Acatalasia** (deficiency of catalase in the blood) **(Takahara's disease)** is an autosomal disease that is usually asymptomatic, but in some cases, oral ulcerations and gangrene occur.

C.   At the active sites of enzymes, **substrates bind** and are recognized with high specificity for a given substrate and are then converted to products and released. **The transition state is a high-energy reactive conformation of reactant(s)** where the probability is very high that the necessary **structural rearrangement of bond(s)** will occur to produce the product(s) of the reaction.

D.   Enzymes are highly specific for their substrates and products.

> *cc* **3.8** The nucleoside analogs **valacyclovir** and **valganciclovir** are valine ester **prodrugs** of the antiviral **acyclovir** (treating herpes simplex 1 and 2 and varicella zoster infections) and **ganciclovir** (treating cytomegalovirus retinitis in patients with acquired immunodeficiency syndrome [AIDS]), **respectively.** This new therapeutic approach involves a "prodrug" that is activated and converted by hepatic and intestinal enzymes to an active drug with higher bioavailability and efficacy. **Famciclovir** is another acyclovir compound used for shingles and recurrent outbreaks of herpes simplex 2.

1. Many enzymes recognize only a single compound as a substrate.
2. Some enzymes (e.g., proteases that hydrolyze proteins to peptides), such as those involved in digestion, are less specific.

> *cc* **3.9** **Enzymes as drug targets account for ~30% of pharmacotherapeutic agents.** Many of the newer agents are designed with the aid of complex protein structure information, which allows researchers to design drugs based on such approaches. Such a strategy is known as **rational drug design.**

E. **Many enzymes require** small organic molecules, or **cofactors** (often called **coenzymes**), that frequently are **metal ions** or derivatives of **vitamins.**

F. **Enzymes decrease the energy of activation (Ea)** for a reaction, and hence speed up the rate of **reactions.**

1. They **do not** affect the thermodynamics (ΔG) of the reaction (net free energy change for the reaction or equilibrium concentrations of the substrates and products).
2. The **thermodynamics of the reaction remains UNCHANGED** (Figure 3-1).

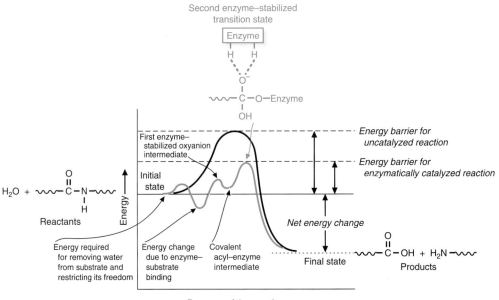

Figure 3-1 Free energy of activation (Ea) and the action of catalysts for a proteolytic reaction catalyzed by chymotrypsin. Enzymes decrease the energy of activation for a reaction; however, it does not change the energy level of the substrates or products.

3. The transition state is at the apex (the top) of the energy diagram between reactants and products.

4. The difference in the average free energy of the reactants and the average free energy of the transition state is the **activation energy barrier (free energy of activation; Ea).**

II. Dependence of Velocity on Enzyme and Substrate Concentrations, Temperature, and pH

A. The **velocity** of a reaction, **v, increases with the enzyme concentration, [E],** if the **substrate concentration, [S],** is constant.

1. If [E] is constant, v increases with [S] until the **maximum velocity, V_{max}** (a measure of the maximum enzyme activity), is attained.

2. At V_{max}, all the **active sites** of the enzyme are **saturated** with substrate.

B. The velocity of a reaction **increases with temperature** until a maximum (usually 37°C in humans) is reached, after which, the velocity decreases due to denaturation of the enzyme (Figure 3-2A).

C. Each enzyme-catalyzed reaction has an **optimal pH** (not always physiological pH).

1. The optimal pH is the pH at which the enzyme and substrate are charged for most efficient interaction and the velocity is at a maximum.

> *cc 3.10* The **optimal pH for pepsin is 2,** reflecting its need as a digestive enzyme in the acidic gastric juice of the **stomach;** whereas the **optimal pH for alkaline phosphatase is 9,** reflecting the basic environment in **bone.**

2. Changes in the pH can alter these charges so that the reaction proceeds at a slower rate. If the pH is too high or too low, the enzyme can also undergo **denaturation** (Figure 3-2B).

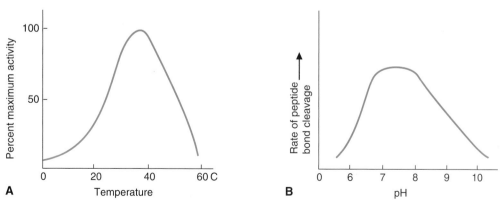

Figure 3-2   The effects of varying reaction conditions on enzyme catalyzed reactions. **(A)** Effects of temperature are illustrated. **(B)** Example of how pH changes the reaction rate. The exact shape of the curve is determined by the ionization states (pK_a) of the amino acids in the active site. The descending portion of the curve reflects the loss of catalytic activity as proteins are denatured at high temperatures.

III. The Michaelis-Menten Equation

A. If, during a reaction, an **enzyme–substrate complex** is formed that **dissociates** (to re-form the free enzyme and the substrate) or **reacts** (to release the product and regenerate the free enzyme), then:

$$E+S \underset{k_2}{\overset{k_1}{\rightleftharpoons}} ES \overset{k_3}{\rightarrow} E+P$$

where E is the enzyme; S the substrate; ES the enzyme–substrate complex; P the product; and k_1, k_2, and k_3 are rate constants.

B. From this concept, the **Michaelis-Menten equation** was derived:

$$v = V_{max}[S]/K_m + [S]$$

where $K_m = (k_2 + k_3)/k_1$ and V_{max} **is the maximum velocity,** or how fast the enzyme can go at full "speed."

C. The rate of formation of products (the velocity of the reaction) is related to the **concentration of the enzyme–substrate complex:**

$$v = k_3[ES]$$

V_{max} **is reached when all of the enzyme is in the enzyme–substrate complex.**

 3.11 The drug **isoniazid,** which is used in the treatment of tuberculosis, is acetylated by an **N-acetyltransferase.** A polymorphism of the enzyme exists, and individuals are classified into two groups: the fast acetylators/metabolizers clear the drug from blood ~300% faster than the other group of individuals, the slow acetylators/poor metabolizers, in whom the presence of drug is prolonged, causing hepatotoxicity and neuropathy. The K_m (affinity of isoniazid substrate) is **normal,** but the V_{max} of "fast" N-acetyltransferase, is **three times normal.**

D. K_m is the **substrate concentration** at which $v = \frac{1}{2} V_{max}$.

1. K_m approximately describes the **affinity** of the substrate for the enzyme. The lower the value of K_m, the higher the affinity for substrate.
2. When $[S] = K_m$, substitution of K_m for $[S]$ in the Michaelis-Menten equation yields $v = \frac{1}{2} V_{max}$.

---

cc **3.12** **Hypersensitivity to alcohol** exists in some people of Asian descent, in whom drinking small amounts of alcohol causes facial flushing and tachycardia. Alcohol dehydrogenase generates acetaldehyde, which is converted to acetate by **aldehyde dehydrogenase.** The latter enzyme exists in two forms, a high-affinity (low K_m) form and a low-affinity (high K_m) form. Those **sensitive to alcohol lack the high-affinity form,** resulting in excess acetaldehyde and, hence, vasodilation.

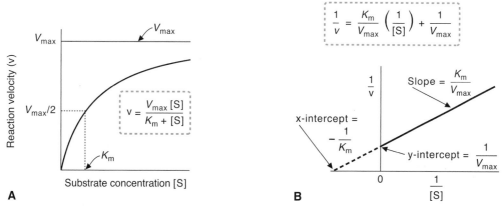

Figure 3-3 The velocity of an enzyme-catalyzed reaction that exhibits Michaelis-Menten kinetics. **(A)** Velocity (v) versus substrate concentration ([S]); **(B)** Lineweaver-Burk plot. Note the points on each plot from which V_{max} and K_m can be determined. V_{max} = maximum velocity, and K_m = the substrate concentration at $\frac{1}{2} V_{max}$.

E. When the velocity is plotted versus [S], a hyperbolic curve is produced (Figure 3-3A).

1. **At low substrate** concentration (left part of the curve, below K_m), the reaction rate increases sharply with increasing substrate concentration because there is abundant free enzyme available (E) to bind added substrate.
2. **At high substrate** concentration, the reaction rate reaches a plateau (V_{max}) as the enzyme active sites are saturated with substrate (ES complex), and there is no free enzyme to bind the added substrate.

IV.   The Lineweaver-Burk Plot (Figure 3-3B)

A.   Because of the difficulty of exactly determining V_{max} from a hyperbolic curve, the Michaelis-Menten equation was transformed by Lineweaver and Burk into an equation for a straight line.

B.   This is a double reciprocal plot of 1/V versus 1/[S].

V.   Inhibitors

Inhibitors are molecules that interact with enzymes, decreasing the rate of enzymatic reactions. Inhibitors can be substrate analogs, toxins, drugs, or metal complexes.

A.   Competitive inhibitors compete with the substrate for binding at the active site of the enzyme and form an enzyme–inhibitor complex, EI, with the free enzyme only (Figure 3-4A). Structurally, these inhibitors are similar to substrate, since they compete for the same site.

1. Competitive inhibition is reversed by increasing [S].
2. V_{max} remains the same, but the **apparent K_m (K_m') is increased.**
3. For Lineweaver-Burk plots, **lines** for the inhibited reaction **intersect on the Y-axis** with those for the uninhibited reaction.

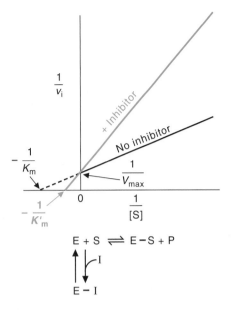

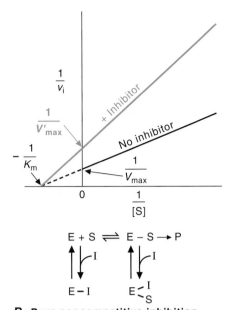

A Competitive inhibition

B Pure noncompetitive inhibition

Figure 3-4 Effect of inhibitors on Lineweaver-Burk plots. **(A)** Competitive inhibition. **(B)** Pure non-competitive inhibition (in which the inhibitor binds to E and ES with the same affinity). If the affinities differ, the lines will not intersect on the X-axis and the apparent K_m (K'_m) will differ from K_m. V'_{max} = the apparent V_{max}.

> *cc* **3.13** Drugs such as **physostigmine, a competitive reversible inhibitor of acetylcholinesterase,** are used to treat a variety of diseases such as glaucoma (increased intraocular pressure) and myasthenia gravis (an autoimmune disease acting at the neuromuscular junction).

> *cc* **3.14** Competitive **HIV protease inhibitors** (saquinavir, ritonavir, indinavir, and nelfinavir) target the final step of viral replication and inhibit the active site formed by the enzyme dimer from functioning.

> *cc* **3.15** **Angiotensin-converting enzyme (ACE)** inhibitors, such as **captopril, enalapril, and lisinopril,** are the most commonly used antihypertensive therapies that inhibit formation of angiotensin II, an octapeptide from angiotensin I.

B. **Noncompetitive inhibitors** bind to the enzyme or the enzyme–substrate complex at a site distinct from the active site, decreasing the activity of the enzyme (Figure 3-4B). Thus, **V_{max} is decreased.** Inhibition can **not** be overcome by increasing substrate. Structurally, these inhibitors are **not** similar to substrate.

> *cc* **3.16** A common **noncompetitive inhibitor** is a result of chelation (metal binding) therapy, such as **ethylenediamine tetraacetic acid (EDTA),** resulting in removal of required divalent metal ions from the active site of enzymes. Blood of patients is collected in tubes with EDTA **to inhibit both calcium-activated proteases and the blood coagulation pathway.**

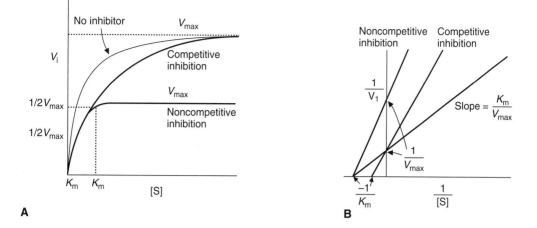

Figure 3-5 Summary of effects of competitive and noncompetitive inhibitors on **(A)** Michaelis-Menten plots, **(B)** Lineweaver-Burk plots, and **(C)** physical interpretation.

C. **Irreversible inhibitors** are enzyme inactivators that bind covalently to the enzyme and **inactivate** it. Their kinetics appear exactly like noncompetitive inhibition—an increase in inhibition with length of exposure and the inability to remove by dilution (since they are covalently bound).

> *cc* **3.17** **Nerve gases,** agents of chemical terrorism such as tabun and sarin, and **alkyl-phosphate insecticides** (malathion) are **irreversible inhibitors of acetylcholine esterase.** These compounds are also termed **"suicide" inhibitors,** creating a reactive group irreversibly reacting in the active site forming an extremely stable intermediate.

D. A summary of various forms of inhibition (graphical) representations are presented in Figure 3-5.

VI. Allosteric Enzymes

A. Virtually every metabolic pathway is subject to feedback control, and allosteric enzymes are used. This is a component of **feedback inhibition, where the concentration of the end product** of a pathway is **"monitored" to shut off the first (usually an allosteric) enzyme in a pathway** to prevent unwanted and wasted production of intermediates.

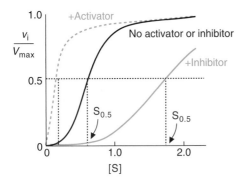

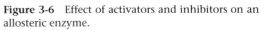

Figure 3-6 Effect of activators and inhibitors on an allosteric enzyme.

B. Allosteric enzymes are oligomeric (multiple subunits) and, through conformational changes, **bind activators or inhibitors** at sites other than (but interacting with) the active substrate binding sites (Figure 3-6).

C. Sigmoidal curves are generated by plots of v versus [S]. Allosteric enzymes do **not** obey Michaelis-Menten kinetics, and a Lineweaver-Burk plot is not interpretable.

1. An allosteric enzyme has two or more subunits, each with **substrate-binding sites** that exhibit **cooperativity**. Binding of a substrate molecule at one site facilitates binding of other substrate molecules at other sites.
   a. **Allosteric activators** cause the enzyme to bind substrate more readily.
   b. **Allosteric inhibitors** cause the enzyme to bind substrate less readily.
2. Similar effects occur during O_2 binding to **hemoglobin** (see Figure 2-7).

VII. Regulation of Enzyme Activity by Post-Translational (Covalent) Modification

A. Enzyme activity may increase or decrease after the covalent addition of a chemical group.

B. Phosphorylation affects many enzymes.

1. Pyruvate dehydrogenase and glycogen synthase are inhibited by phosphorylation, while glycogen phosphorylase is activated.
2. Phosphatases that remove the phosphate groups alter the activities of these enzymes.

C. Proenzyme

1. Inactive, precursor protein (also called **zymogen**) with an additional peptide attached

cc 3.18 **C-peptide** links the insulin A and B chains in proinsulin. The peptide is removed by proteolytic processing via **carboxypeptidase E, yielding active insulin.** Mutations in the enzyme rendering it inactive or lowering its activity may cause **hyperproinsulinism and diabetes** in the homozygous state.

VIII. Regulation by Protein–Protein Interactions

A.   Proteins can bind to enzymes, altering their activity. For example, regulatory subunits inhibit the activity of protein kinase A. When these regulatory subunits bind cyclic adenosine monophosphate (cAMP) and are released from the enzyme, the catalytic subunits become active.

B.   Enzymes can be arranged as **enzyme cascades**, exponentially amplifying the availability/activity of products in the path (e.g., hormone activation, blood clotting).

> *cc* *3.19*   **Hemostasis and thrombosis** are mediated by enzymes along cascading steps of the blood coagulation pathway(s). Inherited **deficiencies of clotting factors result in uncontrolled bleeding. Factor VIII deficiency** causes **Hemophilia A,** an X-linked disease rife in some European royal families.

IX.   Isoenzymes

A.   Isoenzymes (or isozymes) are enzymes comprised of different combinations of at least two nonidentical subunits that catalyze the same reaction but differ in their amino acid sequence and, therefore, in many of their physical properties.

B.   Tissues contain characteristic isozymes or mixtures of isozymes. Enzymes such as lactate dehydrogenase (LDH) and creatine kinase (CK) differ from one tissue to another. Knowing which isozyme is elevated can be indicative of specific tissue damage.

1. **Lactate dehydrogenase** contains four subunits. Each subunit may be either of the heart (H) or the muscle (M) type. Five isozymes exist (HHHH, HHHM, HHMM, HMMM, and MMMM).

> *cc* *3.20*   Increase in serum LDH isoforms has been an important marker of disease. For instance, **LDH-2 is the predominant form found in serum,** mostly due to turnover of **immune cells.** LDH-1 (HHHH) becomes elevated in cases of **myocardial infarction** (MI), over the normal levels of LDH-2, the so called **LDH-flip.** However, this is more of historical significance because better markers, such as CK and troponins, have replaced LDH in the diagnosis of MI. However, LDH does still have some value in diagnosing lymphomas, as well as **determining the etiology of pleural effusions.**

2. **Creatine kinase** contains two subunits. Each subunit may be either of the muscle (M) or the brain (B) type. Three isozymes exist (MM, MB, and BB). The MB fraction is most prevalent in heart muscle.

> *cc* *3.21*   With regard to isozyme distribution, CK-MM comprises 99% of skeletal muscle and ~75% of myocardium. CK-MB comprises ~25% of myocardium, but it is **not found in any other tissues,** so **CK-MB is a significant marker for MI.** CK-MB levels begin to rise **within a few hours of an MI** and remain elevated for up to 3 days.

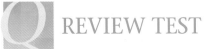

Directions: *Each of the numbered questions or incomplete statements in this section is followed by answers or by completions of the statement. Select the **one** lettered answer or completion that is **best** in each case.*

1. The relationship between an enzyme and a reactant molecule can best be described as:

(A) a temporary association.
(B) an association stabilized by a covalent bond.
(C) one in which the enzyme is changed permanently.
(D) a permanent mutual alteration of structure.
(E) noncomplementary binding.

2. The main function of a coenzyme is to:

(A) extend the number of chemical reactions that can occur in the enzyme's active site.
(B) stabilize the tertiary state.
(C) increase the enzyme K_m.
(D) decrease the enzyme V_{max}.
(E) regulate enzymes through feedback inhibition.

3. An enzymatic reaction proceeds with maximal velocity (V_{max}) when:

(A) the substrate concentration is equal to that of a competitive inhibitor.
(B) allosteric effectors are present.
(C) the enzyme substrate complex is maximal.
(D) the substrate concentration exceeds that of a noncompetitive inhibitor.
(E) all of the substrate is bound to the enzyme.

4. A competitive inhibitor of an enzyme is usually:

(A) a highly reactive compound.
(B) a metal ion such as Hg^{2+} or Pb^{2+}.
(C) structurally similar to the substrate.
(D) water insoluble.
(E) a poison.

5. Allosteric enzymes catalyze reactions by which of the following?

(A) Inhibiting the conversion of product to substrate
(B) Driving thermodynamically unfavorable equilibria
(C) Lowering activation energies
(D) Generating sigmoidal plots of V versus S
(E) Stabilizing the energies of products

6. Isocitrate dehydrogenase catalyzes the reaction:

$$\text{Isocitrate} + \text{NAD}^+ \rightarrow \alpha\text{-ketoglutarate}$$
$$+ CO_2 + \text{NADH} + H^+$$

The curves illustrated below are obtained when the initial velocity (v) of the reaction is plotted against isocitrate concentration in the presence of various levels of ADP and excess NAD^+. Which of the following statements about this system is correct?

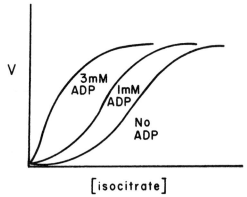

[isocitrate]

(A) Isocitrate dehydrogenase exhibits simple Michaelis-Menten kinetics in the absence of ADP.
(B) ADP increases the K_m of the enzyme for isocitrate.
(C) ADP increases the V_{max} of the enzyme.

(D) ADP activates the enzyme.

(E) ADP is a suicide inhibitor.

7. A series of enzymes catalyze the reaction $X \rightarrow Y \rightarrow Z \rightarrow A$. Product "A" binds to the enzyme that converts X to Y at a position remote from its active site. This binding decreases the activity of the enzyme. Product "A" functions as:

(A) a competitive inhibitor.

(B) a coenzyme.

(C) the substrate.

(D) an intermediate.

(E) an allosteric inhibitor.

Questions 8 and 9

Refer to the following graph when answering questions 8 and 9.

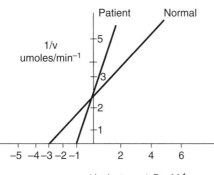

An infant was admitted to the hospital with vomiting, diarrhea, and jaundice. An extract of red blood cells (RBCs) was analyzed for galactose-1-phosphate uridyl transferase at varying concentrations of galactose-1-P.

8. The most likely problem with the transferase in the patient is which of the following?

(A) A noncompetitive inhibitor in RBCs

(B) An irreversible inhibitor in red cells

(C) A mutation in the binding site for galactose-1-P

(D) A mutation in the binding site for UDP-glucose

(E) A mutation in a residue involved in catalysis

9. What is the K_m for the normal enzyme (in mM)?

(A) 0.2

(B) 0.5

(C) 1

(D) 3

(E) 0.33

10. A 10-year-old boy presents with vomiting, sweating, drooling, and a decreased heart rate. His friends state that he was in a corn field when it was sprayed by a crop duster. The pesticide causing his symptoms is an organophosphate that covalently binds to acetylcholinesterase and inactivates the enzyme. What type of inhibition is this?

(A) Competitive

(B) Noncompetitive

(C) Irreversible

(D) Feedback

(E) Allosteric

11. A teenager finishes eating a hot fudge sundae and a milkshake. As her blood sugar rises, the liver recruits both glucokinase ($K_m = 10.0$ mM) and hexokinase ($K_m = 0.10$ mM) to metabolize the glucose. Which of the following is a correct statement about the kinetics of these two enzymes?

(A) Hexokinase will metabolize 100× more glucose molecules.

(B) Hexokinase will lower the energy of activation more than glucokinase.

(C) Hexokinase will have a higher V_{max} than glucokinase.

(D) Hexokinase has a much greater attraction to glucose than glucokinase.

(E) Hexokinase will shut down glucokinase through feedback inhibition.

12. A 64-year-old man complains of an acute onset of unilateral eye pain and reduction in visual acuity. On physical exam, you notice conjunctival injection (eye redness) and a mid-dilated and nonreactive pupil. Funduscopic exam reveals cupping of the optic disc. Recognizing the signs and

symptoms as glaucoma, you administer the medication acetazolamide to decrease the production of aqueous fluid and lower the intraocular pressure. Acetazolamide is a noncompetitive inhibitor of carbonic anhydrase and, therefore, will cause:

(A) an increase in K_m.
(B) a decrease in K_m.
(C) an increase in V_{max}.
(D) a decrease in V_{max}.
(E) a decrease in both K_m and V_{max}.

13. An emergency room physician sees several patients with a wide range of morbidities. The cause of which of the following ailments is most likely caused by enzyme denaturation?

(A) A 34-year-old man diagnosed with a gastrinoma complaining of diarrhea for 2 weeks
(B) A 58-year-old man with chest pain and shortness of breath with increased activity
(C) An 18-year-old boy presenting with a sore throat and fever of 101° F; he has small minimally tender anterior cervical lymph nodes and a red pharynx
(D) An 18-month-old male with a 4-day history of symptoms of an upper respiratory infection presenting with fever, irritability, and pulling at his left ear for the past 24 hours
(E) A 48-year-old female complaining of knee pain after twisting her leg playing tennis

14. A 43-year-old man with a history of hypertension and hyperlipidemia is now diagnosed with type 2 diabetes mellitus. This constellation of morbidities has been shown to increase the risk of coronary artery disease and has been coined "the metabolic syndrome." A promising new drug for this disorder inhibits the enzyme tyrosine phosphatase 1B via binding to multiple, non–substrate-binding sites, producing a conformational change, with subsequent decreased catalytic capacity. Which of the following choices best describes the inhibition of the new drug?

(A) Competitive
(B) Noncompetitive
(C) Allosteric
(D) Feedback
(E) Irreversible

Questions 15–16

An 8-year-old girl presents with precocious puberty, short stature, and large macules the color of coffee with milk. Further history finds the patient to have McCune-Albright syndrome, a result of estrogen production due to an excess aromatase from ovarian follicular cysts. As a research project, you synthesize a compound that inhibits aromatase and will treat the precocious puberty component of her illness. Use the table below to evaluate your new drug.

[Substrate] With Inhibitor	Rate of Reaction (mol/L/s)	[Substrate] Without Inhibitor	Rate of Reaction (mol/L/s)
5 mM	5×10^{-7}	5 mM	8×10^{-7}
10 mM	0.5×10^{-6}	10 mM	1.2×10^{-6}
20 mM	1.0×10^{-6}	20 mM	1.8×10^{-6}
40 mM	1.6×10^{-6}	40 mM	1.9×10^{-6}
80 mM	2.0×10^{-6}	80 mM	2.0×10^{-6}

15. Which answer choice best describes the inhibitor that has been synthesized?

(A) Competitive
(B) Noncompetitive
(C) Allosteric
(D) Feedback
(E) Irreversible

16. A 3-year-old boy in good health began having seizures that consisted of a sudden turning of the head to the left, tonic posturing of the left arm, and loss of awareness for 1 to 2 minutes. The patient was successfully treated with the anticonvulsant phenytoin (Dilantin). Dilantin is a substrate that binds to and is metabolized by an enzyme in the liver. Why doesn't the rate of metabolism by the liver enzyme increase when the level of Dilantin increases?

(A) Enzyme–product complexes prevent further binding of more substrate.

(B) All of the active sites of the enzyme are saturated with substrate at high substrate concentrations.

(C) Substrate–substrate interactions at high concentrations become strong.

(D) None of the enzyme is found in the ES complex.

(E) Significant product formation results in inhibition of the reaction.

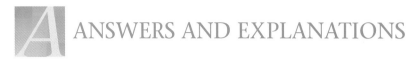

ANSWERS AND EXPLANATIONS

1–A. The ES (enzyme–substrate) complex is a *transient* and highest energy state at the apex of the energy diagram (see Figure 3-1) that collapses to form product (forward direction) or substrate (backward). Therefore, there is neither a covalent bond formed (choice B) nor a permanent change in the enzyme (choice C)/substrate (choice D) alone. ES complex is highly complementary for optimal, productive binding (choice E).

2–A. The purpose of coenzymes (cofactors that are metals or vitamins) is to make the enzyme more efficient in activity. A quick glance at choice B might cause one to mistake *tertiary* state as *transition* state. Choices C and D are changes that would make the enzyme *less efficient*. Choice E pertains to allosteric enzymes only.

3–C. At V_{max} (see Figure 3-3A), the maximum velocity of the reaction depicted on the right part of the curve, the enzyme is working "at full steam" and fully occupied with substrate and thus virtually always in the enzyme–substrate (ES) complex. This question has nothing to with any type of inhibitors or allosteric effectors (choices A, B, and D), and choice E is correct only in the case where substrate concentration is exceedingly high (greater than $20 \times K_m$).

4–C. In general, competitive inhibitors are structurally similar to their substrate, since they compete (hence the name) for the same active site of the enzyme and can be displaced by higher concentrations of the substrate. Because the enzymes are in aqueous milieus, the inhibitors are soluble (choice D). The rest of the choices (A, B, and E) involve irreversible inhibitors that permanently alter enzymes.

5–C. All enzymes, whether allosteric or obeying Michaelis-Menten kinetics, catalyze efficiently by lowering the energy of activation (Ea). Because formation of product is the goal, neither choice A nor choice E is correct. The shape of the V versus S curve does not matter with respect to catalysis. Finally, ΔG determines the equilibrium, not Ea (choice B).

6–D. Without ADP, the curve is sigmoidal, thus Michaelis-Menten kinetics are not exhibited. V_{max} is the same at all ADP concentrations shown. The substrate concentration at $\frac{1}{2} V_{max}$ decreases as the ADP concentration increases; therefore, ADP decreases the K_m, activating the enzyme. (The velocity is higher at lower substrate concentrations in the presence of ADP.)

7–E. This question involves a metabolic pathway and feedback inhibition, where the end product of a pathway is "monitored" to shut off the first (allosteric) enzyme in a pathway to prevent unwanted and wasted production of intermediates. All of the other choices involve single, monomeric enzymes (A, B, and C) or an ambiguous answer (D).

8–C. This is a double reciprocal, Lineweaver-Burk plot, with V_{max} remaining the same and K_m differing in the patient enzyme. This is a competitive inhibitor (A and B represent the noncompetitive kinetic case). Because K_m reflects **affinity** for substrate, choices D and E are also incorrect.

9–E. K_m for the normal enzyme is on the 1/S axis (here 1/galactose 1-P) is 11/Km or $-1/-3$ or $\frac{1}{3} = 0.33$.

10–C. The term "covalent" in the question indicates inhibition, if one forgets about organophosphate toxicity. Irreversible inhibition binds tightly to the target enzyme and inactivates it. Choices A, B, and E do not involve covalent inhibitor binding, and choice D is related to regulation.

11–D. K_m is a measure of the attraction, or affinity, an enzyme has for a specific substrate. Mathematically, the K_m is the concentration of substrate at which the reaction velocity reaches $\frac{1}{2}$ V_{max}.

12–D. A noncompetitive inhibitor forms a covalent bond with an enzyme at a different site than the substrate. Therefore, the number of enzymes capable of catalyzing the reaction is decreased, resulting in a decrease in V_{max}. The inhibitor binds at a different site than the substrate and can even bind the enzyme substrate complex, so increasing the substrate concentration will not affect the reaction rate. Consequently, K_m remains unchanged.

13–A. Factors that cause protein unfolding include heat, chemical denaturants, and changes in pH. A gastrinoma is a neuroendocrine tumor that secretes excessive gastrin, resulting in increased gastric acid secretion. This, in turn, results in a paradoxical acidic environment in the duodenum and denaturation of the pancreatic digestive enzymes. The diarrhea is a result of an osmotic pull due to the undigested nutrients' inability to be absorbed in the gut. Although a fever (choice C) included an increase in temperature, most proteins are denatured above 50°C, a temperature well above the normal body temperature of 37°C.

14–C. Allosteric inhibition is similar to noncompetitive inhibition, in that the inhibitor binds to a site different from the substrate-binding site, but the question states "multiple, non–substrate-binding sites" and, therefore, inhibition is allosteric. However, noncompetitive inhibition exhibits an "on or off" effect on binding, whereas an allosteric inhibitor usually shows cooperativity with multiple binding sites, with a graded effect on enzyme catalytic activity. Furthermore, allosteric inhibition is generally noncovalent (not irreversible) and induces a conformational change of the catalytic site, subsequently affecting the reaction rate.

15–A. Competitive inhibitors will reach the same V_{max} as the uninhibited reaction once the substrate concentration increases and out-competes the inhibitor for the enzyme catalytic site. Noncompetitive and irreversible inhibitors will never reach V_{max} because the portion of the enzyme they are bound to will be taken out of the total. The lack of a sigmoidal curve rules out allostery or feedback regulation.

16–B. The rate of an enzyme-catalyzed reaction will generally increase exponentially with respect to substrate concentration until the substrate concentration exhausts the catalytic sites of the enzyme population. Once this occurs, the rate of reaction remains the same regardless of an increase of substrate since all enzymes are saturated. Substrate cannot bind to enzyme–product complexes (binding sites are all occupied). Substrate–substrate interactions are the same regardless of concentration. Product formation does not inhibit the reaction.

Bioenergetics

I. Metabolic Fuels and Dietary Components

A. Fuels

1. When **fuels** are metabolized (via **catabolism**) in the body, **heat** is generated, and adenosine triphosphate (**ATP**) is synthesized.
2. **Energy** is produced by oxidizing fuels to the final products CO_2 and H_2O.
   a. **Carbohydrates** produce about 4 kcal/g.
   b. **Proteins** produce about 4 kcal/g.
   c. **Fats** produce more than twice as much energy (**9 kcal/g**) as proteins and carbohydrates.
   d. **Alcohol**, present in many diets, produces about **7 kcal/g**.
3. Physicians and nutritionists often use the term "calorie" (cal) in place of the physicist's kilocalorie (kcal).
4. **Heat** generated by fuel oxidation **is used to** maintain body temperature.
5. **ATP** generated by fuel metabolism is used for biochemical reactions, muscle contraction, and other energy-requiring processes.

B. Composition of body fuel stores (Figure 4-1)

1. *Triacylglycerol* (triglyceride)
   a. **Adipose triacylglycerol** is the major fuel store of the body.
   b. Adipose tissue stores fuel very efficiently. It has **more stored calories per gram and less water** (15%) than other fuel stores, like an anhydrous oil droplet with little water. (Muscle tissue is about 80% water.)
2. **Glycogen** stores are hydrated and, although small, are extremely important.
   a. **Liver glycogen** is used to maintain blood glucose during the early stages of fasting.
   b. **Muscle glycogen** is oxidized for muscle contraction.
3. **Protein** is inefficiently degraded, unlike carbohydrate and fat.
   a. Almost all of the nitrogen of protein metabolism is excreted as urea, which is not fully oxidized. Thus, some energy remains unreleased.
   b. Approximately 70% of the energy from protein is available as "fuel."
   c. If too much protein is oxidized for energy, body functions can be severely compromised.

C. Respiratory quotient (R.Q.) is the ratio of CO_2 produced to O_2 (CO_2/O_2) used by a tissue, organism, or complete in vivo oxidation of a foodstuff.

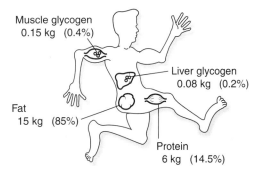

Figure 4-1 Fuel composition of the average 70-kg man after an overnight fast (in kilograms and as a percentage of total calories).

1. For a typical **carbohydrate:**

   $$C_6H_{12}O_6 + 6O_2 \rightarrow 6CO_2 + 6H_2O$$
   (glucose)

   The oxidation of carbohydrate produces 1 mole CO_2/mole of O_2 used. Thus, the R.Q. for carbohydrate is 6/6 or 1.0.

2. For a typical **fat:**

   $$C_{57}H_{110}O_6 + 81.5O_2 \rightarrow 57CO_2 + 55H_2O$$

   Thus, the R.Q. for fat is $57/81.5 = 0.7$.

3. For a typical **protein:**
   An average R.Q. for protein is approximately 0.8.

4. The R.Q. for a **tissue:**
   a. **R.Q. of an arm at rest is ~0.7** because resting muscle uses fat, not carbohydrate.
   b. **R.Q. for the brain is near 1.0** because this organ uses glucose, the principal energy source under all conditions except *prolonged* starvation.
   c. **The R.Q. for the entire body at rest is about 0.82, indicating that about 50% fat and 50% carbohydrate is used.** This value is above 0.7 (for arm or leg only) because the brain and erythrocytes use glucose under all conditions.
   d. Exercise will push the R.Q. to 1.0, indicating a switch to carbohydrate metabolism.
   e. Although one obtains energy from protein (R.Q. ~0.8), little energy is derived in the postabsorptive state (that time after digestion and absorption of a meal is complete, about 12 hours after eating) of amino acid metabolism.

D. **Daily energy expenditure** is the amount of energy required each day.

   1. *Basal metabolic rate (BMR)* is an estimate of the rate of metabolism determined by measuring the volume of respiratory gases generated during a period of time. BMR can vary under different states of health and disease (Table 4-1).

TABLE 4-1	*Basal Metabolic Rate (BMR) Varies Through Life and in Health and Disease*	
	Factor	Effect
cc *4.1*	Sex	Males have a higher BMR than females for all ages
cc *4.2*	Age	Elderly individuals have decreased BMRs

(continued)

TABLE 4-1	*Basal Metabolic Rate (BMR) Varies Through Life and in Health and Disease (Continued)*	
	Factor	**Effect**
cc 4.3	Height	Tall, thin people have higher BMRs
cc 4.4	Growth	Children and pregnant women have increased BMRs
cc 4.5	Body composition	The leaner the tissue, the greater the BMR
cc 4.6	Body temperature	Fever can raise the BMR 14%/°C
cc 4.7	Hormones	Thyroid hormone increases BMR

> *cc 4.8* Reducing metabolism can be achieved by **hypothermia** (reducing temperature). This method is used during open-heart surgery to prevent organ damage while the circulation is interrupted. Organs are stored hypothermically prior to transplantation.

    a. An estimate of basal **BMR = 24 kcal/kg body weight per day.**
    b. To determine an **average calorie expenditure** (or **total metabolic rate**) with normal physical activity, **add 50%** to the basal BMR data.
    c. Strenuous exercise such as running or swimming can use up 600 cal/hour for a 70-kg individual.

> *cc 4.9* **Thyroid dysgenesis/hypothyroidism** is the most frequent cause of **congenital hypothyroidism,** accounting for 85% of cases. This has a significant effect on **lowering BMR.** Congenital hypothyroidism can cause severe neurologic, mental, and motor damage.

  2. *Diet-induced thermogenesis (DIT),* formerly known as **specific dynamic action (SDA),** is the elevation in metabolic rate that occurs during digestion and absorption of foods. Its value is usually unknown and probably small (less than 10% of total energy).
  3. *Physical activity*
    a. The number of calories that physical activity contributes to the daily energy expenditure varies considerably. A person can expend about 5 calories each minute while walking, but 20 calories while running.
    b. The daily energy requirement for an extremely sedentary person is about 30% of BMR. For a more active person, it exceeds 50% of BMR.

E. Energy reserves: fasting versus starvation (long term)

  1. The **principal energy reserve** used for long-term food deprivation **is adipose tissue (fat)** as triglycerides for *both the lean and obese individual.*
  2. The contribution of **carbohydrate to total energy reserves is very small,** yet it is the **energy source called upon** *first* with heavy energy expenditures.

TABLE 4-2	*Fuels Available in the Human Body for Long-Term Fasting*			
	Normal Man		**Obese Man**	
Fuel Reserve	*kg*	*kcal*	*kg*	*kcal*
Fat (adipose triglycerides)	15.0	141,000 (85%)	80.0	752,000 (96%)
Protein (mainly muscle)	6.0	24,000 (14%)	8.0	32,000 (4%)
Glycogen: Muscle	0.120	480	0.160	640
Liver	0.070	280	0.070	280
Glucose (extracellular fluid)	0.020	80	0.025	100
Total available energy	165,840		785,020	

> ## cc *4.10*
> A normal person (Table 4-2) refers to a 70-kg individual who has a fuel reserve of 30% by weight. The **increased reserve of the obese individual is mostly fat.** Several **complete fasts** indicate that one can live with water **for about 60 days without food** (theoretically 165,840/2520 cal/day = 65 days). Death ensues when certain essential proteins (e.g., from brain, heart) start to be used for energy.

F. **Nutrients versus end products**

  1. *The nutrients—carbohydrates, fats, and protein—*are transformed into cellular materials used for growth, "turnover," or energy storage (Figure 4-2).

    a. Nutrients are oxidized, reduced, polymerized, depolymerized, and rearranged.

    b. The final end products of eventual metabolism are: CO_2, H_2O, and urea.

  2. *Catabolism vs anabolism* (Table 4-3)

    a. **Catabolism:** degradative pathways, some of which yield useful energy.

> ## cc *4.11*
> For patients with **severe trauma, burns, overwhelming infections,** or underlying diseases associated with excess protein **catabolism,** support such as **parenteral nutrition** is initiated. **Cancer** produces progressive rapid emaciation and **cachexia** (anorexia, fat and muscle tissue wasting, and psychological distress).

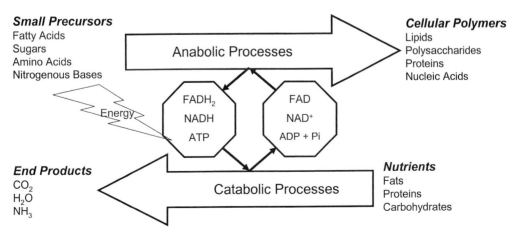

Figure 4-2 The catabolism/anabolism cycle.

TABLE 4-3	*Comparison of Catabolism and Anabolism*		
		Catabolism	**Anabolism**
The Process	Goal	Generate energy	Form compounds
	Type of Process	Oxidative, degradative	Reductive, synthetic
	Net Energetics	Yield energy	Requires energy
The Participants	Starting materials	Complex and variable	Simple and few
	Final Products	Simple and few	Complex and variable
	Representative mediators	$NAD^+ \rightarrow NADH$	$NADPH \rightarrow NADP^+$
		$AD + Pi \rightarrow ATP$	$ATP \rightarrow ADP + Pi$

   b. Anabolism: biosynthetic pathways that make cellular materials. Intuitively, anabolic pathways require energy.

> *cc 4.12*   Examples of **anabolic** processes include **growth and increase in muscle mass and mineralization of bone. Body building** takes anabolic metabolism to an extreme.

  3. Nitrogen balance
    a. Proteins in the body undergo constant turnover; they are degraded to amino acids and are resynthesized.
    b. The **nitrogen balance** is the difference between dietary N (nitrogen ingested) and excreted N (urine, sweat, feces).
      (1) Nitrogen balance: A normal healthy adult.

        dietary N = excreted N

      (2) Positive nitrogen balance: Periods of growth and development

        dietary N ≫ excreted N

> *cc 4.13*   Both children and pregnant women go through a physiologic **positive nitrogen balance** to provide adequate amino acids for growth and development.

      (3) Negative nitrogen balance: Dietary deficiency of protein/amino acids (disease).

        dietary N ≪ excreted N

II.   Bioenergetics

A.   The change in free energy in biologic systems

  1. The **change in free energy** (the energy available to do **useful work** at constant pressure and temperature) is defined by the equation:

    $\Delta G = \Delta H - T\Delta S$

where ΔG is the change in Gibbs free energy; ΔH is the change in enthalpy (heat content); ΔS is the change in entropy (randomness or disorder); and T is the absolute temperature in degrees Kelvin (K).

2. For a biochemical reaction, the change in free energy can be used to predict the **direction** in which the reaction will proceed.
3. For the reaction in which

$$aA + bB \leftrightarrows cC + dD$$

(where the uppercase letters symbolize the molecule, and the lowercase letters indicate the number of molecules), the free energy change depends on the concentrations of substrates and products and on the value of the constant $\Delta G^{\circ\prime}$.

$$\Delta G = \Delta G^{\circ\prime} + RT \ln [C]^c [D]^d/[A]^a [B]^b$$

where $\Delta G^{\circ\prime}$ **is the standard free energy change at pH 7**; R is the gas constant; T is the absolute temperature; and [ ] means concentration.

4. If the value of ΔG
   a. is **negative**, the reaction will proceed spontaneously with the release of energy.
   b. is **positive**, the reaction will not proceed spontaneously.
   c. is = **0**, the reaction is at equilibrium, and, although substrates react to form products and products react to form substrates, there is no net change in the concentrations.

B. **The equilibrium constant and the change in free energy**

1. At equilibrium, $\Delta G = 0$ and

$$\Delta G^{\circ\prime} = -RT \ln [C]^c [D]^d/[A]^a [B]^b$$

2. The **equilibrium constant** (K_{eq}) is related to the **concentrations** of substrates and products **at equilibrium**,

$$K_{eq} = [C]^c [D]^d/ [A]^a [B]^b$$

Therefore, $\Delta G^{\circ\prime} = -RT \ln K_{eq}$.
   a. If $K_{eq} = 1$, $\Delta G^{\circ\prime} = 0$.
   b. If $K_{eq} > 1$, $\Delta G^{\circ\prime}$ is negative.
   c. If $K_{eq} < 1$, $\Delta G^{\circ\prime}$ is positive.

3. The larger and more negative the $\Delta G^{\circ\prime}$, the less substrate relative to product is required to produce a negative ΔG (i.e., the more likely the reaction is to proceed spontaneously).
4. For a sequence of reactions that have common intermediates, the **standard free energy changes are additive** (Table 4-4).

C. **The relevance of free energy changes to biologic systems**

1. The rate of a reaction is not related to its free energy change.
   a. A reaction with a large negative free energy change does not necessarily proceed rapidly.

TABLE 4-4	Free Energy for Transferring Phosphate from ATP to Glucose
glucose + P_i → glucose-6-P + H_2O	$\Delta G^{\circ\prime} = +3.3$ kcal/mole
ATP + H_2O → ADP + P_i	$\Delta G^{\circ\prime} = -7.3$ kcal/mole
Sum: glucose + ATP → glucose-6-P + H_2O	$\Delta G^{\circ\prime} = -4.0$ kcal/mole

    b. The **speed** of a reaction depends on the properties of the **enzyme** that catalyzes
       the reaction.
       (1) An enzyme increases the rate at which a reaction reaches equilibrium.
       (2) It does not affect K_{eq} (the relative concentrations of substrates and prod-
             ucts at equilibrium).
 2. Most biochemical reactions exist in pathways; therefore, other reactions are con-
    stantly adding substrate and removing product.
    a. The relative activities of the enzymes that catalyze the individual reactions of
       a pathway differ.
    b. Some reactions are near equilibrium ($\Delta G = 0$). Their direction can be readily
       altered by small changes in the concentrations of their substrates or products.
    c. Other reactions are far from equilibrium. Allosteric factors that alter the activ-
       ity of these enzymes can change the overall flux through the pathway.

III. Biological Oxidations

A. **Energy is generated in the oxidation of substances in the body.**

 1. For a complete reaction, there is an **oxidant (electron acceptor)** and a **reduc-
    tant (electron donor)**.
 2. The **ultimate electron acceptor of biologic oxidations is oxygen**, which is con-
    verted into water.

B. The **reduction potential** of a compound, **ΔE**, is the **tendency to acquire electrons**
(and thus be reduced).

 1. The more positive the reduction potential, the greater the affinity for electrons
    and tendency to be reduced (the stronger the oxidant). Conversely, the more
    negative the reduction potential, the stronger the reductant.
 2. The loss of electrons (oxidation) is coupled to a gain of electrons (reduction).
    These occur in **redox pairs.**

C. The **standard reduction potential**, ΔE°, is the reduction potential measured under
standard conditions (25°C, a 1M concentration for each ion in the reaction, a partial
pressure of 1 atm for each gas in the reaction).

D. ΔE° is related to the standard energy change ΔG°. $\Delta G^{\circ} = -nF\Delta E^{\circ}$, where n = no. of
electrons, F = Faraday constant, ΔG° = change in standard free energy, and ΔE° = change
in standard reduction potential.

 1. A large *negative* ΔG is associated with an **exergonic reaction.**
 2. **The larger the *positive* value for ΔE, the larger the *negative* value for ΔG.** Thus,
    a positive ΔE indicates an energetically favorable process.

IV. Properties of Adenosine Triphosphate (the principal "downhill" reaction in vivo)

A. The structure of ATP

1. ATP, one of the four nucleotides comprising DNA, consists of the base **adenine,** the sugar **ribose,** and **three phosphate groups** (Figure 4-3).
2. **Adenosine** (a nucleoside) contains the base adenine linked to D-ribose.
3. Adenosine monophosphate (**AMP**) is a nucleotide that contains adenosine with a phosphate group esterified to the 5′-hydroxyl of the sugar.
4. Adenosine diphosphate (**ADP**) contains a second phosphate group attached by an anhydride bond.
5. **ATP** contains a third phosphate group.

B. The functions of ATP

1. ATP plays a central role in **energy exchanges** in the body.

> *cc 4.14* A **myocardial infarction** results in **ischemia** or an attenuated oxygen supply by occlusion of a coronary artery. With **damage in mitochondria,** there is a **decrease in cellular levels of ATP** and creatine phosphate, another high-energy phosphate compound.

2. ATP is constantly being consumed and regenerated during catabolism and anabolism, respectively (see Fig 4-2 and Table 4-3).
   a. It is consumed by processes such as muscular contraction, active transport, and biosynthetic reactions.
   b. It is regenerated by the oxidation of foodstuffs.
3. The **free energy** released when ATP is hydrolyzed "drives" unfavorable reactions that require energy.
   a. ATP can be hydrolyzed to **ADP** and inorganic phosphate (**P$_i$**) or to **AMP** and pyrophosphate (**PP$_i$**). ATP, ADP, and AMP are interconverted by the adenylate kinase reaction.

$$ATP + AMP \leftrightarrows 2ADP$$

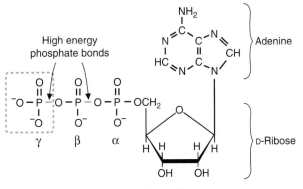

Adenosine 5′–triphosphate

ATP

Figure 4-3 The structure of adenosine triphosphate (ATP).

b. Other nucleoside triphosphates (GTP, UTP, and CTP; guanosine, uridine, and cytosine triphosphates, respectively) are sometimes used to likewise mediate energy exchange in biochemical reactions. They can be derived from ATP.

4. For the **hydrolysis of ATP to ADP and P_i, $\Delta G^{o\prime} = -7.3$ kcal/mole.**
   a. The acid anhydride bonds of ATP are termed "high-energy bonds."
   b. $\Delta G^{o\prime}$ **is large,** however, not because a single bond is broken, but because the products of hydrolysis are more stable than ATP.

5. **ATP** can transfer phosphate groups to compounds such as glucose, with ADP as a product.

6. **ADP** can accept phosphate groups from compounds with a larger ΔG such as phosphoenolpyruvate, phosphocreatine, or 1,3-bisphosphoglycerate, forming ATP.

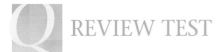 REVIEW TEST

*Directions: Each of the numbered questions or incomplete statements in this section is followed by answers or by completions of the statement. Select the **one** lettered answer or completion that is **best** in each case.*

1. A reaction is at equilibrium when:

(A) the $\Delta G^{\circ\prime}$ is negative.
(B) the ΔG is negative.
(C) the $\Delta G^{\circ\prime}$ is positive.
(D) the ΔG is positive.
(E) the ΔG is zero.

2. The basal metabolic rate (BMR) is:

(A) elevated by an all-carbohydrate diet.
(B) higher in women than men of the same age.
(C) lower in an 80-year-old man than a 20-year-old man.
(D) higher in a 12-year-old girl than a 12-year-old boy.
(E) determined by measuring expired CO_2.

3. During starvation, what percentage of the total caloric stores is provided by carbohydrate for a normal nonobese individual?

(A) 85%
(B) 50%
(C) 25%
(D) 14%
(E) Less than 2%

4. A sleeping student in the library uses 18 L of O_2 per hour. Under these conditions, what is the approximate CO_2 output in liters per hour?

(A) 14
(B) 9
(C) 36
(D) 18
(E) 22

5. Which of the following statements is correct concerning catabolism?

(A) Photosynthesis would be an example.
(B) Electrons are removed from NADH to form NAD^+.
(C) The production of protein from amino acids would be an example.

(D) Energy is released and captured to form ATP.
(E) More than one of the above statements are true of catabolism.

6. The Gibbs free energy, ΔG, is negative for:

(A) exergonic processes.
(B) endergonic processes.
(C) nonspontaneous processes.
(D) temperature-independent processes.
(E) concentration of reactants and products <1.0 M.

7. Given the following information: (T = 298°K; R = 1.98×10^{-3} kcal/mole), the standard free energy ($\Delta G^{\circ\prime}$) for the hydrolysis of ATP is −7.3 kcal/mole. If this reaction can be coupled to a reaction with $\Delta G^{\circ\prime}$ + 3.3 kcal/mole, what is the overall $\Delta G^{\circ\prime}$?

(A) −10.6 kcal/mole
(B) +8 kcal/mole
(C) −4 kcal/mole
(D) +4
(E) +4 kcal/mole

8. Blood gas consumption and production was measured in a resting leg. O_2 consumed in 1 hour was 4.0 L. What is the expected volume in liters of released CO_2?

(A) 5.6
(B) 4.0
(C) 3.4
(D) 2.8
(E) 2.0

9. For reaction x → y, the ΔG° is −3 kcal/mole. For the reaction y → x, the:

(A) reaction favors product x.
(B) ΔG is −3 kcal/mole.
(C) equilibrium constant is less than 1.
(D) reaction is exergonic.
(E) ΔG° is equal to ΔH°.

10. For two coupled reactions, the overall process will be exergonic if:

(A) at least one reaction is spontaneous.
(B) both reactions have $\Delta G° > 0$.
(C) at least one reaction generates no heat.
(D) $\Delta G1 + \Delta G2 < 0$.
(E) the second reaction is faster than the first.

11. If the K_{eq} of a reaction is 10, then the K_{eq} of the reverse reaction is:

(A) 0.01.
(B) 0.1.
(C) 1.0.
(D) 10.0.
(E) Cannot be determined without a calculator.

12. If the $\Delta E°$ of a reaction is negative, then:

(A) no products are present at equilibrium.
(B) no reactants are present at equilibrium.
(C) products are present at equilibrium, but at a lower concentration than that of reactants.
(D) reactants are present at equilibrium, but at a lower concentration than that of products.
(E) it can be made positive by increasing the temperature.

13. A 35-year-old man with normal daily activity and who weighs 80 kg comes to you because he just lost 20 pounds and feels he is at his optimal weight. What is the approximate percentage of daily caloric requirement provided by his diet of 200 g carbohydrate, 100 g fat, and 100 g protein?

(A) 50%
(B) 60%
(C) 75%
(D) 90%
(E) 125%

Questions 14 and 15

14. A 33-year-old woman is being treated with thyroid hormone for Hashimoto's thyroiditis, a disease causing hypothyroid- ism. Her treatment now affords her a daily energy expenditure of 2200 calories a day. If 20% of her calories are derived from protein, how many grams of protein should she eat to maintain her weight?

(A) 55 g
(B) 100 g
(C) 110 g
(D) 165 g
(E) 220 g

15. The same woman has been counseled by her doctor to lose 10 pounds to reduce her risk of heart disease. How many kilo-calories will she have to "burn off"? Assume the 10 pounds (~4500 g) consists mainly of fat.

(A) 900 kcal
(B) 4,500 kcal
(C) 9,000 kcal
(D) 18,000 kcal
(E) 40,500 kcal

16. A 22-year-old man has started to work out twice a day with the goal of competing in an upcoming bodybuilding competition. Despite his strict workout routine, he continues eating a diet of fast food hamburgers and french fries. After a gain of 15 pounds, it is likely he is in a:

(A) vitamin overload.
(B) negative nitrogen balance.
(C) positive nitrogen balance.
(D) state of decreased BMR.
(E) state of increased BMR.

17. A 58-year-old man complains of fatigue and a 20-pound weight loss over the past 3 months. The patient's father and grand-father both died of colon cancer. Colonos-copic examination is significant for several sites of cancerous growth, but no adeno-mas are appreciated. You diagnose him with "hereditary nonpolyposis colon can-cer," which results from a mismatch repair defect. One common cause of mismatch mutations is the spontaneous conversion of cytosine to thymine due to deamina-tion. To assure this reaction is spontaneous, which of the following criteria are needed?

(A) Negative enthalpy, positive entropy
(B) Negative enthalpy, negative entropy
(C) Positive enthalpy, positive entropy
(D) Positive enthalpy, negative entropy
(E) None of the above due to temperature dependence

18. A medicinal chemist is synthesizing a new medication. One of the products of the reaction is water, which is removed during the reaction through evaporation. By decreasing the concentration of the product, which of the following values would change?

(A) ΔG°
(B) ΔG
(C) ΔH
(D) ΔS
(E) K_{eq}

19. A 14-year-old dizygotic twin is referred to a nutritionist. He is 5′4″ and weighs 187 lb. His twin sister, however, is 5′5″ and weighs 88 lb. The nutritionist empathizes with the child and explains that even with the same exercise and diet, people have different basal metabolic rates (BMRs). Which of the following would most readily change the boy's BMR?

(A) Running up a flight of stairs
(B) Eating a meal high in fiber
(C) Weight lifting program
(D) Undergoing gastric bypass surgery
(E) Undergoing a thyroidectomy

20. A 70-kg distance runner trains by running 6 hours/day at a rate that consumes 7 kcal/(kg hr). He walks [2 kcal/(kg hr)] for an additional 2 hours, stands or sits [0.5 kcal/(kg hr)] for 8 hr/day, and sleeps during the remainder (assume full basal energy expenditure for sleep). He eats 5000 kcal/day. How many kilocalories does he use in a day?

(A) 3500 kcal
(B) 5180 kcal
(C) 5348 kcal
(D) 6180 kcal
(E) 7000 kcal

Questions 21 and 22

Please answer questions 21 and 22 from the following information.

A 34-year-old woman has suffered from anorexia nervosa for 8 years. She was admitted to a hospital for treatment. She is 62″ tall and weighs 72 lb, approximately 40% less than ideal weight. She was sedentary and appeared depressed. Her hemoglobin was 9 g/dL (anemic). She was fed by gavage through a nasogastric tube with 3 L/day nutrient solution providing 1000 kcal/L with protein (egg white homogenate), fat (triglyceride), carbohydrate (starch and sucrose), vitamins, and minerals.

21. What is happening with respect to the patient's weight after almost 3 weeks?

(A) The weight decrease has slowed down.
(B) No significant change yet, metabolism takes awhile to reset.
(C) A few pounds have been gained.
(D) A significant amount of weight has been gained.
(E) The patient exhibited hyperthyroidism and lost weight until corrected.

22. What is the status of the nitrogen balance in this patient?

(A) Nitrogen balance equals 1, homeostasis.
(B) Negative nitrogen balance, proteins take many weeks to be resynthesized.
(C) Negative nitrogen balance, there is hyperexcretion with large gavage volume.
(D) Positive nitrogen balance, proteins are replenished.
(E) Positive nitrogen balance, excretion is diminished with egg whites and minerals.

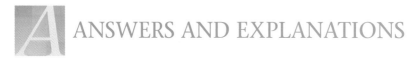

ANSWERS AND EXPLANATIONS

1–E. ΔG is the change in free energy. $\Delta G^{\circ\prime}$ is the standard free energy change at pH 7. At equilibrium, $\Delta G = 0$, and there is no net formation of products or reactants. If ΔG is negative, the reaction will proceed spontaneously to form products. If ΔG is positive, the reaction will not proceed spontaneously.

2–C. The basal metabolic rate is higher in younger than older people of a given gender and higher in males than females at a given age. It is not elevated with a carbohydrate diet; this is confusing BMR with respiratory quotient, and it is determined by inspired O_2, **not** expired CO_2.

3–E. Eighty-five percent of the fuel reserve in a nonobese individual resides in fat, approximately 14% in protein, and the remaining in carbohydrate (glycogen in muscle and liver) and glucose in extracellular fluid are less than 2%.

4–A. This question concerns the respiratory quotient (or R.Q.). The R.Q. is the ratio of CO_2 produced to O_2 used (CO_2/O_2) by a tissue, by an organism, or by the complete in vivo oxidation of a given foodstuff. An individual **at rest** has a relatively low R.Q. (about **0.8**), while a run up a flight of stairs will push the R.Q. close to 1.0, indicating a switch to carbohydrate metabolism. The CO_2 produced to O_2 used by the student = 14/18 = ~0.8.

5–D. **Catabolisms** are degradative pathways, some of which harvest useful energy from breaking down complex polymers. This is where the energy released is converted into generating ATP. Conversely, **anabolism** consists of biosynthetic pathways that make cellular materials. Intuitively, anabolic pathways require energy input. Photosynthesis, electron removal ($NADH \rightarrow NAD^+$), and amino acids producing proteins are all facets of anabolism.

6–A. $\Delta G < 0$ represents an exergonic process, not endergonic or nonspontaneous. Furthermore, $\Delta G = \Delta H - T\Delta S$ exhibits temperature dependence, and the concentration of reactants and products is unknown.

7–C. The reactions are additive (–7.3 kcal/mole + 3.3 kcal/mole = –4 kcal/mole). The other answers are variations of the sign (+ or –), subtracting, adding, or omitting the units. The information about temperature (T) and the gas constant (R) were distracters.

8–D. The R.Q. is the ratio of CO_2 produced to O_2 used (CO_2/O_2). The value for inspired O_2 is given. The R.Q. of a leg at rest would be close to 0.7 (2.8/4.0) because resting muscle uses fat instead of carbohydrate. The other answers involve glucose utilization (4.0/4.0), a ratio = 1 (B) and a ratio >1 (A); or 0.5 (E), which is nonsense; or an intermediate value that does not apply (C).

9–C. $\Delta G^\circ = -RT \ln K_{eq} = -RT \ln$ [products]/[reactants]. For $x \rightarrow y$, ΔG° is negative (–3 kcal/mol) and $K_{eq} > 1$. Therefore, the reaction occurs spontaneously, and the equilibrium favors products. In the reverse reaction, $y \rightarrow x$, ΔG° is positive and $K_{eq} < 1$. Therefore the reverse reaction does not occur spontaneously, and the equilibrium favors reactants. There is not enough information to know if ΔG is –3 kcal/mol as well, or if ΔG° is equal to ΔH°. A reaction is exergonic when a reaction proceeds spontaneously and releases energy.

10–D. For reactions that are coupled, **their ΔGs are additive. Exergonic**, or downhill reactions, release energy, and their **net ΔG << 0.** Therefore, ΔG1 + ΔG2 < 0 is true. Both reactions with ΔG° > 0 is the case for an endergonic reaction, and the remaining choices, while describing one of the reactions, give no information on the second reaction. One needs to know the ΔG of the second reaction since it is the **net ΔG << 0.**

11–B. K_{eq} = [products]/[reactants]. If we are given that the forward reaction is 10 or 10/1, then the reverse of K_{eq} = [reactants]/[products]. Thus, the reverse of K_{eq} is 1/10 or 0.1.

12–C. Consider **ΔG° = −nFΔE°.** If ΔE° is negative, then ΔG° must be positive, and the reaction favors reactants. This eliminates choices A, B, and D. Although at first, there appears to be no temperature term in the equation, ΔG° = –RT ln K_{eq}, so an increase in temperature would make ΔE° more negative (choice E).

13–C. We estimate the caloric requirements to be kcal = weight in kg × hour = 80 kg × 24 hr = 1920, and add another 50% for normal levels of activity since we are not at the recumbent, postabsorptive, physically rested state where BMR is measured. Therefore, 1920 + 960 (50%) = 2880 calories is the daily caloric requirement. The caloric values for carbohydrate, fat, and protein are 4, 9, and 4 kcal/g, respectively. Therefore the intake was (200 × 4) + (100 × 9) + (100 × 4) = 800 + 900 + 400 = 2100. The caloric intake/caloric requirement = 2100/2880 = 73%.

14–B. To maintain her weight and if protein calories will comprise 20% of her diet (0.20 × 2200 = 440 calories), she should consume 440/4 kcal/g, which equals 110 g of protein per day.

15–E. To lose 4500 g of fat, she must burn 4500 × 9 kcal/g, or an additional 40,500 kcal of energy. This is roughly equivalent to 50 hours of moderate to extreme exercise. Although an overwhelming number, this problem should stress the importance of a lifestyle that includes a healthy diet and exercise.

16–C. Although his diet is not optimal, his weight gain most likely includes newly formed muscle. A person's basal metabolic rate (BMR) is proportional to lean body mass, which has most likely increased in this individual despite a probable gain in adipose tissue as well. Unfortunately, fast food lacks leafy green vegetables, a primary source of vitamins.

17–A. To establish if a reaction is spontaneous, the value of Gibbs free energy (ΔG) must be determined. The equation, ΔG = ΔH — TΔS, where ΔH and ΔS represent enthalpy and entropy, respectively, must result in a negative value to conclude the reaction is spontaneous. Because temperature (T) is evaluated in the Kelvin temperature scale, the value is always positive.

18–B. Gibbs free energy can be expressed by the following two reactions:

ΔG = ΔG° + RT ln Keq ([products]/[reactants]) or ΔG = ΔH + TΔS. Therefore, as the product (P) is removed, the natural log (ln) value is decreased, resulting in a decrease of ΔG. All of the remaining answer choices are constants in which the values are established under a standard set of conditions.

19–C. The basal metabolic rate is the rate at which your body burns calories while you rest. The BMR can only be accurately measured after 12 hours of fasting and while the person is at complete rest. Examples that **do** increase the BMR are illness, hyperthyroidism, and increased lean muscle mass.

20–C. The runner's use of energy: running + walking + resting, can be calculated as follows:

$$\left(\frac{7kcal}{kg*hour}\times\frac{70kg\times6hr}{1}\right)+\left(\frac{2kcal}{kg*hour}\times\frac{70kg\times2hr}{1}\right)+\left(\frac{0.5kcal}{kg*hours}\times\frac{70kg\times8hr}{1}\right)=3500kcal$$

The BMR and the DIT must then be added to this value as follows:

BMR = 24/kcal/kg × day) × 70 kg = 1680 kcal; 10% of 1680 kcal = 168 kcal. 1680 kcal + 168 kcal = 1848 kcal.

Total kilocalories are: 3500 kcal + 1848 kcal = 5348 kcal.

21–D. The patient gained a significant amount of weight because the energy in the gavage solution was much greater than the energy expenditure required for the present weight. The patient's BMR = 32.7 kg × 24 kcal/kg = 785 kcal. Accounting for increases in activity (sedentary in the hospital, so we factor in 33%), activity = 790 × 0.33 = 260 kcal (<0.5). Even if you say she has normal activity and we add 50%, that is only an additional 393 kcal to add to the basal BMR. The intake is 3l × 1000 kcal/L = 3000 kcal. So the total of 1178 kcal expended is far less than the 3000 kcal taken in. After 3 weeks, the patient had a significant increase in body weight.

22–E. No complications arose, and with the proteins taken in, there is weight gain and muscle mass is increasing; protein synthesis resumes quickly. Any answer with excretion is obviously not the case since her weight gain means more nitrogen intake. Positive nitrogen balance indicates proteins are being synthesized and there is a net accumulation of protein. With the positive nitrogen balance, one can conclude that the nutrients were used for tissue synthesis. In a healthy individual, there is an equilibrium between dietary and urinary nitrogen.

CHAPTER 5

The Biochemistry of Digestion

I. Digestion of Carbohydrates

A. **Dietary carbohydrates** (mainly starch, sucrose, and lactose) constitute about 50% of the calories in the average diet in the United States.

1. *Starch,* the storage form of carbohydralants, is similar in structure to glycogen (Figure 5-1).
    a. Starch contains amylose (long, unbranched chains with glucose units linked to α-1,4)
    b. Starch also contains amylopectin (α-1,4–linked chains with α-1,6–linked branches). Amylopectin has fewer branches than glycogen.
2. *Sucrose* (a component of table sugar and fruit) contains glucose and fructose residues linked via their anomeric carbons (see Figure 1-8).
3. *Lactose* (milk sugar) contains galactose-linked β-1,4 to glucose (see Figure 1-8).

B. **Digestion of dietary carbohydrates in the mouth** (Figure 5-2)

1. In the mouth, **salivary α-amylase** cleaves starch by breaking α-1,4 linkages between glucose residues within the chains (see Figure 5-1).
2. Dextrins (linear and branched oligosaccharides) are the major products that enter the stomach.

C. **Digestion of carbohydrates in the intestine** (see Figure 5-2)

1. The stomach contents pass into the intestine where **bicarbonate** (HCO_3^-) secreted by the pancreas neutralizes the stomach acid, raising the pH into the optimal range for the action of the intestinal enzymes.
2. Digestion by **pancreatic enzymes** (see Figure 5-2)
    a. The pancreas secretes an **α-amylase** that acts in the lumen of the small intestine and, like salivary amylase, cleaves α-1,4 linkages between glucose residues.

> *cc 5.1* Serum **amylase** is elevated in cases of **pancreatitis,** and the test to measure amylase is often ordered in patients to evaluate such a condition. However, serum **lipase** is another marker of **pancreatitis** that demonstrates higher sensitivity and specificity as compared to **amylase.**

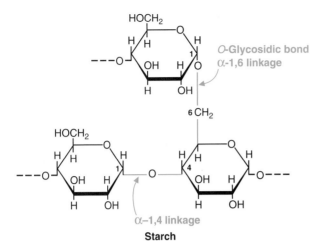

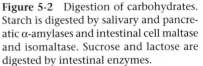

Figure 5-1 α-1,4 and α-1,6 linkages between glucose residues in starch and glycogen.

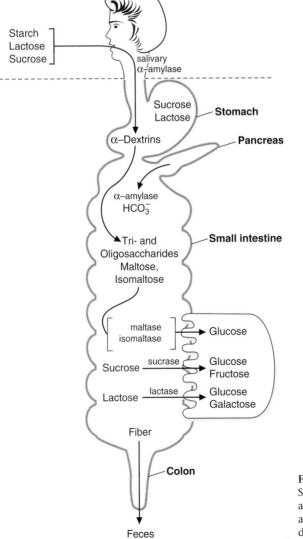

Figure 5-2 Digestion of carbohydrates. Starch is digested by salivary and pancreatic α-amylases and intestinal cell maltase and isomaltase. Sucrose and lactose are digested by intestinal enzymes.

b. The products of pancreatic α-amylase are the disaccharides maltose and iso-maltase, trisaccharides, and small oligosaccharides containing α-1,4 and α-1,6 linkages.

3. Digestion by **enzymes of intestinal cells**
   a. **Complexes of enzymes,** produced by intestinal epithelial cells and located in their **brush borders,** continue the digestion of carbohydrates (see Figure 5-2).
   b. **Glucoamylase** (an **α-glucosidase**) and other **maltases** cleave glucose residues from the nonreducing ends of oligosaccharides and also cleave the α-1,4 bond of maltose, releasing the two glucose residues.

> *cc* **5.2** **Acarbose, an α-glucosidase inhibitor,** works in the intestine, slowing down digestion of carbohydrates and lengthening the time it takes for carbohydrates to be converted to glucose, which facilitates **better postdigestive blood glucose control.**

   c. **Isomaltase** cleaves α-1,6 linkages, releasing glucose residues from branched oligosaccharides.
   d. **Sucrase** converts sucrose to glucose and fructose.
   e. **Lactase** (a β-galactosidase) converts lactose to glucose and galactose.

> *cc* **5.3** **Lactase deficiency** occurs in more than 80% of Native, African, and Asian Americans. Lactose is not digested at a normal rate and accumulates in the gut, where it is metabolized by bacteria. **Bloating, abdominal cramps,** and **watery diarrhea** result.

D. **Carbohydrates that cannot be digested**

1. Indigestible polysaccharides are part of the **dietary fiber** that passes through the intestine into the feces.
2. For example, because enzymes produced by human cells **cannot cleave the β-1,4 bonds of cellulose,** this polysaccharide is indigestible.

> *cc* **5.4** Because **insoluble fiber** aids digestion and adds bulk to stool, it hastens passage of fecal material through the gut, thus helping to prevent or alleviate constipation. Fiber also may help reduce the risk of **diverticulosis,** a condition in which small pouches form in the colon wall. Studies also show that **high-fiber diets** are associated with a decreased incidence of various cancers.

E. **Absorption of glucose, fructose, and galactose**

1. **Glucose, fructose, and galactose**—the final products generated by digestion of dietary carbohydrates—can be absorbed by intestinal cells by **two forms of transport,** facilitated transport and active transport.
2. By **facilitated transport,** monosaccharides move into cells on transport proteins, moving down a concentration gradient.
3. Glucose also moves into cells by **secondary active transport,** in which sodium ions are carried along with glucose. A Na^+-K^+ ATPase pumps Na^+ into the blood, and glucose moves down a concentration gradient from the cell into the blood.

II. Digestion of Dietary Triacylglycerol

A. **Dietary triacylglycerols** are digested in the **small intestine** by a process that requires bile salts and secretions from the pancreas (Figure 5-3). Normally, 95% of lipids

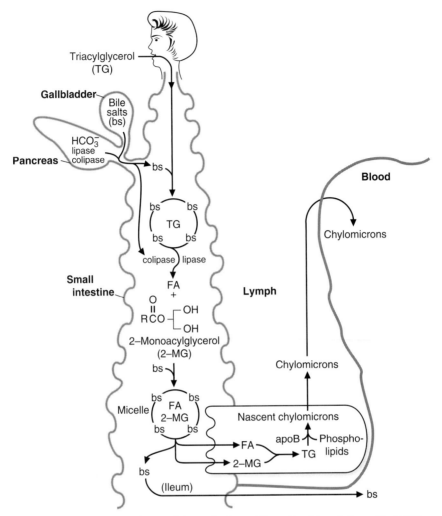

Figure 5-3 Digestion of triacylglycerols. bs = bile salts; FA = fatty acid; 2-MG = 2-monoacylglycerol; TG = triacylglycerols.

are absorbed. Major digestion of all lipids occurs in the lumen of the duodenum/jejunum.

 Steatorrhea occurs when excess lipids are excreted into the feces due to lipid malabsorption from impaired lipolysis, micelle or chylomicron formation, or chylomicron transport.

1. **Bile salts** are synthesized in the liver from cholesterol and are secreted into the bile. Bile is stored in the **gall bladder** and is released in response to hormones. Bile then passes into the intestine, where it **emulsifies the dietary lipids.**
2. The **pancreas** secretes digestive enzymes and bicarbonate, which neutralizes stomach acid, raising the pH into the optimal range for the digestive enzymes.
3. **Pancreatic lipase,** with the aid of colipase, digests the triacylglycerols to 2-monoacylglycerols and free fatty acids, which are packaged into micelles. The micelles, which are tiny microdroplets emulsified by bile salts, also contain other dietary lipids such as cholesterol and the fat-soluble vitamins.

> *cc* **5.6** The anti-obesity drug, **orlistat,** inhibits pancreatic and gastric lipase, resulting in ~30% blockage of dietary fat from digestion and absorption, leading to **reduction in body weight in some patients.**

4. The **micelles** travel to the microvilli of the intestinal epithelial cells, which absorb the fatty acids, 2-monoacylglycerols, and other dietary lipids.

> *cc* **5.7** **Olestra** is an artificial fat composed of a sucrose polyester and fatty acids. It is neither degraded by gastric nor pancreatic lipases and **passes through the body undigested and unabsorbed.** Excess use in foods may interfere with absorption of fat-soluble vitamins.

5. The **bile salts are resorbed in the terminal ileum,** recycled by the liver, and secreted into the gut during subsequent digestive cycles.

B. **Synthesis of chylomicrons**

1. In intestinal epithelial cells, the **fatty acids** from micelles are **activated** by fatty acyl coenzyme A (CoA) synthetase (thiokinase) to form fatty acyl CoA.
2. A **fatty acyl CoA** reacts with a 2-monoacylglycerol to form a **diacylglycerol.** Then another fatty acyl CoA reacts with the diacylglycerol to form a **triacylglycerol.**
3. The triacylglycerols pass into the lymph packaged in **nascent (newborn) chylomicrons,** which eventually enter the blood.

III. Protein Digestion and Amino Acid Absorption

A. **Digestion of proteins** (Figure 5-4)

1. The 70 to 100 g of **protein consumed** each day and an equal or larger amount of protein that enters the digestive tract as **digestive enzymes** or in **sloughed-off cells** from the intestinal epithelium are converted to amino acids by **digestive enzymes.**

> *cc* **5.8** **Nontropical sprue** (adult **celiac disease**) results from a **reaction to gluten,** a protein found in grains. Intestinal epithelial cells are damaged, and **malabsorption** results. Common symptoms are steatorrhea, diarrhea, and weight loss.

2. In the **stomach,** pepsin is the major proteolytic enzyme. It cleaves proteins to smaller polypeptides (Figure 5-5).
   a. **Pepsin** is produced and secreted by the chief cells of the stomach as the inactive zymogen **pepsinogen.**
   b. **Hydrochloric acid (HCl)** produced by the parietal cells of the stomach causes a conformational change in pepsinogen that enables it to cleave itself (autocatalysis), forming **active pepsin.**

> *cc* **5.9** Patients with **achlorhydria,** which is the lack of ability to produce HCl (usually due to autoimmune destruction of gastric parietal cells), have **deficiencies in protein digestion and absorption.**

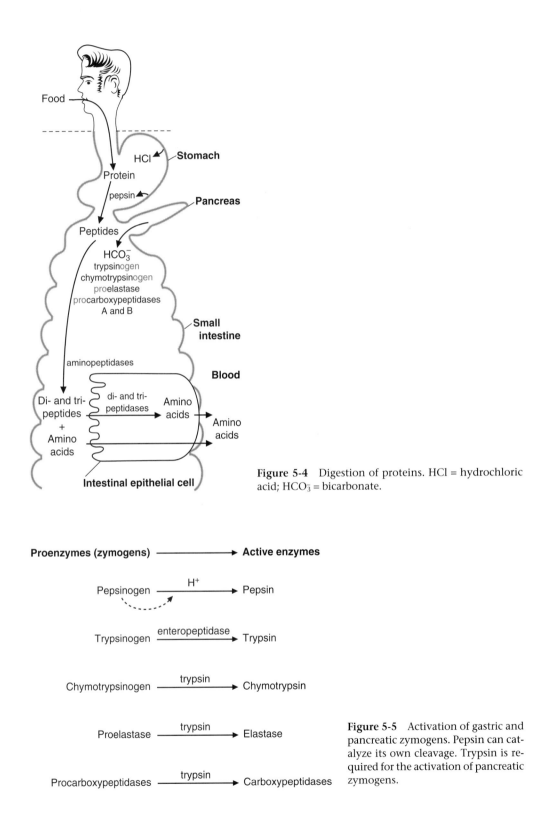

Figure 5-4   Digestion of proteins. HCl = hydrochloric acid; HCO_3^- = bicarbonate.

Figure 5-5   Activation of gastric and pancreatic zymogens. Pepsin can catalyze its own cleavage. Trypsin is required for the activation of pancreatic zymogens.

> *cc 5.10* Some individual have a condition known as **gastroesophageal reflux disease (GERD),** which results from reflux of HCl back into the esophagus. This condition creates a **burning sensation in the chest,** along with cough and even shortness of breath.

   c. **Pepsin** has a **broad specificity** but tends to cleave peptide bonds in which the carboxyl group is contributed by the aromatic amino acids or by leucine.

3. In the **intestine,** the partially digested material from the stomach encounters **pancreatic secretions,** which include bicarbonate and a group of proteolytic enzymes.

   a. **Bicarbonate** neutralizes the stomach acid, raising the pH of the contents of the intestinal lumen into the optimal range for the digestive enzymes to act.

> *cc 5.11* **Bicarbonate is released** from the pancreas in response to the hormone **secretin,** which is synthesized by the cells lining the duodenum. Failure to fully neutralize the acidic gastric contents results in **peptic ulcers** in the duodenum.

   b. **Endopeptidases** from the pancreas cleave peptide bonds within protein chains (see Figure 5-5).

     (1) **Trypsin** cleaves peptide bonds in which the carboxyl group is contributed by **arginine** or **lysine.**

       (i) **Trypsin is secreted as the inactive zymogen** trypsinogen. Trypsinogen is cleaved to form trypsin by the enzyme **enteropeptidase (enterokinase),** which is produced by intestinal cells. Trypsinogen may also undergo autocatalysis by trypsin.

> *cc 5.12* Hereditary **deficiency of enterokinase** has been reported. Deficiency of this important zymogen activator results in diarrhea, failure to thrive, and hypoproteinemia and is managed during infancy with pancreatic enzyme supplementation. When patients become adults, they no longer need such supplementation, due to the decreased anabolic demands and the autocatalysis of digestive enzymes.

     (2) **Chymotrypsin** usually cleaves peptide bonds at the carboxyl group of **aromatic amino acids** or by **leucine. Chymotrypsinogen,** the inactive zymogen, is cleaved to form active chymotrypsin by trypsin (see Figure 5-5).

     (3) **Elastase** cleaves at the carboxyl end of amino acid residues with small, uncharged side chains such as alanine, glycine, or serine. **Proelastase,** the inactive zymogen, is cleaved to active elastase by trypsin (see Figure 5-5).

> *cc 5.13* **Elastase** has many important functions outside of digestion. It is an important molecule in neutrophil function, and deficiency of the molecule can result in **congenital neutropenia.** Untowardly actions of elastase in the lung, normally inhibited by the serum protein α_1-**antitrypsin,** can contribute to the development of **chronic obstructive pulmonary disease (COPD).**

   c. **Exopeptidases** in the pancreas (carboxypeptidases A and B) cleave one amino acid progressively from the C-terminus end of the peptide.

     (1) The carboxypeptidases are produced as inactive **pro-carboxypeptidases,** which are cleaved to their active form by trypsin.

     (2) **Carboxypeptidase** A cleaves **aromatic** amino acids from the C-terminus.

        (3) **Carboxypeptidase B** cleaves the **basic** amino acids, lysine and arginine, from the C-terminal terminus.

    d. **Proteases** produced by **intestinal epithelial cells** complete the conversion of dietary proteins to peptides and finally to amino acids.

        (1) **Aminopeptidases** are exopeptidases produced by intestinal cells, cleaving one amino acid at a time from the N-terminus of peptides.

        (2) **Dipeptidases** and **tripeptidases** associated with the intestinal cells produce amino acids from dipeptides and tripeptides.

B. Transport of amino acids from the intestinal lumen into the blood

  1. Amino acids are absorbed by intestinal epithelial cells and released into the blood by two types of transport systems.

  2. At least seven different carrier proteins transport different groups of amino acids.

  3. *Sodium-amino acid carrier system*

    a. The major transport system involves cellular uptake by the cell of a **sodium ion** and an **amino acid** by the same carrier protein on the luminal surface.

    b. The **sodium ion** is pumped out of the cell into the blood by the Na^+-K^+ ATPase, while the **amino acid** travels down its concentration gradient into the blood.

    c. Thus, amino acid transport from the intestinal lumen to the blood is driven by hydrolysis of adenosine triphosphate ATP (**secondary active transport**).

> *cc 5.14* In **cystinuria,** transport of cysteine is defective. Cysteine is synthesized in the body and oxidized to cystine, which can crystallize, forming kidney stones.

> *cc 5.15* In **Hartnup's disease,** transport of neutral amino acids is defective, resulting in **deficiencies of essential amino acids** because they are not absorbed from the diet.

  4. *γ-Glutamyl cycle*

    a. An amino acid in the lumen reacts with **glutathione** (γ-glutamyl-cysteinyl-glycine) in the cell membrane, forming a γ-glutamyl amino acid and the dipeptide cysteinyl-glycine.

    b. The amino acid is carried across the cell membrane attached to **γ-glutamate** and released into the cytoplasm. The γ-glutamyl moiety is used in the resynthesis of glutathione.

> *cc 5.16* Translocation of amino acids in the γ-glutamyl cycle is mediated **by γ-glutamyl transferase (GGT). Elevated serum levels** of GGT often occur in intra- and posthepatic **biliary obstructions,** indicating cholestasis, and in some primary neoplasms as well as **pancreatic cancer and alcohol-induced liver disease.**

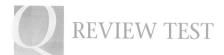

Directions: Each of the numbered questions or incomplete statements in this section is followed by answers or by completions of the statement. Select the **one** lettered answer or completion that is **best** in each case.

1. After digestion of a piece of cake that contains flour, milk, and sucrose as its primary ingredients, the major carbohydrate products entering the blood are:

(A) glucose.
(B) fructose and galactose.
(C) galactose and glucose.
(D) fructose and glucose.
(E) glucose, fructose, and galactose.

2. In cystic fibrosis, the pancreatic ducts become obstructed by viscous mucus. Consequently, digestion of which of the following substances would be most impaired?

(A) Starch
(B) Fat
(C) Lactose
(D) Sucrose
(E) Maltose

3. A gallstone that blocked the upper part of the bile duct would cause an increase in:

(A) the formation of chylomicrons.
(B) the recycling of bile salts.
(C) the excretion of bile salts.
(D) the excretion of fat in the feces.
(E) incomplete protein digestion.

4. Which of the following is the best marker for the diagnosis of pancreatitis?

(A) Lactase
(B) Amylase
(C) Lipase
(D) Bicarbonate
(E) γ-Glutamyl transferase

5. The pancreas is the source of the proteolytic enzyme trypsin. The reason that the trypsin does not digest the tissue in which it is produced is that trypsin is:

(A) only active at the pH of the intestine and not at the pH of the pancreatic cells.

(B) synthesized in an inactive phosphorylated form.
(C) inactive until its regulatory protein, calmodulin, binds calcium.
(D) synthesized as an inactive zymogen, which requires proteolysis for activation.
(E) bound to a carrier protein that releases the active enzyme when denatured.

Questions 6–8

A molecule of palmitic acid, attached to carbon 1 of the glycerol moiety of a triacylglycerol, is ingested and digested.

6. Which of the following molecular complexes in the blood carries the palmitate residue from the lumen of the gut to the surface of the gut epithelial cell?

(A) Very low–density lipoprotein
(B) Chylomicron
(C) Bile salt

7. Which of the following molecular complexes in the blood carries the palmitate residue from the gut epithelial cell to the blood?

(A) Very low–density lipoprotein
(B) Chylomicron
(C) Bile salt

8. Which of the following molecular complexes in the blood carries the palmitate residue from the intestine through the blood to a fat cell?

(A) Very low–density lipoprotein
(B) Chylomicron
(C) Bile salt
(D) Lipase

9. Which of the following enzymes digests dietary proteins in the stomach?

(A) Pepsin
(B) Trypsin
(C) Carboxypeptidase A
(D) Enteropeptidase

10. Which of the following enzymes is synthesized by intestinal cells?

(A) Pepsin
(B) Trypsin
(C) Carboxypeptidase A
(D) Enteropeptidase

11. Which of the following enzymes cleaves bonds at the carboxyl end of the arginine and lysine residues within a polypeptide chain?

(A) Pepsin
(B) Trypsin
(C) Carboxypeptidase A
(D) Enteropeptidase

12. Which of the following enzymes acts as an exopeptidase?

(A) Pepsin
(B) Trypsin
(C) Carboxypeptidase A
(D) Enteropeptidase

13. Which of the following enzymes is produced by the action of HCl on its precursor?

(A) Pepsin
(B) Trypsin
(C) Carboxypeptidase A
(D) Enteropeptidase

14. As an experiment, a high school professor convinces each of his students to put a soda cracker in their mouths and not swallow it. After several minutes, some of the students report a sweet taste. Which of the following enzymes is responsible for this phenomenon?

(A) Amylase
(B) Sucrase
(C) Lactase
(D) Maltase
(E) Isomaltase

15. A 38-year-old man gets bloated and has episodes of diarrhea after eating his favorite ice cream. It also occurs when he consumes yogurt, cheese, and other milk-containing products. The enzyme responsible for the digestion of this sugar cleaves which of the following bonds?

(A) Glucose-α (1→4) glucose
(B) Glucose-α (1→2) fructose
(C) Galactose-β (1→4) glucose
(D) Glucose-α (1→6) glucose
(E) Peptide bond

16. A 65-year-old man expresses his concern about developing colon cancer to his physician. He states that his father as well as grandmother died of colon cancer. After performing a physical exam and observing negative Hemoccult tests and unremarkable colonoscopy, the physician recommends a diet low in fat and high in fiber. The doctor explains that studies have shown a decreased risk of colon cancer with insoluble fiber consumption. Which of the following bonds is responsible for the fiber's inability to be digested?

(A) α (1→4)
(B) α (1→6)
(C) β (1→4)
(D) α (1→ β 2)
(E) α (4→6)

17. A 55-year-old man has been attempting to lose weight using a low-carbohydrate diet. After 2 months of little success, he confides in his son that he does add glucose to his coffee in the morning and after dinner but feels only some of this will be absorbed and should not be the cause of his limited success. The son, a medical school student, states that glucose is almost completely absorbed from the gut. What type of transport does glucose utilize for gastrointestinal absorption?

(A) Passive
(B) Facilitated
(C) Active
(D) Passive and facilitated
(E) Active and facilitated

18. A 33-year-old, nonalcoholic man is referred to a gastroenterologist for a newly diagnosed liver disease. A liver biopsy reveals α_1-antitrypsin deficiency. This enzyme normally inhibits the enzyme trypsin that cleaves proteins at which of the following sites?

(A) The carboxyl side of arginine or lysine
(B) The carboxyl side of aromatic amino acids
(C) The carboxyl side of uncharged amino acids
(D) Aromatic amino acids from the carboxy-terminus
(E) Basic amino acids from the carboxy-terminus

19. A newborn is seen by a neonatologist for failure to thrive. The nurses in the pediatric intensive care unit note that the child has diarrhea every time he feeds. In addition, laboratory studies suggest severe hypoproteinemia. The neonatologist sends for a panel of tests, which indicate a congenital deficiency of enterokinase. This enzyme normally activates which zymogen?

(A) Trypsin
(B) Secretin
(C) Trypsinogen
(D) Proelastase
(E) Chymotrypsinogen

20. A morbidly obese woman decides to see her physician to begin a weight loss program. He tells her that diet and exercise play an essential role in her program. She is concerned that does not have the time to devote to exercise and wants to know if there is any pharmacologic treatment for her. The physician decides to start her on orlistat, which directly inhibits which step in the absorption of fats?

(A) Bile salt formation
(B) Micelle formation
(C) Pancreatic and gastric lipases
(D) Absorption of free fatty acids
(E) Chylomicron formation

21. A 57-year-old alcoholic is transported to the emergency room after sustaining an injury in a motor vehicle accident. A comprehensive metabolic panel and a serum γ-glutamyl transferase (GGT) level are ordered. The GGT is shown to be dramatically elevated. This enzyme is important for which of the following digestive processes?

(A) Recycling of bile salts
(B) Absorption of carbohydrates
(C) Digestion of triglycerides
(D) Absorption of amino acids
(E) Digestion of carbohydrates

22. A 65-year-old woman is evaluated by a gastroenterologist for progressive signs and symptoms of malnutrition. Throughout her workup, she is found to have significantly decreased stomach acid. She is also found to have antibodies to gastric parietal cells, which are normally responsible for the production of acid. Why is hydrochloric acid important in digestion?

(A) It stimulates the cleavage of trypsinogen to trypsin.
(B) It is required for the activity of α-amylase.
(C) It drives secondary active transport of amino acids.
(D) It converts pepsinogen to pepsin.
(E) It is required for lipid digestion.

23. A 23-year-old man develops steatorrhea, weight loss, and a bloody diarrhea. He notes that the diarrhea is worse when he eats breads or cereals. A gastroenterologist performs a biopsy during a colonoscopy, which reveals celiac disease. This disorder is most directly due to which of the following?

(A) Excess lipids in the feces
(B) Deficiency of enterokinase
(C) Defective transport of the amino acid cysteine
(D) A defect in the transport of neutral amino acids
(E) Hypersensitivity to the protein gluten

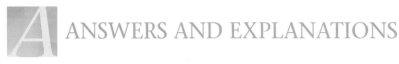
ANSWERS AND EXPLANATIONS

1–E. The cake contains starch, lactose (milk sugar), and sucrose (table sugar). Digestion of starch produces glucose. Lactase cleaves lactose to galactose and glucose, and sucrase cleaves sucrose to fructose and glucose.

2–B. Lactose, maltose, and sucrose are digested by disaccharidases on the brush border of intestinal epithelial cells. Starch is digested by salivary and pancreatic α-amylase. Therefore, its digestion would be less affected by a lack of pancreatic juice than fat, which is digested mainly by pancreatic lipase. A common finding in cystic fibrosis is steatorrhea (fatty stools).

3–D. In this situation, bile salts could not enter the digestive tract. Therefore, recycling and excretion of bile salts, digestion of fats, and formation of chylomicrons would all decrease. As a consequence, fat in the feces would increase (steatorrhea). The digestion of protein does not require bile salts.

4–C. Although both lipase and amylase are elevated in pancreatitis, lipase demonstrates higher sensitivity and specificity compared to amylase. Lactase is found in the brush boarder of enterocytes. Bicarbonate is a product of the pancreas as well. γ-Glutamyl transferase is found in the intestine as well as the liver and is a marker of alcoholic liver disease.

5–D. There are various ways that enzyme activity is regulated. For digestive proteases such as trypsin, chymotrypsin, pepsin, and matrix metalloproteases, there is a larger, **inactive** precursor that is cleaved to form a shorter, active enzyme. All of the other choices involve other modes of regulation but are not applicable to trypsin activation.

6–C. A palmitate residue attached to carbon 1 of a dietary triacylglycerol is released by pancreatic lipase and carried from the intestinal lumen to the gut epithelial cell in a bile salt micelle.

7–B. Palmitate is absorbed into the intestinal cell and used to synthesize a triacylglycerol, which is packaged in a nascent chylomicron and secreted via the lymph into the blood.

8–B. The chylomicron, containing the palmitate, travels through the blood to a fat cell.

9–A. Pepsin acts in the stomach.

10–D. Enteropeptidase, which is produced by intestinal cells, cleaves trypsinogen to trypsin.

11–B. Trypsin is an endopeptidase that cleaves polypeptide chains at arginine and lysine residues.

12–C. Carboxypeptidases A and B are pancreatic exopeptidases, which cleave one amino acid at a time from the C-terminal end of a polypeptide chain.

13–A. Pepsin is produced as pepsinogen (a zymogen), which autocatalyzes its own cleavage to pepsin when exposed to HCl.

14–A. One of the first enzymes in the process of digestion occurs in the mouth with salivary α-amylase. This enzyme is rendered inactive in the stomach due to the acidic environment, being replaced by pancreatic α-amylase secreted into the duodenum. The enzyme specifically cleaves the α-1,4 bonds between the glucosyl residues of starch, resulting in glucose polysaccharides of varying number of residues. The other glycosidases are associated with the brush border of enterocytes of the intestine.

15–C. The vignette is a classic presentation of lactase deficiency. Lactase is an enzyme that cleaves the galactose-β (1→4) glucose bond of the disaccharide lactose. Sucrase cleaves the glucose-α (1→2) fructose bond. Maltase cleaves glucose-α (1→4) glucose bonds, whereas isomaltase cleaves glucose-α (1→6) glucose bonds. Proteins are not substrates for any of these glycosidases.

16–C. The enzyme β (1→4) endoglucosidase is required to digest the polysaccharides found in cellulose, the carbohydrate storage found in plants. Humans lack this enzyme. However, humans do possess enzymes that can digest disaccharides, such as galactose, that possess the same β (1→4) bond. The (α 1→β 2) bond is exemplified in table sugar, sucrose. The α (1→4) glycosidic bonds make up the primary chain of glycogen. The α (1→6) linkage creates the unbranched component of glycogen. An α (4→6) linkage is formed during the formation of branches in glycogen.

17–E. Glucose absorption in the small intestine occurs via two types of transport. The first is facilitated transport (a form of passive transport in which molecules move down a concentration gradient with the assistance of transport proteins). The second is active transport (requires ATP to move against a concentration gradient), in which sodium ions are carried along with glucose into cells. A Na^+-K^+ ATPase pumps Na^+ into the blood, and glucose moves down a concentration gradient into the blood.

18–A. α_1-Antitrypsin inhibits the action of trypsin, which normally cleaves a peptide on the carboxyl side of arginine or lysine. Chymotrypsin has the ability to cleave a peptide on the carboxyl side of aromatic amino acids. Elastase is actually another enzyme inhibited by α_1-antitrypsin that cleaves peptides on the carboxyl side of uncharged amino acids. Carboxypeptidase A cleaves aromatic amino acids from the carboxy-terminus, whereas carboxypeptidase B cleaves basic amino acids from the carboxy-terminus.

19–C. Enterokinase cleaves the zymogen trypsinogen to the active enzyme trypsin. Trypsinogen is also capable of autoactivation. Trypsin, in turn, cleaves the zymogens proelastase to elastase and chymotrypsinogen to chymotrypsin. Secretin is a hormone that stimulates the release of bicarbonate into the small intestine so that these enzymes have the proper pH to become biologically active.

20–C. Orlistat inhibits pancreatic and gastric lipase, preventing the release of free fatty acids covalently attached to the triacyl backbone of triglycerides and, therefore, the absorption of such fatty acids. The normal sequence of digestion is that triacylglycerols are emulsified by bile salts from the gall bladder. These micelles are then acted on by lipases. Liberation of fatty acids results in the absorption of free fatty acids by enterocytes, which are then packaged into chylomicrons.

21–D. γ-Glutamyl transferase (GGT) is a key enzyme in the γ-glutamyl cycle used for the absorption of many free amino acids into the intestinal enterocytes. Recycling of bile salts occur in the terminal ileum. Digestion of carbohydrates is performed by many glycosidases, and transport into cells is by secondary active transport. Triacylglycerides are digested by lipases with the help of colipase, once they have been emulsified by bile salts.

22–D. The acidic environment of the stomach stimulates the conversion of pepsinogen to pepsin, the major proteolytic enzyme of the stomach. Patients with achlorhydria, as in this case, have deficiencies in protein digestion as well as vitamin B_{12} absorption (as the same parietal cells make intrinsic factor). Amylase is inactivated by acid, as are lipases and other proteases, and that is why bicarbonate from the pancreas is secreted into the duodenum, where such enzymes act. The conversion of pepsinogen to pepsin is aided by the enzyme enterokinase.

23–E. Celiac disease, or nontropical sprue, results from hypersensitivity to the grain protein gluten. Biopsy of the intestine demonstrates destruction of the absorptive cells of the gut, as gluten stimulates an inflammatory response in the gut. Excess lipids in the feces does result in steatorrhea, which is an effect, not a cause, of celiac disease. Defective transport of cysteine in the kidney leads to kidney stones, a condition known as cystinuria. Defects in the transport of neutral amino acids results in Hartnup's disease.

Glycolysis

I.   General Overview

A.   Glycolysis is the **principle route of metabolism for glucose** as well as fructose, galactose, and other dietary carbohydrates.

B.   The enzymes and transporters of the pathway **demonstrate stereo-specificity** for naturally occurring **D-isomers.**

C.   The reactions of glycolysis take place within the **cytoplasm.**

D.   Glycolysis can provide adenosine triphosphate (ATP) in the **absence of oxygen.**

> *cc 6.1*   **Red blood cells (RBCs),** which **lack mitochondria,** are nearly **completely reliant on glycolysis** as a source of energy. As such, many of the deficiencies of glycolytic enzymes have a profound effect on RBC function.

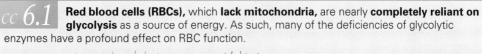

hexokinase, glucose-phosphate isomerase, aldolase,
triosephosphate isomerase, phosphate glycerate kinase,
enolase, pyruvate kinase

II.   Transport of Glucose into Cells

A.   Glucose travels across the cell membrane on a **transport protein.**

B.   Insulin stimulates glucose transport into muscle and adipose cells by causing glucose transport proteins (GLUT-4) within cells to move to the cell membrane (Table 6-1).

C.   Insulin does not significantly stimulate the transport of glucose into tissues such as liver, brain, and RBCs.

> *cc 6.2*   **Hereditary deficiency of GLUT-1, an insulin-independent transporter,** results in decreased glucose in the **cerebral spinal fluid.** Patients manifest with intractable seizures in infancy and developmental delay.

III.   Reactions of Glycolysis (Figure 6-1)

A.   Glucose is converted to glucose 6-phosphate in a reaction that uses ATP and produces adenosine diphosphate (ADP).

TABLE 6-1	Properties of the GLUT-1 to GLUT-5 Isoforms of the Glucose Transport Proteins	
Transporter	Tissue Distribution	Comments
GLUT-1	Human erythrocyte Blood–brain barrier Blood–retinal barrier Blood–placental barrier Blood–testis barrier	Expressed in cell types with barrier function; a high-affinity glucose transport system
GLUT-2	Liver Kidney Pancreatic β-cell Serosal surface of intestinal mucosal cells	A high-capacity, low-affinity transporter; may be used as the glucose sensor in the pancreas
GLUT-3	Brain (neurons)	Major transporter in the central nervous system; a high-affinity system
GLUT-4	Adipose tissue Skeletal muscle Heart muscle	Insulin-sensitive transporter; in the presence of insulin, the number of GLUT-4 transporters increases on the cell surface; a high-affinity system
GLUT-5	Intestinal epithelium Spermatozoa	This is actually a fructose transporter

Genetic techniques have identified additional GLUT transporters (GLUT-7 through GLUT-12), but the roles of these transporters have not yet been fully described.
Adapted, with permission, from Smith C, Marks A, Lieberman M. *Marks' Basic Medical Biochemistry: A Clinical Approach,* 2nd ed. Philadelphia: Lippincott, Williams & Wilkins, 2005:505.

    1. Enzymes: **hexokinase** in all tissues and, in the liver, **glucokinase.** Both of these enzymes are subject to regulatory mechanisms.
    2. Unlike glucose, which can diffuse through the transporters on the cell membranes, **glucose 6-phosphate is obligated to the intracellular compartment.**

B. Glucose 6-phosphate is isomerized to fructose 6-phosphate.

    • Enzyme: phosphoglucose isomerase

C. Fructose 6-phosphate is phosphorylated by ATP, forming fructose 1,6-bisphosphate and ADP.

    1. Enzyme: **phosphofructokinase 1 (PFK1)**
    2. PFK1 is regulated by a number of effectors.
    3. The first committed step of glycolysis.

D. Fructose 1,6-bisphosphate is cleaved—with the enzyme **aldolase**—to form the triose phosphates, glyceraldehyde 3-phosphate and dihydroxyacetone phosphate (DHAP).

cc 6.3   Absence of the A isoform of **aldolase** has been reported. The disorder presents with a nonspherocytic **hemolytic anemia.** Patients also have episodes of **rhabdomyolysis** (destruction of muscle cells) following febrile illness.

E. Dihydroxyacetone phosphate is isomerized—by the enzyme **triose phosphate isomerase**—to glyceraldehyde 3-phosphate.

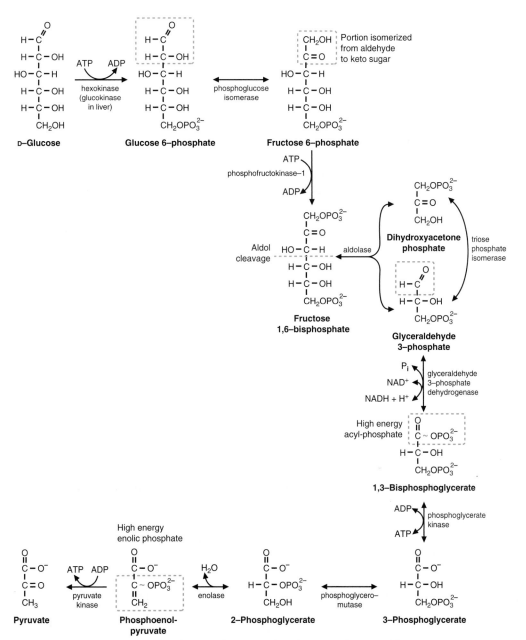

Figure 6-1 The reactions of glycolysis. High-energy phosphates are shown in blue.

Note: Two moles of glyceraldehyde 3-phosphate are formed from 1 mole of glucose.

cc 6.4 Patients with **triose phosphate isomerase (TPI)** deficiency have neonatal onset **hemolytic anemia** as well as progressive **neurologic involvement**. Children have progressive hypotonia with eventual diaphragm paralysis that requires ventilation and as well as **cardiomyopathy.**

F. **Glyceraldehyde 3-phosphate** is oxidized by NAD^+ and reacts with inorganic phosphate (P_i) to form 1,3-bisphosphoglycerate and $NADH + H^+$.

   1. Enzyme: **glyceraldehyde 3-phosphate dehydrogenase**
   2. The aldehyde group of glyceraldehyde 3-phosphate is oxidized to a carboxylic acid, which forms a high-energy anhydride with P_i.

G. **1,3-Bisphosphoglycerate** reacts with ADP—using the enzyme **phosphoglycerate kinase**—to produce 3-phosphoglycerate and **ATP**.

H. **3-Phosphoglycerate** is converted—via enzyme **phosphoglyceromutase**—to 2-phosphoglycerate by transfer of the phosphate group from carbon 3 to carbon 2.

I. **2-Phosphoglycerate** is dehydrated—using the enzyme **enolase**—to phosphoenolpyruvate (PEP), which contains a high-energy enol phosphate.

> cc **6.5** The enzyme **enolase** is inhibited by **fluoride.** To prevent ongoing glycolysis in patient's blood samples collected for sensitive **glucose tolerance tests,** blood is collected in tubes containing fluoride.

J. **Phosphoenolpyruvate** reacts with ADP to form **pyruvate** and **ATP** in the last reaction of glycolysis.

   1. Enzyme: **pyruvate kinase**
   2. Pyruvate kinase is more active in the fed state than in the fasting state.

IV. Special Reactions in Red Blood Cells

A. In RBCs, 1,3-bisphosphoglycerate can be converted to **2,3-bisphosphoglycerate** (BPG), a compound that decreases the affinity of hemoglobin for oxygen.

B. BPG is dephosphorylated to form inorganic phosphate and 3-phosphoglycerate, an intermediate that re-enters the glycolytic pathway.

> cc **6.6** **Fetal hemoglobin (HbF),** composed of 2 α subunits and 2 γ subunits, has a lower affinity for BPG than does HbA, and therefore, HbF has a higher affinity for O_2. This difference in maternal and fetal hemoglobin facilitates the unloading of O_2 at the maternal/fetal interface, i.e., the placenta.

V. Regulatory Enzymes of Glycolysis (Figure 6-2)

A. **Hexokinase** is found in most tissues and is geared to provide glucose 6-phosphate for ATP production even when blood glucose is low.

   1. Hexokinase has a **low K_m** for glucose (about 0.1 mM). Therefore, it is working near its maximum rate (V_{max}), even at fasting blood glucose levels (about 5 mM).
   2. Hexokinase is **inhibited** by its product, **glucose 6-phosphate.** Therefore, it is most active when glucose 6-phosphate is being rapidly utilized.

insulin → ⊖ phosphatases
glucagon → ⊕ PKA

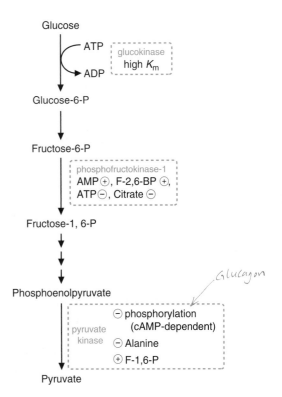

Figure 6-2   Regulation of glycolysis. In muscle, PFK1 is the key enzyme. It is activated (⊕) by AMP and inhibited (⊖) by ATP and citrate. In liver, glucokinase, PFK1 (activated by fructose 2,6-bisphosphate [F-2,6-P]), and pyruvate kinase are the key enzymes.

---

cc **6.7**   **Maturity onset diabetes of the young (MODY)** type 2 is an autosomal dominant disorder involving mutations in the **hexokinase gene.** Patients have **nonprogressive hyperglycemia** that is usually asymptomatic at diagnosis and is usually managed with diet alone.

B.   **Glucokinase** is found in the **liver** and actively functions at a significant rate only after a meal (when blood glucose is high).

    1.   Glucokinase has a **high K_m** for glucose (about 6 mM). Therefore, it is very **active after a meal,** when glucose levels in the hepatic portal vein are high, and it is inactive during the postabsorptive state or fasting, when glucose levels are low.

    2.   Glucokinase is **induced** when insulin levels are high.   (Fed - state)

    3.   Glucokinase is not inhibited by its product, glucose 6-phosphate, at physiologic concentrations.

C.   **Phosphofructokinase 1 (PFK1)** is an allosteric enzyme regulated by several factors. It functions at a rapid rate in the liver when blood glucose is high or in cells such as muscle when there is a need for ATP.

---

cc **6.8**   **Phosphofructokinase deficiency** (a form of **glycogen storage disease** [type VII] in which glycogen accumulates in muscles) results in inefficient use of glucose stores by red blood cells and muscles. Patients experience **hemolytic anemia** as well as **muscle cramping.**

1. PFK1 is **activated by fructose 2,6-bisphosphate** (F-2,6-P), an important regulatory mechanism in the liver (Figure 6-3).
   a. After a meal, F-2,6-P is formed from fructose 6-phosphate by **phosphofructokinase 2 (PFK2)**. (Step 1)
   b. F-2,6-P activates PFK1, and **glycolysis** is **stimulated**. The liver is using glycolysis to produce fatty acids for triacylglycerol synthesis. (Step 2)
   c. **In the fasting state** (when glucagon is elevated), **PFK2** is phosphorylated by **protein kinase A**, which is activated by cyclic adenosine monophosphate (cAMP). (Step 3)
   d. Phosphorylated PFK2 converts F-2,6-P to fructose 6-phosphate. F-2,6-P levels fall, and **PFK1** is **less active**. (Step 4)
   e. **In the fed state, insulin** causes **phosphatases** to be stimulated. A phosphatase dephosphorylates PFK2, causing it to become more active in forming F-2,6-P from fructose 6-phosphate. F-2,6-P levels rise, and **PFK1** is **more active**. (Step 5)
   f. Thus, **PFK2** acts as a **kinase** (in the **fed state** when it is dephosphorylated) and as a **phosphatase** (in the **fasting state** when it is phosphorylated). PFK2 catalyzes two different reactions.
2. PFK1 is **activated by AMP**, an important regulatory mechanism in **muscle** (see Figure 6-2).
   a. In muscle during **exercise**, AMP levels are high, and ATP levels are low.
   b. Glycolysis is promoted by a more active PFK1, and ATP is generated.
3. PFK1 is **inhibited** by ATP and **citrate**, which are important regulatory mechanisms in **muscle**.
   a. When ATP is high, the cell does not need ATP, and glycolysis is inhibited.

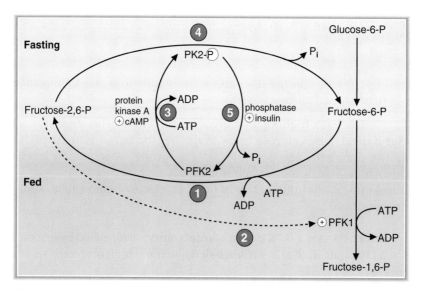

Figure 6-3 Regulation of fructose 2,6-bisphosphate (F-2,6-P) levels in the liver. F-2,6-P is an activator of phosphofructokinase 1 (PFK1), which converts fructose 6-phosphate to fructose 1,6-bisphosphate. Phosphofructokinase 2 (PFK2) acts as a kinase in the fed state and as a phosphatase during fasting. It regulates the cellular levels of fructose 2,6-phosphate. The *circled numbers* correspond with steps 1 to 5 under V C 1 a-e in the text.

   b. High levels of citrate indicate that adequate amounts of substrate are entering the tricarboxylic acid (TCA) cycle. Therefore, glycolysis slows down.

D. Pyruvate kinase

   1. Pyruvate kinase is **activated** by **fructose 1,6-bisphosphate** and **inhibited by alanine** and by **phosphorylation** in the liver **during fasting** when glucagon levels are high (see Figure 6-2).
      a. Glucagon, via cAMP, activates **protein kinase A**, which phosphorylates and inactivates pyruvate kinase.
      b. The inhibition of pyruvate kinase promotes gluconeogenesis.
   2. Pyruvate kinase is **activated in the fed state.** Insulin stimulates phosphatases that dephosphorylate and activate pyruvate kinase.

   > cc *6.9* Deficiency of **pyruvate kinase** causes decreased production of ATP from glycolysis. RBCs have insufficient ATP for their membrane pumps, and a **hemolytic anemia** results.

VI. The Fate of Pyruvate (Figure 6-4)

A. Conversion to lactate

   1. Pyruvate can be reduced in the cytosol by NADH, forming **lactate** and regenerating NAD^+.
   2. NADH, which is produced by glycolysis, must be reconverted to NAD^+ so that carbons of glucose can continue to flow through glycolysis.
   3. **Lactate dehydrogenase (LDH)** converts pyruvate to lactate. LDH consists of four subunits that can be either of the muscle (M) or the heart (H) type.
      a. Five isozymes occur (MMMM, MMMH, MMHH, MHHH, and HHHH), which can be separated by electrophoresis.
      b. Different tissues have different mixtures of these isozymes.
   4. Lactate is released by tissues (e.g., RBCs or **exercising muscle**) and is used by the liver for gluconeogenesis or by tissues such as the heart and kidney, where it is converted to pyruvate and oxidized for energy.

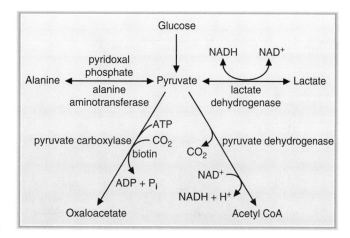

Figure 6-4 The fate of pyruvate.

cc *6.10* An increase of lactate levels in the blood causes an acidosis, resulting from hypoxia or alcohol ingestion. Lack of oxygen slows the electron transport chain, resulting in increased NADH levels. High NADH levels cause pyruvate to be converted to lactate. High NADH levels from alcohol metabolism also cause increased conversion of pyruvate to lactate.

     5. The **LDH reaction** is **reversible.**

B. Conversion to acetyl coenzyme A (CoA)

     1. Pyruvate can enter mitochondria.
     2. There it can be converted by **pyruvate dehydrogenase** to acetyl CoA, which can enter the TCA cycle.

C. Conversion to oxaloacetate

     1. Pyruvate can be converted to oxaloacetate by **pyruvate carboxylase,** which is found in tissues such as the liver and brain but not in muscle.
     2. This reaction serves to **replenish intermediates of the TCA cycle** as well as **provide substrates for gluconeogenesis.**
     3. The enzyme is activated by acetyl CoA.

D. Conversion to alanine

     1. Pyruvate can be transaminated to form the amino acid **alanine.**
     2. The enzymes involved are pyridoxal phosphate and alanine aminotransferase.

VII. Generation of ATP by Glycolysis

A. Production of ATP and NADH in the glycolytic pathway

     1. One mole of glucose yields 2 moles of pyruvate.
     2. Two moles of ATP are used in this pathway, and 4 moles of ATP are produced, for a **net yield of 2 moles of ATP.**
     3. In addition, 2 moles of cytosolic NADH are generated.

B. Energy generated by conversion of glucose to lactate (Figure 6-5)

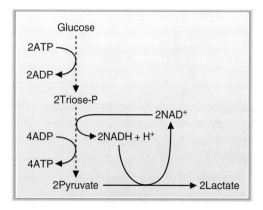

Figure 6-5 Conversion of 1 molecule of glucose to lactate produces 2 molecules of adenosine triphosphate (ATP) (net). The NADH produced by glycolysis is used to convert pyruvate to lactate.

- If the NADH generated by glycolysis is used to reduce pyruvate to lactate, the net yield is 2 moles of ATP per mole of glucose converted to lactate.

C. **Energy generated by conversion of glucose to CO_2 and H_2O** (Figure 6-6)

1. When glucose is oxidized completely to CO_2 and H_2O, approximately 36 or 38 moles of ATP are generated.
2. Two moles of ATP and 2 moles of NADH are generated from the conversion of 1 mole of glucose to 2 moles of pyruvate.
3. The 2 moles of pyruvate enter the mitochondria and are converted to 2 moles of acetyl CoA, producing 2 moles of NADH, which generate approximately 6 moles of ATP by oxidative phosphorylation.
4. The 2 moles of acetyl CoA are oxidized in the TCA cycle, generating approximately 24 moles of ATP.
5. NADH, produced in the cytosol by glycolysis, cannot directly cross the mitochondrial membrane. Therefore, the electrons are passed to the mitochondrial electron transport chain by two shuttle systems.
   a. **Glycerol phosphate shuttle** (Figure 6-7, *left side*)
      (1) Cytosolic DHAP is reduced to glycerol-3-phosphate by NADH.
      (2) Glycerol-3-phosphate reacts with a flavin adenine dinucleotide (FAD)–linked dehydrogenase in the inner mitochondrial membrane. DHAP is regenerated and re-enters the cytosol.
      (3) Each mole of $FADH_2$ that is produced generates approximately 2 moles of ATP via oxidative phosphorylation.
      (4) Because glycolysis produces 2 moles of NADH per mole of glucose, approximately **4 moles of ATP are produced by this shuttle.**
   b. **Malate-aspartate shuttle** (see Figure 6-7, *right side*)
      (1) Cytosolic oxaloacetate is reduced to malate by NADH. The reaction is catalyzed by cytosolic malate dehydrogenase.

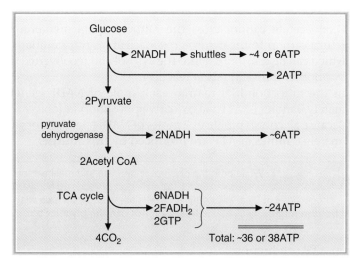

Figure 6-6 Adenosine triphosphate (ATP) produced by conversion of glucose to CO_2. The ATP produced by oxidative phosphorylation is approximate (indicated by ~).

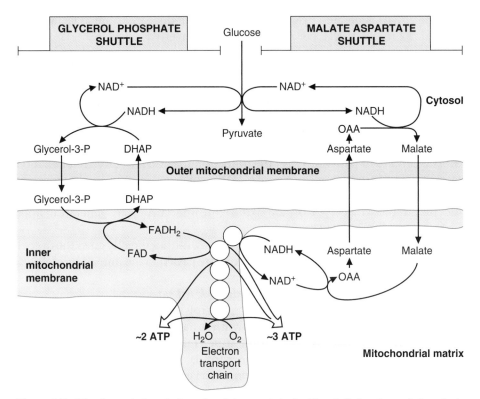

Figure 6-7 The glycerol phosphate and malate-aspartate shuttles. *Left,* the glycerol phosphate shuttle produces $FADH_2$, each of which generates approximately 2 ATP by oxidative phosphorylation. *Right,* the malate-aspartate shuttle produces NADH, each of which generates approximately 3 ATP. DHAP = dihydroxyacetone phosphate; OAA = oxaloacetate.

    (2) Malate enters the mitochondrion and is re-oxidized to oxaloacetate (OAA) by the mitochondrial malate dehydrogenase, generating NADH in the matrix.

    (3) Oxaloacetate cannot cross the mitochondrial membrane. In order to return carbon to the cytosol, oxaloacetate is transaminated to aspartate, which can be transported into the cytosol and reconverted to oxaloacetate by another transamination reaction.

    (4) In the mitochondrial matrix, each mole of NADH generates approximately 3 moles of ATP via oxidative phosphorylation.

    (5) Because glycolysis produces 2 moles of NADH per mole of glucose, approximately **6 moles of ATP are produced by this shuttle.**

> *cc* **6.11** While both the glycerol phosphate and malate-aspartate shuttle systems exist for the transport of reducing equivalents into the mitochondria, they are not equally used. For instance, **tissues with high metabolic demands,** such as the **heart, do not use the glycerol phosphate shuttle.**

6. Maximal ATP production

    a. Overall, when 1 mole of glucose is oxidized to CO_2 and H_2O, approximately **36 moles of ATP** are produced if the **glycerol phosphate shuttle** is used.

    b. If the **malate-aspartate shuttle** is used, **38 moles** of ATP are produced.

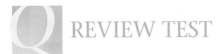

*Directions: Each of the numbered questions or incomplete statements in this section is followed by answers or by completions of the statement. Select the **one** lettered answer or completion that is **best** in each case.*

1. In which compartment of the cell does glycolysis occur?

(A) Mitochondrion
(B) Nucleus
(C) Soluble cytoplasm (cytosol)
(D) Rough endoplasmic reticulum
(E) Smooth endoplasmic reticulum

2. What type of bond is formed between phosphate and carbon 1 of 1,3-bisphosphoglycerate?

(A) Anhydride
(B) Ester
(C) Phosphodiester
(D) Amide
(E) Ether

3. See figure below. During glycolysis, the conversion of compound I to compound II:

$$CH_2OH \qquad\qquad CO_2^-$$
$$|\qquad\qquad\qquad\quad |$$
$$C=O \qquad\qquad\quad C=O$$
$$|\qquad\qquad\qquad\quad |$$
$$CH_2OPO_3^{-2} \qquad\quad CH_3$$

Compound I   Compound II

(A) requires a dehydrogenase.
(B) releases inorganic phosphate.
(C) produces 1 molecule of ATP per molecule of product.
(D) is catalyzed by a phosphatase.
(E) requires 2 molecules of NADH.

4. Which of the following statements about glycolysis is correct?

(A) Glucokinase catalyzes the conversion of glucose to glucose 6-phosphate in the liver.
(B) Phosphofructokinase 1 catalyzes the conversion of fructose 1,6-bisphosphate to dihydroxyacetone phosphate.
(C) When 1 molecule of glucose is converted to pyruvate via glycolysis, 1 molecule of NAD^+ is reduced.

(D) When 1 molecule of glucose is converted to pyruvate via glycolysis, 1 carbon is lost as CO_2.
(E) Hexokinase catalyzes the conversion of fructose 6-phosphate to fructose 1,6-bisphosphate.

5. In an embryo with a complete deficiency of pyruvate kinase, how many net moles of ATP are generated in the conversion of 1 mole of glucose to one mole of pyruvate?

(A) 0
(B) 1
(C) 2
(D) 3
(E) 4

6. A positive allosteric activator of phosphofructokinase 1 in the liver is:

(A) ADP.
(B) acetyl CoA.
(C) fructose 2,6-bisphosphate.
(D) ATP.
(E) citrate.

7. Which of the following is a regulatory mechanism of glycolysis?

(A) Inhibition of phosphofructokinase 1 by AMP
(B) Inhibition of hexokinase by its product
(C) Activation of pyruvate kinase when glucagon levels are elevated
(D) Inhibition of aldolase by fructose 1,6-bisphosphate
(E) Inhibition of glucokinase by fructose 2,6-bisphosphate

8. The only glycolytic enzyme that cleaves a carbon-carbon bond is:

(A) enolase.
(B) triose phosphate isomerase.
(C) phosphoglycerate kinase.
(D) glyceraldehyde 3-phosphate dehydrogenase.
(E) aldolase.

9. Which of the following is an attribute of the shuttle systems?

(A) The glycerol phosphate shuttle is primarily bidirectional and transports reducing equivalents both into and out of mitochondria.
(B) Via the malate-aspartate shuttle, reducing equivalents are transferred from cytosolic NADH to mitochondrial $FADH_2$.
(C) Via the glycerol phosphate shuttle, reducing equivalents are transferred from cytosolic NADH to mitochondrial $FADH_2$.
(D) The malate-aspartate shuttle does not require the participation of mitochondrial transporters.
(E) The malate-aspartate shuttle only operates unidirectionally.

10. The catabolism of 1 mole of glucose to lactate in the glycolytic pathway is accompanied by the reduction of how many moles of O_2?

(A) 0
(B) 2
(C) 4
(D) 8
(E) 16

11. A 47-year-old obese man complains of having to get out of bed three times a night to urinate. He has also noticed that he is constantly thirsty and eating more often. The patient is diagnosed with type 2 diabetes mellitus (DM) due to insulin resistance. If this is a problem at the level of the glucose transporter, which tissues will be most affected?

(A) Red blood cells
(B) Small intestine
(C) Muscle tissue
(D) Brain tissue
(E) Liver tissue

12. A 58-year-old woman is diagnosed with breast cancer. The oncologist orders a positron emission tomography (PET) scan of the brain to rule out metastasis. This imaging modality covalently links a radioactive isotope most commonly to glucose to appreci-ate highly active areas in the body such as a tumor. Which of the following traps the tracer in the cell?

(A) Insulin
(B) GLUT-4
(C) GLUT-1
(D) Glucokinase
(E) Phosphofructokinase

13. An 8-year-old girl presents with polydipsia, polyuria, and fatigue. A urinalysis is significant for glucose. To differentiate between type 1 diabetes mellitus and maturity onset diabetes of the young (MODY) an assay is run in search of one of the six proteins responsible for MODY. Results reveal a missense mutation in exon 7 of the glucokinase gene establishing MODY2. Which of the following is a characteristic of glucokinase?

(A) The K_m is above the fasting concentration of glucose in the blood
(B) Found in many tissues
(C) Stimulated in response to fructose 2,6-bisphosphate
(D) Inhibited by glucose 6-phosphate
(E) Found only in muscle

14. A 36-year-old woman is training for her first marathon. Her coach has her keeping a pace that allows her to stay below her anaerobic threshold. Avoiding anaerobic muscle glycolysis, pyruvate does not accumulate because it is converted to:

(A) ethanol.
(B) lactic acid.
(C) acetyl CoA.
(D) alanine.
(E) oxaloacetate.

15. A patient presents with dizziness, fatigue, and tremors. A fingerstick test indicates a blood glucose of 36 mmol/L. Of the allosteric activators of glycolysis in the liver, which of the following is the most important in maintaining a normal blood glucose level?

(A) Citrate
(B) ATP
(C) Fructose 2,6-bisphosphate

(D) Glucose 6-phosphate

(E) Acetyl CoA

16. A 30-year-old woman is enduring her first trimester of pregnancy. As the mother's hemoglobin relinquishes oxygen to the greater affinity of the fetal hemoglobin, it changes back to the relaxed form. This process also releases the allosteric factor 2,3-bisphosphoglycerate (BPG). If the allosteric factor then enters glycolysis, how much energy will it net by the end of its oxidative pathway?

(A) 0 ATP

(B) 1 ATP

(C) 2 ATP

(D) 4 ATP

(E) 6 ATP

17. A 24-year-old woman complains of intermittent right upper quadrant pain that extends to the inferior tip of her scapula. Ultrasound is relevant for stones in her gallbladder. Cholecystectomy notes pigmented stones in her gallbladder. Measurement of glycolytic intermediates, 2,3-diphosphoglycerol and glucose 6-phosphate, are elevated in her serum. A deficiency of which of the following enzymes most likely led to her gallstones?

(A) Glucose 6-phosphate dehydrogenase

(B) Phosphofructokinase

(C) Pyruvate kinase

(D) Pyruvate dehydrogenase

(E) Pyruvate carboxylase

18. A 33-year-old triathlete is admitted to the hospital with an acute episode of weakness, fatigue, and myalgia. Upon urination, it is noticed that the urine is dark, and there are laboratory findings of hemoglobin and myoglobin with serum lactate dangerously elevated. The destruction of muscle cells indicates rhabdomyolysis. Intravenous hydration rids the body of excess myoglobin, and the patient recovers. The basis for the elevated lactate is:

(A) ATP increase because of lack of oxygen for the muscle.

(B) NADH increase because of lack of oxygen for the muscle.

(C) a defect in the M form of lactate dehydrogenase.

(D) a defect in the H form of lactate dehydrogenase.

(E) a defect in the B form of muscle aldolase.

19. A pediatric hematologist sees an 18-month-old patient with jaundice, splenomegaly, and hemolytic anemia. A blood smear indicates red blood cells that are more rigid in appearance than normal. A diagnosis of pyruvate kinase deficiency is made. Since pyruvate is the last step in the glycolysis that produces ATP, products before the last step of the pathway will build up. What products in the pathway will be made in abnormal amounts?

(A) Acetyl CoA

(B) Glucose

(C) Lactate

(D) Oxaloacetate

(E) Glycogen

20. A 4-year-old girl was referred to a neurologist because of progressive neurologic deficits characterized by spasticity. Upon further workup, a peripheral blood smear indicated that there was a non-spherocytic hemolytic anemia of Dacie's type II (in vitro autohemolysis not corrected by glucose addition). A diagnosis of triose phosphate isomerase deficiency was made. Upon examination of muscle cells, it was found there was an elevated amount of:

(A) 6-carbon glycolytic products.

(B) many 3-carbon glycolytic products.

(C) a component of the glycerol phosphate shuttle.

(D) a component of the malate-aspartate shuttle.

(E) pyruvate.

ANSWERS AND EXPLANATIONS

1–C. All of the reactions of glycolysis occur in the cytosol.

2–A. The carboxylic acid (carbon 1) reacts with phosphoric acid, splitting out H_2O and forming an anhydride. Cleavage of this bond in the next step of glycolysis generates enough energy to produce 1 ATP from ADP and P_i.

3–A. Dihydroxyacetone phosphate (compound I) is isomerized to glyceraldehyde 3-phosphate and converted in a series of steps to pyruvate (compound II). One of the reactions requires glyceraldehyde 3-phosphate dehydrogenase, which uses 1 molecule of inorganic phosphate for each molecule of NADH it produces. In the conversion of 1 molecule of 1,3-bisphosphoglycerate to 1 molecule of pyruvate, 2 molecules of ATP are produced. A phosphatase is not required.

4–A. Glucokinase, a liver enzyme, converts glucose to glucose 6-phosphate. Phosphofructokinase 1 converts fructose 6-phosphate to fructose 1,6-bisphosphate. In glycolysis, 1 molecule of glucose is converted to 2 molecules of pyruvate, and 2 molecules of NADH are produced. No carbons are lost as CO_2.

5–A. Normally, 1 mole of ATP is used to convert 1 mole of glucose to 1 mole of glucose 6-phosphate, and a second mole of ATP is used to convert 1 mole of fructose 6-phosphate to the bisphosphate. Two triose phosphates are produced by cleavage of fructose 1,6-bisphosphate. As the two triose phosphates are converted to pyruvate, 4 ATP are generated: 2 by phosphoglycerate kinase and 2 by pyruvate kinase. The net result is that 2 ATP are produced. If pyruvate kinase is completely deficient, 2 less ATP will be produced, thus net ATP production will be zero.

6–C. Phosphofructokinase 1 (PFK1) is activated by AMP and fructose 2,6-bisphosphate. It is inhibited by ATP and citrate and not directly affected by acetyl CoA or ADP. In the liver, fructose 2,6-bisphosphate is the major activator.

7–B. Hexokinase is inhibited by its product, glucose 6-phosphate. PFK1 is activated by AMP and fructose 2,6-bisphosphate (F-2,6-P). F-2,6-P does not inhibit glucokinase. Aldolase is not inhibited by its substrate, fructose-1,6-P. Pyruvate kinase is inactivated by glucagon-mediated phosphorylation.

8–E. Aldolase cleaves a carbon-carbon bond of a 6-carbon sugar (fructose 1,6-bisphosphate) in half to create two 3-carbon moieties: glyceraldehyde 3-phosphate and dihydroxyacetone phosphate (DHAP). Other enzymes dehydrate (enolase), isomerize (triose phosphate isomerase), phosphorylate (phosphoglycerate kinase), or oxidize an aldehyde to a carboxylate (glyceraldehyde 3-phosphate dehydrogenase) (see Figure 6-1).

9–C. The shuttle systems refer to the glycerol phosphate and malate-aspartate shuttles collectively (see Figure 6-7). The glycerol phosphate shuttle (on the left of the diagram) transfers reducing equivalents from cytosolic NADH to mitochondrial $FADH_2$. The malate-aspartate shuttle (on the right of the diagram) requires a mitochondrial transporter to aid OAA crossing the membrane and is bidirectional.

10–A. Glycolysis provides ATP in the absence of oxygen. One mole of glucose yields 2 moles of lactate, with a yield of 2 ATP through fermentation (incomplete metabolism). In aerobic respiration, via the electron transport chain, O_2 is used as a terminal electron acceptor and is reduced to water. In fermentation, the end products are lactate, CO_2, and alcohol (R-OH); therefore, 0 moles of O_2 are present.

11–C. Both muscle and adipose tissue rely mainly on the glucose transporter GLUT-4, which requires insulin for optimal glucose transport. GLUT-1 is ubiquitously distributed in various tissues. GLUT-2 is present in liver and pancreatic β-cells. GLUT-3 is also found in the intestine with GLUT-1. Finally, GLUT-5 functions primarily as a fructose transporter.

12–D. The conversion of glucose to glucose 6-phosphate by glucokinase traps the labeled glucose within the cell. Glucose is transported into the cell through the insulin-sensitive GLUT-4 transporter or the insulin-independent GLUT-1 transporter. However, until the molecule is phosphorylated, it can diffuse out of the cell. Phosphofructokinase is the first committed step of glycolysis, although not the only pathway from glucose utilization.

13–A. Glucokinase and hexokinase catalyze the same reactions; however, glucokinase has unique qualities for use only when glucose levels are excessive. For example, glucokinase has a low affinity, high K_m, allowing substantial catalytic activity only at high glucose concentration, such as after a meal. Glucokinase also escapes any local regulation, although regulation at the level of transcription is influenced via the hormones insulin and glucagon. Glucokinase is only found in the liver.

14–C. Glycolysis is dependent on NAD^+ as a substrate for the pathway to continue to metabolize glucose. Under aerobic conditions, NAD^+ is generated via the electron transport chain. Under anaerobic conditions, an oxygen deficit limits the electron transport chain, and NAD^+ is generated by the conversion of pyruvate to lactate in mammals and to ethanol in yeast and some micro-organisms.

15–C. The primary step in the regulation of glycolysis is the conversion of fructose 6-phosphate to fructose 1,6-bisphosphate, catalyzed by the enzyme phosphofructokinase 1 (PFK1). PFK1 is activated by both fructose 2,6-bisphosphate and AMP and inhibited by ATP and citrate. Glucose 6-phosphate acts by negative feedback inhibition on hexokinase, whereas acetyl CoA is an inhibitor of the tricarboxylic acid (TCA) cycle.

16–C. Synthesis of 2,3-bisphosphoglycerate (BPG) represents a major reaction pathway in red blood cells (RBCs). When glucose is oxidized by this pathway, the RBC loses the ability to gain 2 moles of ATP by the oxidation of 1,3-BPG to 3-phosphoglycerate via the phosphoglycerate kinase reaction. Instead 2,3-BPG phosphatase converts 2,3-BPG to the next step in glycolysis, resulting in 3-bisphosphoglycerate. The result is 2 moles of ATP per glucose molecule.

17–C. Pyruvate kinase (PK) deficiency is an autosomal recessively inherited disease that causes hemolytic anemia of varying degrees depending on the disparity of PK. The RBCs of affected individuals have a greatly reduced capacity to make ATP and thus do not have sufficient ATP to perform ion pumping and maintain osmotic balance and, therefore, lyse readily. The presence of 2,3-diphosphoglycerol and glucose 6-phosphate rule out the more prevalent glucose 6-phosphate dehydrogenase deficiency.

18–B. Because of the lack of oxygen for the muscles, there is an increase in NADH, leading to more glucose metabolized through glycolysis, causing an increase to pyruvate and thus lactate that is reduced by NADH. In the muscle, there is a concomitant increase in ADP and AMP, not ATP. There is no indication for a change either in the muscle (M form) or in the heart (H form) forms of lactate dehydrogenase. Absence of the A form of aldolase can lead to hemolytic anemia.

19–C. RBCs contain NO mitochondria. Therefore, NO glucose can be derived from acetyl CoA or oxaloacetate, and there are no glycogen deposits. RBCs do have lactate dehydrogenase, so depending on the concentration of pyruvate, lactate is made.

20–C. The concentration a substrate of triose phosphate isomerase, dihydroxyacetone phosphate (DHAP), which is an element of the glycerol phosphate shuttle (not malate-aspartate shuttle), was elevated. There is a metabolic block in the glycolytic pathway leading to accumulated DHAP (not 6-carbon or many 3-carbon products) and an impaired cellular energy supply. There would be no accumulation of downstream pyruvate.

The Tricarboxylic Acid Cycle

I. The Tricarboxylic Acid (TCA) Cycle

A. Overview of the tricarboxylic acid cycle (Krebs cycle, citric acid cycle)

1. Involves the oxidation of acetyl coenzyme A (CoA) along with the reduction of coenzymes, which are subsequently re-oxidized to produce adenosine triphosphate (ATP).

2. The cycle is **amphibolic**, providing carbon skeletons for **gluconeogenesis, fatty acid synthesis, and the interconversion of amino acids.**

3. All the enzymes of the TCA cycle are in the **mitochondrial matrix** except succinate dehydrogenase, which is in the inner mitochondrial membrane.

> *cc 7.1* Given the importance of this pathway in the production of energy, few genetic deficiencies of the enzymes are reported; these mutations would be **incompatible with life.**

B. Entry of pyruvate from glycolysis

1. In order for carbons from glucose to enter the TCA cycle, glucose is first converted to pyruvate by glycolysis, then pyruvate forms acetyl CoA.

2. *Reaction sequence*

   a. Pyruvate dehydrogenase (PDH), a multienzyme complex located exclusively in the mitochondrial matrix, catalyzes the oxidative decarboxylation of pyruvate, forming acetyl CoA.

   b. The reactions catalyzed by the pyruvate dehydrogenase complex (PDHC) are analogous to those catalyzed by the α-ketoglutarate dehydrogenase complex.

> *cc 7.2* **Arsenic** is an odorless and tasteless heavy metal, which has been used throughout the centuries as a **poison.** It inhibits one of the subunits of the **PDHC,** resulting in **impaired** production of acetyl CoA and subsequent oxidative phosphorylation.

3. *Regulation of pyruvate dehydrogenase* (Figure 7-1)

   a. In contrast to α-ketoglutarate dehydrogenase, PDH exists in a phosphorylated (inactive) form and a dephosphorylated (active) form.

   b. A **kinase** associated with the multienzyme complex phosphorylates the pyruvate decarboxylase subunit, inactivating the PDHC.

   (1) The products of the PDH reaction, **acetyl CoA** and **NADH,** activate the kinase

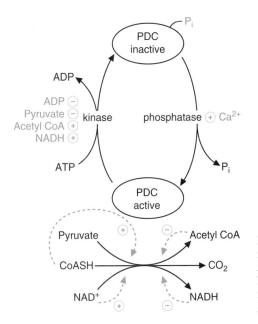

Figure 7-1 Regulation of the pyruvate dehydrogenase complex (PDHC). ADP = adenosine diphosphate; ATP = adenosine triphosphate; CoA = coenzyme A; NAD$^+$ = nicotine adenine dinucleotide; NADH = reduced nicotinamide adenine dinucleotide; P$_i$ = inorganic phosphate.

    (2) The substrates, coenzyme A **(CoA)** and **NAD$^+$**, inactivate the kinase.

    (3) The kinase is also inactivated by adenosine diphosphate (ADP).

  c. A **phosphatase** dephosphorylates and activates the PDHC.

  d. When the concentration of substrates is high, the dehydrogenase is active, and pyruvate is converted to acetyl CoA. When the concentration of products is high, the dehydrogenase is relatively inactive.

> **cc 7.3** **Pyruvate dehydrogenase complex (PDHC) deficiency** is one of the most common **neurodegenerative disorders** associated with abnormal mitochondrial metabolism. Severe forms of the disease are lethal; mild forms exhibit **ataxia and mild psychomotor delay** and nonspecific symptoms (e.g., severe lethargy, poor feeding, tachypnea) related to **lactate buildup,** especially during times of illness, stress, or high carbohydrate intake.

C. The reactions of the TCA cycle (Figure 7-2)

  1. *Acetyl CoA* and **oxaloacetate** condense, forming citrate.

    a. Enzyme: **citrate synthase.**

    b. Cleavage of the high-energy thioester bond in acetyl CoA provides the energy for this condensation.

    c. Citrate (the product) is an inhibitor of this reaction.

  2. *Citrate* is isomerized to isocitrate by a rearrangement of the molecule.

    a. Enzyme: **aconitase.**

    b. Aconitate serves as an enzyme-bound intermediate.

> **cc 7.4** The rat poison **fluoroacetate** reacts with oxaloacetate to form fluorocitrate. Fluorocitrate inhibits **aconitase,** leading to the **accumulation of citrate.** Ingestion may result in convulsions, cardiac arrhythmias, and eventually death.

  3. *Isocitrate* is oxidized to α-ketoglutarate in the first oxidative decarboxylation reaction. CO$_2$ is produced, and the electrons are passed to NAD$^+$ to form NADH + H$^+$.

    a. Enzyme: **isocitrate dehydrogenase.**

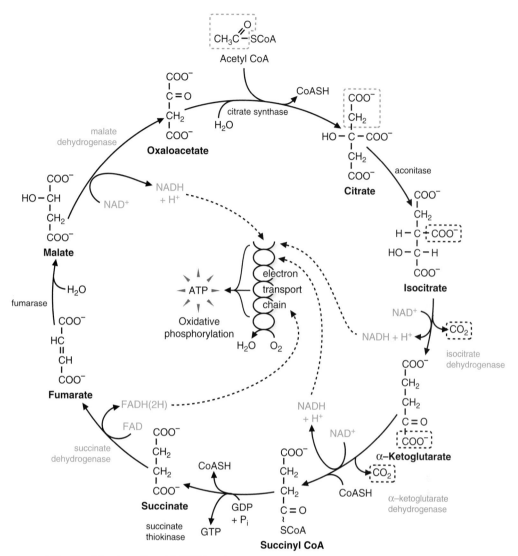

Figure 7-2 The tricarboxylic acid (TCA) cycle.

    b. This key regulatory enzyme of the TCA cycle is allosterically activated by ADP and inhibited by NADH.

  4. *α-Ketoglutarate* is converted to succinyl CoA in a second oxidative decarboxylation reaction. CO_2 is released, and succinyl CoA, NADH, and H^+ are produced.

    a. Enzyme: **α-ketoglutarate dehydrogenase.**

    b. This enzyme requires five cofactors: thiamine pyrophosphate, lipoic acid, CoASH, flavin adenine dinucleotide (FAD), and NAD^+.

  5. *Succinyl CoA* is cleaved to succinate. Cleavage of the high-energy thioester bond of succinyl CoA provides energy for the **substrate level phosphorylation** of GDP to GTP. Because this does not involve the electron transport chain, it is not an oxidative phosphorylation.

    a. Enzyme: **succinate thiokinase.**

    b. The enzyme is also called succinyl CoA synthetase.

6. *Succinate* is oxidized to fumarate. Succinate transfers two hydrogens together with their electrons to FAD, which forms $FADH_2$.
   a. Enzyme: **succinate dehydrogenase.**
   b. This enzyme is present in the inner mitochondrial membrane. The other enzymes of the cycle are in the matrix.

> cc *7.5* The chemical **malonate** decreases cellular respiration. It is a competitive inhibitor of **succinate dehydrogenase** and resembles the substrate succinate, without a $-CH_2-CH_2$ group required for dehydrogenation.

7. *Fumarate* is converted–by the enzyme **fumarase**–to malate by the addition of water across the double bond.
8. *Malate* is oxidized with the help of the enzyme malate dehydrogenase, regenerating **oxaloacetate** and thus completing the cycle. Two hydrogens along with their electrons are passed to NAD^+, producing $NADH + H^+$.

D. **Energy production by the TCA cycle**

1. The NADH and $FADH_2$ (produced by the cycle) donate electrons to the electron transport chain. For each **NADH**, approximately **3 ATP** are generated, and for each **$FADH_2$**, approximately **2 ATP** are generated by the passage of these electrons to O_2 (oxidative phosphorylation). In addition, GTP is produced when succinyl CoA is cleaved. **GTP** produces ATP.

$$(GTP + ADP \leftrightarrows ATP + GDP)$$

2. The **total energy** generated by one round of the cycle, starting with 1 acetyl CoA, is approximately **12 ATP.**

E. **Regulation of the TCA cycle** (Figure 7-3)

1. The TCA cycle is regulated by the **cell's need for energy** in the form of ATP. The TCA cycle acts in concert with the electron transport chain and the ATP synthase in the inner mitochondrial membrane to produce ATP.
2. The cell has limited amounts of adenine nucleotides (ATP, ADP, and adenosine monophosphate [AMP]).
3. When ATP is utilized, ADP and inorganic phosphate (P_i) are produced.
4. **When ADP levels are high** relative to ATP—that is, when the cell needs energy— the reactions of the electron transport chain are accelerated.
   a. NADH is rapidly oxidized; consequently, the **TCA cycle speeds up.**
   b. ADP allosterically activates isocitrate dehydrogenase.
5. **When the concentration of ATP is high**—the cell has an adequate energy supply—the electron transport chain slows down, NADH builds up, and consequently, **the TCA cycle is inhibited.**
   a. **NADH allosterically inhibits isocitrate dehydrogenase.** Isocitrate accumulates, and because the aconitase equilibrium favors citrate, the concentration of citrate rises. **Citrate inhibits citrate synthase**, the first enzyme of the cycle.
   b. High NADH (low NAD^+) levels also affect the reactions of the cycle that generate NADH, slowing the cycle by mass action.
   c. Oxaloacetate (OAA) is converted to malate when NADH is high, and therefore, less substrate is available for the citrate synthase reaction.

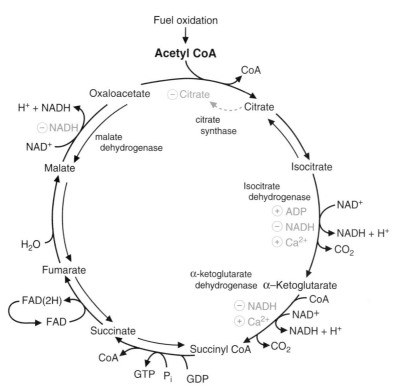

Figure 7-3 Major regulatory interactions of the TCA cycle.

F. **Cofactors and vitamins required for reactions of the TCA cycle**

1. *NAD$^+$* accepts a hydride ion, which reacts with its nicotinamide ring. NAD$^+$ is reduced; the substrate (RH$_2$) is oxidized; and a proton is released.

$$NAD^+ + RH_2 \leftrightarrows NADH + H^+ + R$$

a. NAD$^+$ is frequently involved in oxidizing a hydroxyl group to a ketone.

$$R-\overset{\overset{\displaystyle OH}{|}}{C}H-R_1 + NAD^+ \leftrightarrows R-\overset{\overset{\displaystyle O}{||}}{C}-R_1 + NADH + H^+$$

b. The **nicotinamide ring** of NAD$^+$ is derived from the vitamin **niacin** (nicotinic acid) and, to a limited extent, from the amino acid **tryptophan.**

c. NAD$^+$ is used in the isocitrate dehydrogenase, α-ketoglutarate dehydrogenase, and malate dehydrogenase reactions.

2. *FAD* accepts two hydrogen atoms (with their electrons). FAD is reduced, and the substrate is oxidized.

$$FAD + RH_2 \leftrightarrows FADH_2 + R$$

a. FAD is frequently involved in reactions that produce a double bond.

$$R-CH_2-CH_2-R_1 + FAD \leftrightarrows R-CH=CH-R_1 + FADH_2$$

     b. FAD is derived from the vitamin **riboflavin.**

     c. FAD is the cofactor for **succinate dehydrogenase.** FAD is also required by **α-ketoglutarate dehydrogenase.**

3. *Coenzyme A* (Figure 7-4)

     a. CoA contains a sulfhydryl group that reacts with carboxylic acids to form **thioesters,** such as acetyl CoA, succinyl CoA, and palmityl CoA.

        (1) The $\Delta G°$ for hydrolysis of the thioester bond is −7.5 kcal/mole (a high-energy bond).

        (2) CoA contains the vitamin **pantothenic acid.**

        (3) CoA is used in the α-ketoglutarate dehydrogenase complex.

4. *Thiamine and lipoic acid, cofactors for α-ketoacid dehydrogenases*

     a. **α-Ketoacid dehydrogenases** catalyze **oxidative decarboxylations** in a sequence of reactions involving thiamine pyrophosphate, lipoic acid, CoA, FAD, and NAD^+.

     b. The major α-ketoacid dehydrogenases are:

        (1) **PDH,** the enzyme complex that oxidatively decarboxylates pyruvate, forming acetyl CoA

        (2) **α-Ketoglutarate dehydrogenase,** which catalyzes the conversion of α-ketoglutarate to succinyl CoA

     c. **Thiamine pyrophosphate** (Figure 7-5A) is involved in the **decarboxylation of α-ketoacids.**

        (1) The α-carbon of the α-ketoacid becomes covalently attached to thiamine pyrophosphate, and the carboxyl group is released as CO_2.

        (2) Thiamine pyrophosphate (TPP) is formed from ATP and the vitamin **thiamine.**

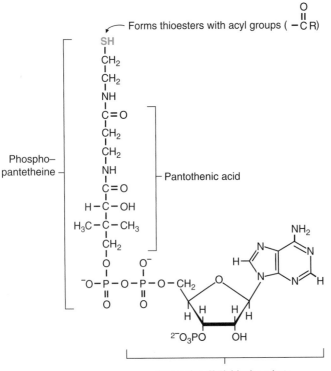

Figure 7-4 The structure of coenzyme A. The *arrow* indicates where acyl (e.g., acetyl, succinyl, and fatty acyl) groups bind to form thioesters.

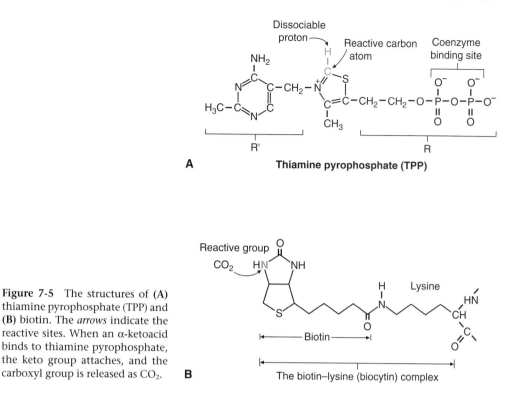

Figure 7-5 The structures of **(A)** thiamine pyrophosphate (TPP) and **(B)** biotin. The *arrows* indicate the reactive sites. When an α-ketoacid binds to thiamine pyrophosphate, the keto group attaches, and the carboxyl group is released as CO_2.

d. Lipoic acid oxidizes the keto group of the decarboxylated α-ketoacid (Figure 7-6).

(1) After an α-ketoacid is decarboxylated, the remainder of the compound is oxidized as it is transferred from TPP to lipoic acid, which is reduced in the reaction.

(2) The oxidized compound, which forms a thioester with lipoate, is then transferred to the sulfur of CoA.

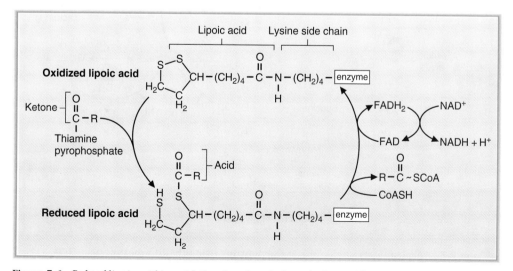

Figure 7-6 Role of lipoic acid in oxidative decarboxylation of α-ketoacids.

(3) Because there is a limited amount of lipoate in the cell, reduced lipoate must be re-oxidized so that it can be re-utilized in these types of reactions. It is re-oxidized by FAD, which becomes reduced to $FADH_2$ and is subsequently re-oxidized by NAD^+.

(4) Lipoic acid is not derived from a vitamin.

e. Biotin is involved in the **carboxylation** of **pyruvate** (which forms oxalo-acetate), **acetyl CoA** (which forms malonyl CoA), and **propionyl CoA** (which forms methylmalonyl CoA). The vitamin biotin is covalently linked to a lysyl residue of the enzyme (Figure 7-5B).

G. **Synthetic functions of the TCA cycle** (Figure 7-7)

1. *Intermediates* of the TCA cycle are used in the fasting state in the liver for the production of **glucose** and in the fed state for the synthesis of **fatty acids**. Intermediates of the TCA cycle are also used to synthesize **amino acids** or to convert one amino acid to another.

2. *Anaplerotic reactions* replenish intermediates of the TCA cycle as they are removed for the synthesis of glucose, fatty acids, amino acids, or other compounds.

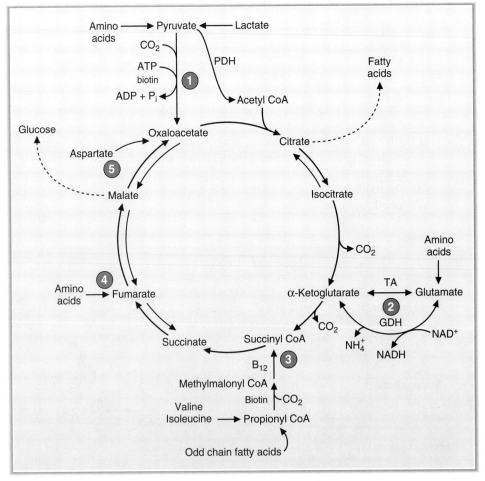

Figure 7-7 Anaplerotic and biosynthetic reactions involving the tricarboxylic acid (TCA) cycle intermediates. Synthetic reactions that form fatty acids and glucose are indicated by *dashed lines*. GDH = glutamate dehydrogenase; PDH = pyruvate dehydrogenase; TA = transamination; ❶ to ❺ = anaplerotic reactions; PC = pyruvate carboxylase.

a. A key anaplerotic reaction is catalyzed by **pyruvate carboxylase,** which carboxylates pyruvate, forming oxaloacetate. (Step 1)
   (1) Pyruvate carboxylase requires **biotin,** a cofactor that is commonly involved in CO_2 fixation reactions.
   (2) Pyruvate carboxylase, found in liver, brain, and adipose tissue (but not in muscle), is **activated by acetyl CoA.**

> *cc* **7.6** **Pyruvate carboxylase deficiency** results in accumulation of **lactic acid** in the blood stream as the conversion of pyruvate to oxaloacetate is blocked. The disorder presents early in life with delayed development, muscle weakness (hypotonia), impaired ability to control voluntary movements (ataxia), seizures, and vomiting.

b. **Amino acids** produce intermediates of the TCA cycle through anaplerotic reactions.
   (1) **Glutamate** is converted to α-ketoglutarate. (Step 2) Amino acids that form glutamate include glutamine, proline, arginine, and histidine.
   (2) **Aspartate** is transaminated to form oxaloacetate. Asparagine can produce aspartate.
   (3) **Valine, isoleucine, methionine,** and **threonine** produce propionyl CoA, which is converted to methylmalonyl CoA and, subsequently, to succinyl CoA, an intermediate of the TCA cycle. (Step 3)
   (4) **Phenylalanine, tyrosine,** and **aspartate** form fumarate. (Step 4)

3. *Synthesis of glucose*
   a. The synthesis of glucose occurs by the pathway of **gluconeogenesis,** which involves intermediates of the TCA cycle.
   b. As glucose is synthesized, **malate or oxaloacetate** is removed from the TCA cycle and replenished by anaplerotic reactions.
      (1) Pyruvate, produced from lactate or alanine, is converted by pyruvate carboxylase to oxaloacetate, which forms malate. (Step 5)
      (2) **Various amino acids that supply carbon for gluconeogenesis** are converted to intermediates of the TCA cycle, which form malate and, thus, glucose.

4. *Synthesis of fatty acids*
   a. The pathway for fatty acid synthesis from glucose includes reactions of the TCA cycle.
   b. From glucose, pyruvate is produced and converted to oxaloacetate (by pyruvate carboxylase) and to acetyl CoA (by pyruvate dehydrogenase).
   c. Oxaloacetate and acetyl CoA condense to form **citrate,** which is used for fatty acid synthesis.
   d. Pyruvate carboxylase catalyzes the anaplerotic reaction that replenishes the TCA cycle intermediates.

5. *Synthesis of amino acids*
   a. Synthesis of amino acids from glucose involves intermediates of the TCA cycle.
   b. **Glucose** is converted to pyruvate, which forms oxaloacetate, which by transamination, forms **aspartate** and, subsequently, **asparagine.**
   c. Glucose is converted to pyruvate, which forms both oxaloacetate and acetyl CoA, which condense, forming citrate. Citrate forms isocitrate and then α-ketoglutarate, producing **glutamate, glutamine, proline,** and **arginine.**

6. *Interconversion of amino acids* involves intermediates of the TCA cycle. For example, the carbons of **glutamate** can feed into the TCA cycle at the α-ketoglutarate level and traverse the cycle, forming oxaloacetate, which may be transaminated to **aspartate.**

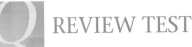

REVIEW TEST

*Directions: Each of the numbered questions or incomplete statements in this section is followed by answers or by completions of the statement. Select the **one** lettered answer or completion that is **best** in each case.*

1. The enzyme pyruvate dehydrogenase (PDH):

(A) contains only one polypeptide chain.
(B) requires thiamine pyrophosphate (TPP) as a cofactor.
(C) produces oxaloacetate from pyruvate.
(D) is converted to an active form by phosphorylation.
(E) is activated when NADH levels increase.

2. The principal function of the tricarboxylic acid (TCA) cycle is to:

(A) generate CO_2.
(B) transfer electrons from the acetyl portion of acetyl coenzyme A (CoA) to NAD^+ and flavin adenine dinucleotide (FAD).
(C) oxidize the acetyl portion of acetyl CoA to oxaloacetate.
(D) generate heat from the oxidation of the acetyl portion of acetyl CoA.
(E) dispose of excess pyruvate and fatty acids.

3. Which of the following vitamins is required for synthesis of a cofactor required for reactions in the oxidation of pyruvate to CO_2 and H_2O?

(A) Biotin
(B) Vitamin K
(C) Pantothenate
(D) Ascorbate
(E) Pyridoxine

4. The reactions of the TCA cycle that oxidize succinate to oxaloacetate:

(A) require coenzyme A.
(B) include an isomerization reaction.
(C) produce one high-energy phosphate bond.
(D) require both NAD^+ and FAD.

(E) produce one GTP from GDP + inorganic phosphate (P_i).

5. In the TCA cycle, thiamine pyrophosphate:

(A) accepts electrons from the oxidation of pyruvate and α-ketoglutarate.
(B) accepts electrons from the oxidation of isocitrate.
(C) forms a covalent intermediate with the α-carbon of α-ketoglutarate.
(D) forms a thioester with the sulfhydryl group of CoASH.
(E) forms a thioester with the sulfhydryl group of lipoic acid.

6. During exercise, stimulation of the TCA cycle results principally from:

(A) allosteric activation of isocitrate dehydrogenase by increased NADH.
(B) allosteric activation of fumarase by increased adenosine diphosphate (ADP).
(C) a rapid decrease in the concentration of four-carbon intermediates.
(D) product inhibition of citrate synthase.
(E) stimulation of the flux through a number of enzymes by a decreased $NADH/NAD^+$ ratio.

7. CO_2 production by the TCA cycle would be increased to the greatest extent by a genetic abnormality that resulted in:

(A) a 50% increase in the concentration of ADP in the mitochondrial matrix.
(B) a 50% increase in the oxygen content of the cell.
(C) a 50% decrease in the V_{max} of α-ketoglutarate dehydrogenase.
(D) a 50% increase in the K_m of isocitrate dehydrogenase.

114

Questions 8 and 9

Refer to the reactions and associated values in the table below when answering questions 8 and 9.

Reaction	Approximate $\Delta G^{\circ\prime}$ (kcal/mole)
Acetate $+ 2\, O_2 \rightarrow 2\, CO_2 + 2\, H_2O$	−243
$NADH + H^+ + \frac{1}{2}\, O_2 \rightarrow NAD^+ + H_2O$	−53
$FADH_2 + \frac{1}{2}\, O_2 \rightarrow FAD + H_2O$	−41
$GTP \rightarrow GDP + P_i$	−8
$ATP \rightarrow ADP + P_i$	−8

8. Of the total energy available from the oxidation of acetate, what percentage is transferred via the TCA cycle to NADH, $FADH_2$, and GTP?

(A) 38%
(B) 42%
(C) 82%
(D) 86%
(E) 100%

9. What percentage of the energy available from the oxidation of acetate is converted to ATP?

(A) 3%
(B) 30%
(C) 40%
(D) 85%
(E) 100%

10. A 58-year-old man is taken to the emergency room after being poisoned with arsenic. Arsenic has several harmful effects, including forming an inactivated complex with alpha-lipoic acid in PDH. As a result of this poisoning, how many ATP equivalents will the oxidation of glucose yield?

(A) 1
(B) 2
(C) 4
(D) 5
(E) 6

11. A biochemistry graduate student isolates all the enzymes of the TCA cycle and adds oxaloacetate and acetyl CoA. He also adds the appropriate energy precursors, cofactors, and water. Which of the following will not be a direct product of his experiment?

(A) ATP
(B) GTP
(C) NADH
(D) CO_2
(E) $FADH_2$

12. A medical student just finished reading the pathology chapter on vitamin deficiencies and has become completely unwound. She drives to the local herbal store and makes a several hundred–dollar purchase of products. The next day, she brags to her nutrition professor of her conscientious investment only to find that a healthy diet would have sufficed. Which of the following cofactors is correctly matched with the vitamin it is derived from?

(A) NADH–vitamin B_2
(B) $FADH_2$–vitamin B_3
(C) Coenzyme A–vitamin B_5
(D) Pyridoxal phosphate–vitamin B_1
(E) TPP–vitamin B_6

13. A 24-year-old woman presents with diarrhea, dysphagia, jaundice, and white transverse lines on the fingernails (Mee's lines). The patient is diagnosed with arsenic poisoning, which inhibits which of the following enzymes?

(A) Citrate synthase
(B) Isocitrate dehydrogenase
(C) Pyruvate dehydrogenase
(D) α-Ketoglutarate dehydrogenase
(E) Succinate dehydrogenase

14. A 3-year-old boy presents to the pediatric clinic with the symptoms of hypotonia, lactic acidosis, and seizures. After an extensive workup, he is diagnosed with pyruvate dehydrogenase complex (PDHC) deficiency, an X-linked recessive disorder. Which of the following cofactors is not required by this enzyme to convert pyruvate to acetyl CoA?

(A) Thiamine
(B) Lipoic acid
(C) Pantothenate
(D) Niacin
(E) Ascorbic acid

15. A medicinal chemist working for a pharmaceutical company is synthesizing the barbiturate, barbital, for a clinical trial. In the following pathway for the synthesis of the barbital, which substrate is most likely to inhibit the only membrane-bound enzyme of the Krebs cycle?

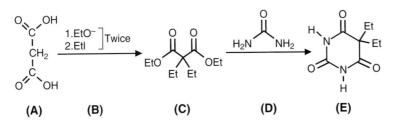

(A)   (B)   (C)   (D)   (E)

16. An 18-month-old child is left unattended while in the kitchen and ingests a small portion of rat poisoning found in the cupboards under the sink. The ingredient fluoroacetate reacts with oxaloacetate to form the enzyme inhibitor fluorocitrate. Which of the following substrates would result in the greatest energy production yet bypass the inhibited enzyme?

(A) Citrate
(B) Malate
(C) Isocitrate
(D) Fumarate
(E) Oxaloacetate

17. A 3-year-old boy presents to the emergency room after having a generalized tonic/clonic seizure. The child has a history of epilepsy, ataxia, and lactic acidosis. When questioned, the parents state that their child was born with the disease, pyruvate carboxylase deficiency. Which of the following products is the fate of pyruvate when the reaction is catalyzed by pyruvate carboxylase?

(A) Lactic acid
(B) Alanine
(C) Acetyl CoA
(D) Oxaloacetate
(E) Acetaldehyde

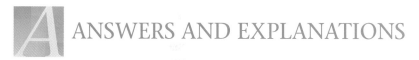

1–B. Pyruvate dehydrogenase (PDH) converts pyruvate to acetyl coenzyme A (CoA). It contains multiple subunits: a dehydrogenase component that oxidatively decarboxylates pyruvate, a dihydrolipoyl transacetylase that transfers the acetyl group to CoA, and a dihydrolipoyl dehydrogenase that re-oxidizes lipoic acid. Thiamine pyrophosphate (TPP), lipoic acid, CoA, NAD$^+$, and flavin adenine dinucleotide (FAD) serve as cofactors for these reactions. In addition, a kinase is present that phosphorylates and inactivates the decarboxylase component. Acetyl CoA and NADH activate this kinase, thus inactivating PDH. A phosphatase dephosphorylates the kinase, thereby reactivating PDH.

2–B. Although the tricarboxylic acid (TCA) cycle produces CO_2 and oxaloacetate and generates heat, these are not its major functions. It does not "dispose" of excess pyruvate and fatty acids; it oxidizes them in a controlled manner to generate energy. The principal function of the cycle is to pass electrons to NAD$^+$ and FAD, which transfer them to the electron transport chain. The net result is the production of adenosine triphosphate (ATP).

3–C. Pantothenate is required for the synthesis of coenzyme A (CoA). CoA is a cofactor for PDH, which converts pyruvate to acetyl CoA. Acetyl CoA enters the TCA cycle to be oxidized to CO_2 and H_2O. α-Ketoglutarate dehydrogenase, which converts α-ketoglutarate to succinyl CoA in the TCA cycle, also requires CoA.

4–D. FAD is required for conversion of succinate to fumarate, and NAD$^+$ is required for conversion of malate to oxaloacetate. Five ATP are generated. CoA is not required, and no isomerization reactions occur. Guanosine triphosphate (GTP) is produced in the previous step of the cycle, when succinyl CoA is converted to succinate.

5–C. Thiamine pyrophosphate forms a covalent intermediate with the α-carbon of α-ketoglutarate.

6–E. NADH decreases during exercise (if it increased, it would slow the cycle). Fumarase is not activated by adenosine diphosphate (ADP). Four-carbon intermediates of the cycle are recycled. Their concentration does not decrease. Product inhibition of citrate synthase would slow the cycle. During exercise, the TCA is stimulated because the NADH/NAD$^+$ ratio decreases and stimulates flux through isocitrate dehydrogenase, α-ketoglutarate dehydrogenase, and malate dehydrogenase.

7–A. If the V_{max} of α-ketoglutarate dehydrogenase decreased, flux through the TCA cycle would decrease; therefore, CO_2 production would decrease. If the K_m of isocitrate dehydrogenase increased, higher concentrations of isocitrate would be required for the cycle to operate at its normal rate. O_2 is normally present in excess and is not rate-limiting. The only change that would increase the rate of CO_2 production by the cycle would be an increase of ADP, which would allosterically activate isocitrate dehydrogenase.

8–D. In the TCA cycle, 3 NADH are produced ($3 \times 53 = 159$ kcal), 1 FADH$_2$ is produced (41 kcal), and 1 GTP is produced (8 kcal). The percentage of the total energy available from oxidation of acetate that is transferred to these compounds is, therefore, 208/243 kcal or 86%.

9–C. About 12 ATP are produced by the TCA cycle (12×8 kcal = 96 kcal). The percentage of the total energy available from oxidation of acetate that is converted to ATP is 96/243, or 40%.

10–C. With the arrest of PDH, glucose will only provide energy gains from glycolysis. Since the glycerol-3-phosphate shuttle is the major shuttle in most tissues, the 2 molecules of NADH produced will yield 4 ATP equivalents. When added to the 2 ATP produced at the substrate level, a total of 4 ATP equivalents will be netted.

11–A. The Krebs cycle produces no substrate level ATP, but rather depends on NADH and $FADH_2$ at the electron transport chain for ATP equivalents. Further energy equivalence includes GTP when succinate is produced. CO_2 results in the production and reduction of isocitrate.

12–C. CoA is generated from pantothenic acid (vitamin B_5); NADH is derived from niacin (vitamin B_3); $FADH_2$ is created from riboflavin (vitamin B_2); pyridoxal phosphate is created from pyridoxine (vitamin B_6); and TPP is derived from thiamine (vitamin B_1).

13–D. Arsenic binds the sulfhydryl groups of lipoic acid, creating an inactive 6-membered ring. Because lipoic acid is one of the three cofactors of PDH, this inactivates the enzyme's ability to synthesize acetyl CoA from pyruvate. The answer choices include the major rate-controlling Krebs cycle enzymes citrate synthase, isocitrate dehydrogenase, and PDH through feedback inhibition by NADH. Finally, succinate dehydrogenase is competitively inhibited by the succinate analogue, malonate.

14–E. Ascorbic acid is a cofactor in the hydroxylases responsible in collagen formation. The pyruvate dehydrogenase complex (PDHC) begins its conversion of pyruvate to acetyl CoA through the decarboxylation of pyruvate, which is bound to the cofactor TPP. The next reaction of the complex is the transfer of the 2-carbon acetyl group from acetyl TPP to lipoic acid, the covalently bound coenzyme of lipoyl transacetylase. The enzyme dihydrolipoyl dehydrogenase, with FAD^+ as a cofactor, catalyzes that oxidation reaction. The final activity of the PDHC is the transfer of reducing equivalents from the $FADH_2$ of dihydrolipoyl dehydrogenase to NAD^+.

15–A. Malonate binds to the active site of succinate dehydrogenase, yet it is not oxidized due to the absence of an ethyl group between the carboxyl groups, as in succinate. Ethyl oxide and ethyl iodine (choice B) act as nucleophiles but have no inhibitory effects on the Krebs cycle. Diethyl ethyl malonate (choice C), urea (choice D), and barbital (choice E), differ greatly from the endogenous substrate succinate and, therefore, would likely not inhibit the enzyme.

16–C. The active ingredient in rat poisoning, fluoroacetate, reacts with oxaloacetate to form fluorocitrate, resulting in the inhibition of the Krebs cycle enzyme, aconitase. Therefore, citrate is not converted to isocitrate. Citrate will accumulate without the catalysis provided by aconitase. Malate, fumarate, and oxaloacetate will bypass the inhibited aconitase. Unfortunately, they will also bypass the Krebs cycle steps, which involve the synthesis of NADH, GTP, and $FADH_2$.

17–D. Pyruvate carboxylase is a biotin-dependent mitochondrial enzyme that converts pyruvate to oxaloacetate. Pyruvate is converted to lactic acid by lactate dehydrogenase. The amino acid alanine is formed when the enzyme aminotransferase transfers an amino group to pyruvate. PDH converts pyruvate to acetyl CoA. Finally, pyruvate decarboxylase converts pyruvate to acetaldehyde.

The Electron Transport Chain and Oxidative Metabolism

I. Electron Transport Chain and Oxidative Phosphorylation

A. Overview of the electron transport chain (ETC) (Figure 8-1)

1. **NADH** (reduced nicotinamide adenine dinucleotide) **and FADH$_2$** (the reduced form of flavin adenine dinucleotide) are produced by glycolysis, β-oxidation of fatty acids, the tricarboxylic acid (TCA) cycle, and other oxidative reactions. NADH and FADH$_2$ pass electrons to the components of the ETC, which are located in the inner mitochondrial membrane.

2. **NADH** freely diffuses from the matrix to the membrane, while **FADH$_2$** is tightly bound to enzymes that produce it within the inner mitochondrial membrane.

3. **Mitochondria** are separated from the cytoplasm by two membranes. The soluble interior of a mitochondrion is called the **matrix.** The matrix is surrounded by the inner membrane, which contains vast infoldings to increase surface area, known as **cristae.**

4. The **transfer of electrons** from NADH to oxygen (O$_2$) occurs in **three stages**, each of which involves a large protein complex in the inner mitochondrial membrane.

5. Some of the genes for the large protein complexes are encoded by **nuclear DNA,** while others are coded for by **mitochondrial DNA (mtDNA).**

> *cc 8.1* **Fatal infantile mitochondrial myopathy** involves decreased activity of the **mtDNA**-encoded **respiratory chain complexes (I, III, IV, and V).** Patients have early progressive **liver failure** and **neurologic abnormalities, hypoglycemia,** and increased lactate in body fluids.

6. Each complex uses the energy from electron transfer to **pump protons** to the cytosolic side of the membrane.

7. An **electrochemical potential** or proton-motive force is generated, and adenosine triphosphate (ATP) is produced as the protons enter back into the matrix through the **ATP synthase** complex.

8. During the transfer of electrons through the ETC, **some** of the **energy is lost as heat.**

9. The electron transport chain has a large negative $\Delta G°'$, thus electrons flow from NADH (or FADH$_2$) toward O$_2$.

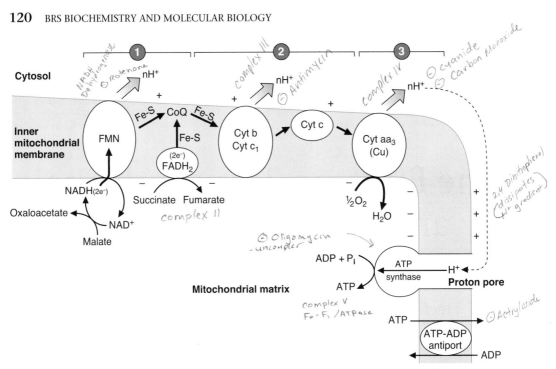

Figure 8-1 The electron transport chain and oxidative phosphorylation. *Heavy arrows* indicate the flow of electrons. CoQ = coenzyme Q (ubiquinone); Cyt = cytochrome; Fe-S = iron-sulfur centers; FMN = flavin mononucleotide. nH⁺ indicates that an undetermined number of protons are pumped from the matrix to the cytosolic side. The *numbers* at the top of the figure correspond with the three major stages of electron transfer described in the text (under I C).

B. Components of the electron transport chain

  1. The reduced cofactors, NADH (Figure 8-2) and $FADH_2$ (Figure 8-3), transfer electrons to the ETC.
  2. **Flavin mononucleotide (FMN)** receives electrons from NADH and transfers them through iron-sulfur (Fe-S) centers to coenzyme Q (Figure 8-4). FMN is derived from **riboflavin.**
  3. **Coenzyme Q** (CoQ) receives electrons from FMN and also through Fe-S centers from $FADH_2$.
     a. $FADH_2$ is not free in solution like NAD^+ and NADH; it is tightly bound to enzymes.
     b. CoQ can be synthesized in the body. It is not derived from a vitamin.

> cc 8.2 Nutritional supplements containing **coenzyme Q** have shown some promise in the treatment of **Parkinson's disease** and other **neurodegenerative diseases,** mitochondrial myopathies, and congestive heart failure and diabetes.

  4. **Cytochromes** receive electrons from the reduced form of CoQ.
     a. Each cytochrome consists of a **heme** group (Figure 8-5) associated with a protein.
     b. The **iron** of the heme group is reduced when the cytochrome accepts an electron.

  $$Fe^{3+} \leftrightarrows Fe^{2+}$$

     c. Heme is synthesized from glycine and succinyl coenzyme A (CoA) in humans. It is not derived from a vitamin.

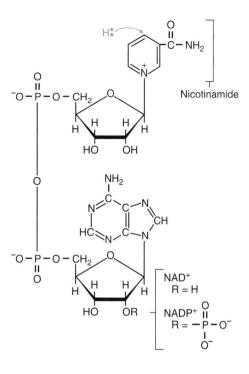

Figure 8-2 The structure of NAD+ and NADP+. R differs for NAD+ and NADP+ as indicated. The *arrow* shows the position where a hydride ion (H-; H:) covalently binds when NAD+ or NADP+ is reduced. NAD+ = the oxidized form of nicotinamide adenine dinucleotide; NADP+ = the oxidized form of nicotinamide adenine dinucleotide phosphate.

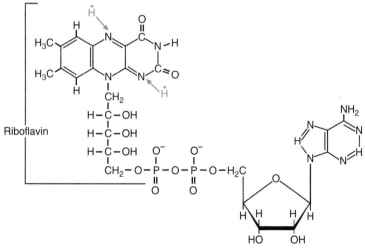

Figure 8-3 The structure of flavin adenine dinucleotide (FAD). *Arrows* indicate positions where hydrogens (Ḣ) covalently bind when FAD is reduced to $FADH_2$. Flavin mononucleotide (FMN) consists only of the riboflavin moiety plus one phosphate.

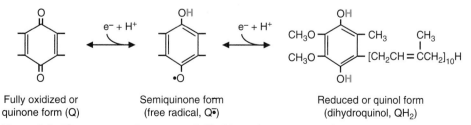

Fully oxidized or quinone form (Q)

Semiquinone form (free radical, Q•)

Reduced or quinol form (dihydroquinol, QH_2)

Figure 8-4 The structure of coenzyme Q (CoQ), or ubiquinone. Hydrogen atoms can bind, one at a time, as indicated by the *arrows*.

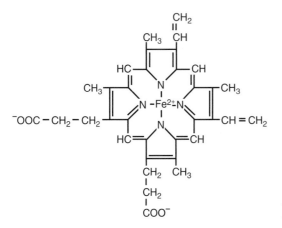

Figure 8-5 The general structure of the heme group, which is present in hemoglobin, myoglobin, and the cytochromes b, c, and c_1.

5. O_2 ultimately receives the electrons at the end of the electron transport chain and is reduced to water (H_2O).

C. **The three major stages of electron transport** (see Figure 8-1)

1. *Transfer of electrons from NADH to coenzyme Q*
   a. **NADH** passes electrons via the **NADH dehydrogenase complex** to FMN.
      (1) NADH is produced by the α-ketoglutarate dehydrogenase, isocitrate dehydrogenase, and malate dehydrogenase reactions of the TCA cycle, by the pyruvate dehydrogenase reaction that converts pyruvate to acetyl CoA, by β-oxidation of fatty acids, and by other oxidation reactions.
      (2) NADH produced in the mitochondrial matrix diffuses to the inner mitochondrial membrane where it passes electrons to FMN, which is tightly bound to a protein. (Stage 1)

   > *cc* **8.3** **Rotenone,** a fish poison, **complexes with NADH dehydrogenase,** causing NADH to accumulate. It does not block the transfer of electrons to the chain from $FADH_2$.

   > *cc* **8.4** The barbiturate sedative, **Amytal,** also **blocks complex I** of the ETC.

   b. **FMN** passes the electrons through a series of Fe-S protein complexes to **CoQ**, which accepts electrons one at a time, forming first the semiquinone and then ubiquinol.
   c. The energy produced by these electron transfers is used to pump protons to the cytosolic side of the inner mitochondrial membrane.
   d. As the protons flow back into the matrix through pores in the ATP synthase complex, approximately 1 ATP is generated for each NADH that transfers electrons to CoQ. (Stage 2)

   > *cc* **8.5** Mutations in the mitochondrial encoded gene for **NADH:ubiquinone oxidoreductase (complex I)** results in the disorder **MELAS.** MELAS is an acronym for the clinical manifestations of the disease **mitochondrial encephalopathy, lactic acidosis,** and **stroke.**

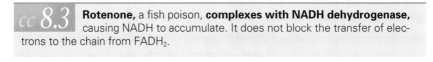

Handwritten margin notes:
- Mt inheritance
- Exercise intolerance
- Fluctating lactic acidosis
- Tx: Succinate (bypass)

2. *Transfer of electrons from CoQ to cytochrome c*
   a. **CoQ** passes electrons through Fe-S centers to **cytochromes b and c_1 (complex III)**, which transfer the electrons to **cytochrome c**. The protein complex involved in these transfers is called **cytochrome reductase**.

   > *cc* **8.6**   **Antimycin,** a fungal antibiotic, blocks the passage of electrons through the **cytochrome b-c_1 complex.**

   (1) These cytochromes each contain heme as a prosthetic group but have different apoproteins.
   (2) In the **ferric (Fe^{3+})** state, the heme iron can accept one electron and be reduced to the **ferrous (Fe^{2+})** state.
   (3) Because the cytochromes can only carry one electron at a time, two molecules in each cytochrome complex must be reduced for every molecule of NADH that is oxidized.

   > *cc* **8.7**   Some patients with the **mtDNA** disorder known as **Leber's hereditary optic neuropathy (LHON)** have point mutations in the gene for **cytochrome reductase.** Patients are typically males in their 20s to 30s who develop **loss of central vision.**

   b. The energy produced by the transfer of electrons from CoQ to cytochrome c is used to pump protons across the inner mitochondrial membrane.
   c. As the protons flow back into the matrix through pores in the ATP synthase complex, approximately **one ATP is generated for every $CoQH_2$ that transfers two electrons to cytochrome c.**
   d. Electrons from $FADH_2$ **(complex II)**, produced by reactions such as the oxidation of succinate to fumarate by succinate dehydrogenase, **enter** the electron transport chain **at the CoQ level** (see Figure 8-1).

   > *cc* **8.8**   Some patients with the mtDNA defect known as **Kearns-Sayre syndrome** have mutations in complex II of the ETC. These patients manifest with short stature, complete external **ophthalmoplegia, pigmentary retinopathy,** ataxia, and **cardiac conduction defects.**

3. *Transfer of electrons from cytochrome c to oxygen*
   a. **Cytochrome c** transfers electrons to the **cytochrome aa_3 complex (complex IV)**, which transfers the electrons to molecular O_2, reducing it to H_2O. **Cytochrome oxidase** catalyzes this transfer of electrons. (Stage 3)

   [handwritten: Cyt C oxidase]

   [handwritten:
   - hypotonia
   - growth retardation
   - cardiomyopathy
   - encephalopathy
   - liver failure
   - lactic acidosis]

   > *cc* **8.9**   Patients with **Leigh's disease,** an **mtDNA** disorder, present with **lactic acidemia, developmental delay,** seizure, **extraocular palsies,** and hypotonia. The disorder is usually **fatal by the age of 2,** with some patients exhibiting mutations in **cytochrome oxidase.**

   (1) Cytochromes a and a_3 each contain a heme and two different proteins that each contain **copper.**
   (2) **Two electrons are required to reduce 1 atom of O_2;** therefore, for each NADH that is oxidized, $\frac{1}{2} O_2$ is converted to H_2O.
   b. The energy produced by the transfer of electrons from cytochrome c to O_2 is used to pump protons across the inner mitochondrial membrane.

    c. As the protons flow back into the matrix, approximately **one ATP is generated for every two electrons** that are transferred from **cytochrome c to oxygen**—that is, for every $\frac{1}{2} O_2$ that is reduced to H_2O.

> **cc 8.10**   **Cyanide and carbon monoxide,** which are poisons sometimes used for suicide, combine with **cytochrome oxidase** and block the transfer of electrons to O_2.

D. ATP production

  1. As elements of the ETC pass electrons from complex I to IV, an **electrochemical potential** or proton-motive force is generated.
    a. The electrochemical potential consists of both a **membrane potential** and a **pH gradient.**
    b. The cytosolic side of the membrane is more acidic (i.e., has a higher $[H^+]$) than the matrix.
  2. The protons can re-enter the matrix only through the ATP synthase complex (**complex V, the F_0–F_1/ATPase**), causing ATP to be generated.
    a. The inner mitochondrial membrane is **impermeable to protons.**

> **cc 8.11**   **2-4-Dinitrophenol** is an **ionophore** that allows protons from the cytosol to re-enter the matrix without going through the pore in the ATP synthase complex. Thus, they **uncouple electron transport** and ATP production.

    b. The **(F_0) component forms a channel** in the inner mitochondrial membrane, through which protons can flow.
    c. The **(F_1) is the ATP-synthesizing head**, projecting into the mitochondrial matrix that is connected to the F_0 portion via a **stalk.**

> **cc 8.12**   **Oligomycin** is a drug that **binds to the stalk of the ATP synthase,** preventing proton re-entry into the mitochondrial matrix. It is an **uncoupler, increasing** the rate of O_2 consumption (respiration), **electron transport,** the **TCA** cycle, and CO_2 production, while **generating heat, rather than energy.**

> **cc 8.13**   In **genetically prone individuals,** the use of **inhalation anesthetics (halothane, ether,** and **methoxyflurane)** triggers a reaction termed **malignant hyperthermia.** It results in the **uncoupling of oxidative phosphorylation from electron transport.** ATP production decreases; heat is generated; and the temperature rises markedly. The TCA cycle is stimulated, and excessive CO_2 production leads to respiratory acidosis.

  3. *Total ATP production*
    a. **For every NADH that is oxidized,** $\frac{1}{2} O_2$ is reduced to H_2O and approximately **3 ATP are produced.**
    b. For every **FADH$_2$ that is oxidized,** approximately **2 ATP are generated** because the electrons from $FADH_2$ enter the chain via CoQ, bypassing the NADH dehydrogenase step.

E. The ATP-ADP antiport. ATP produced within mitochondria is transferred to the cytosol in exchange for ADP by a transport protein in the inner mitochondrial membrane known as the ATP-ADP antiport (see Figure 8-1).

The plant toxin **atractyloside** inhibits the **ATP-ADP antiport,** resulting in depletion of mitochondrial ADP and the eventual termination of ATP synthesis.

II.   Reactive Oxygen Species (ROS)

A. Oxygen radicals (Figure 8-6)

1. Molecules with **extra electrons on the oxygen** are **free radicals.**
2. They often result as a **byproduct** of normal metabolic pathways of **oxidative metabolism.**

B. Sources of reactive oxygen species

1. *CoQ of the ETC*
   a. CoQ occasionally loses an electron in the transfer of reducing equivalents though the electron chain.
   b. This **electron is transferred** to dissolved O_2 for the production of **superoxide.**
   c. CoQ is the major source of superoxide within the cell.
2. *Production of ROS in the peroxisome*
   a. **Fatty oxidation** occurs within these organelles with the transfer of **2 electrons** from **FADH$_2$** to O_2.
   b. H_2O_2, **hydrogen peroxide** is formed within the peroxisome.
3. *Cytochrome P450 mono-oxygenases*
   a. This group of enzymes is involved in the **detoxification of various drugs** that enter the body.

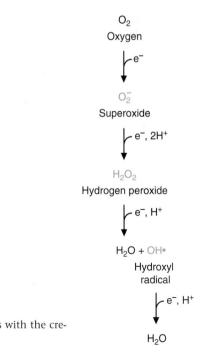

Figure 8-6   The reduction of oxygen by four 1-electron steps with the creation of reactive oxygen species along the pathway.

b. The enzyme catalyses the transfer of electrons from **NADPH** (the reduced form of nicotinamide adenine dinucleotide phosphate) to O_2 and the various substrates to be detoxified.

c. Free radical intermediates in these conversions are often created by **"leakage" of electrons** as the reactions take place.

> *cc* **8.15** **Consumption of alcohol and certain drugs induces expression of various cytochrome mono-oxidases.** Patients who abuse such substances are more prone to the **deleterious effects of ROS species** formed by these **P450** enzymes.

4. *NADPH oxidase* (Figure 8-7)

a. This enzyme is embedded in the membrane of the **phagolysosome within immune cells.**

b. Electrons are transferred from **NADPH to O_2** to form **superoxide.**

c. The superoxide is used to **kill engulfed microbes** within the cell.

> *cc* **8.16** **Chronic granulomatous disease (CGD)** results from a deficiency of **NADPH oxidase** and the inability to effectively kill engulfed microbes, especially bacteria. Patients with CGD present with **serious recurrent bacterial infections.**

5. *Myeloperoxidase (MPO)* (see Figure 8-7)

a. This enzyme, too, is an important enzyme in immune cells, particularly **neutrophils.**

b. It catalyzes the formation of hypochlorous acid (HOCl) from **H_2O_2** in the presence of a halide ion, such as **chloride.**

> *cc* **8.17** The **H_2O_2-MPO-halide system** is one of the **most effective mechanisms for killing bacteria** within neutrophils. However, patients with defects in this system have **near-normal immune function** because bacteria are killed, albeit slower, by **superoxide** produced by the action of **NADPH oxidase.**

6. *Ionizing radiation*

a. High-energy cosmic rays and man-made x-rays can deliver enough energy to split water into hydroxyl and hydrogen radicals.

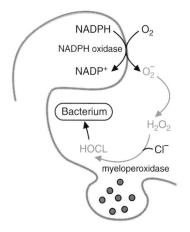

Figure 8-7 The generation of superoxide (O_2-) and hypochlorous acid (HOCl) by NADPH oxidase and myeloperoxidase, respectively, within a neutrophil. Cl⁻ = chloride; NAD⁺ = the oxidized form of nicotinamide adenine dinucleotide; NADPH = the reduced form of nicotinamide adenine dinucleotide phosphate.

b. These radicals go on to damage tissue in mechanisms described below.

> cc *8.18*   The use of **radiation in the treatment of cancer** has greatly improved the management of patients with cancer. Radiation is given in doses and intervals that seek to take advantage of the **decreased ability of cancer cells to repair radiation damage to cells.** The field of radiation oncology plays an important role in the management of cancers of the **breast, prostate, head and neck, and brain;** as well as **lymphoma** and many other cancers.

C. Deleterious effects of ROS (Figure 8-8)

1. ROS chemically modify various biomolecules within the cell, causing deleterious effects and even cell death.
2. *Damage to lipids*
    a. Free radicals can cause peroxidation of lipids.
    b. Lipid membranes become damaged, leading to increased cell permeability, influx of calcium (an important cofactor for proteolytic enzymes), and cell swelling.

> cc *8.19*   The organic solvent **carbon tetrachloride** (CCl_4) is used in the **dry cleaning industry.** The P450 cytochrome system converts CCL_4 to the free radical species **$CCl_3\cdot$.** This highly reactive species causes a chain reaction of **lipid peroxidation,** particularly in the liver, that leads to **hepatocellular necrosis.**

3. *Peptide and protein damage*
    a. ROS species react with iron and sulfur moieties of proteins including sulfhydryl groups, methionine, ferredoxin, and heme.
    b. Oxidative decarboxylation, deamination of proteins, and cleavage of peptide bonds can occur.

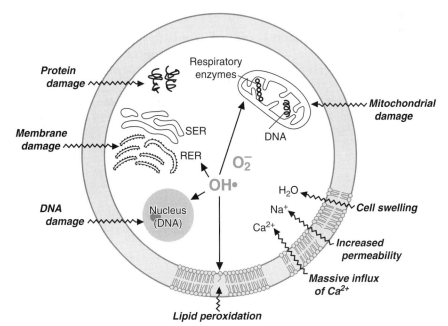

Figure 8-8   Free radical–induced cellular injury. Ca^{2+} = calcium; Na^+ = sodium; O_2^- = super-oxide; $OH\bullet$ = hydrogen radical.

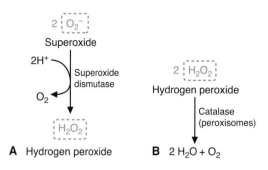

Figure 8-9 Antioxidant enzymes that degrade reactive oxygen species. (**A**) Superoxide dismutase. (**B**) Catalase.

4. *Damage to DNA*
    a. ROS cause alteration in the nucleotide bases of the DNA molecule.
    b. ROS cause **breaks in the deoxyribose backbone.**
    c. DNA damage, if not repaired, often results in programmed cell death.

D. **Antioxidants, the cell's defense against ROS**

1. The cell has developed enzymes and other molecules to help protect itself from the deleterious effects of ROS.
2. *Superoxide dismutase (SOD)* (Figure 8-9A)
    a. Isozymes of this enzyme are found in the mitochondria, cytosol, and even extracellularly.
    b. Catalyzes the conversion of superoxide anion to H_2O_2 **and O_2.**

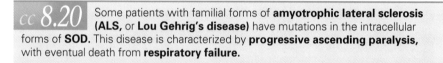

cc 8.20 Some patients with familial forms of **amyotrophic lateral sclerosis (ALS, or Lou Gehrig's disease)** have mutations in the intracellular forms of **SOD.** This disease is characterized by **progressive ascending paralysis,** with eventual death from **respiratory failure.**

3. *Catalase* (Figure 8-9B)
    a. This enzyme promotes the conversion of H_2O_2 to H_2O and O_2.
    b. This enzyme is mainly found within **peroxisomes,** where it protects the cell from the **endogenous production of hydrogen peroxide.**

cc 8.21 Many **bacterial pathogens,** such as *Staphylococcus,* produce **catalase.** These pathogens are of particular concern in patients **who lack NADPH oxidase,** as hydrogen peroxide kills phagocytosed bacteria. Thus, infections involve catalase-positive organisms.

4. *Glutathione*
    a. Glutathione is a **tripeptide** that is oxidized in order to **donate reducing equivalents** to **regenerate oxidized cellular molecules.**
    b. Glutathione is generated as part of the γ-glutamyl cycle (see Chapter 5). It is most concentrated in the liver.

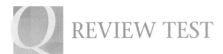

*Directions: Each of the numbered questions or incomplete statements in this section is fol-lowed by answers or by completions of the statement. Select the **one** lettered answer or com-pletion that is **best** in each case.*

1. Which of the following statements is true concerning cytochrome P450?

(A) As an oxidase, molecular oxygen is a substrate of P450.
(B) Reduction-oxidation of P450 is coupled to the pumping out of protons.
(C) It is inhibited by antimycin.
(D) It is a mono-oxygenase.
(E) It is a component of the mito-chondrial electron transport chain (ETC).

2. Which of the following sentences de-scribes oligomycin?

(A) It uncouples oxidation from phosphorylation.
(B) It inhibits NADH dehydrogenase.
(C) It can combine with the F1 ATPase.
(D) It can inhibit adenosine triphosphate (ATP) synthase activity of isolated submitochondrial particles.
(E) It stimulates respiration if adenosine diphosphate (ADP) is added to mitochondria.

3. The importation of ADP into the mito-chondrial matrix:

(A) depends on a shuttle mechanism located in the outer mitochondrial membrane.
(B) is stimulated by atractyloside.
(C) is an active transport process.
(D) is directly inhibited by valinomycin.
(E) is accompanied by ATP departing from the mitochondrial matrix.

4. Which is a component of succinate de-hydrogenase in the mitochondrial ETC?

(A) Cytochrome b
(B) Cytochrome c
(C) Flavin adenine dinucleotide (FAD)
(D) Flavin mononucleotide (FMN)
(E) Coenzyme Q

5. All of the individual steps of the ETC are:

(A) energetically favorable reactions.
(B) coupled to ATP synthesis.
(C) coupled to proton translocation.
(D) inhibited with dinitrophenol (DNP).
(E) uncoupled in the presence of oligomycin.

6. What catalyzes the conversion of hydro-gen peroxide to water?

(A) Catalase
(B) Superoxide dismutase
(C) O_2
(D) A dioxygenase
(E) Cytochrome P450

7. A site along the electron transport chain that is not coupled to ATP synthesis is:

(A) NADH-coenzyme Q (CoQ) reductase.
(B) succinate-CoQ reductase.
(C) cytochrome b/c_1 reductase.
(D) cytochrome oxidase.
(E) NADH-cytochrome c reductase.

8. Uncouplers of oxidative phosphory-lation:

(A) uncouple ATP synthesis with phosphoenolpyruvate.
(B) uncouple ATP/ADP translocation.
(C) uncouple ATP synthesis with phosphoglycerate.
(D) uncouple electron transport from oxygen reduction.
(E) uncouple electron transfer with ATP synthesis.

9. What is the correct arrangement of the components of the ETC of electrons streamed into the mitochondria? (Cyt = cytochrome)

(A) FAD → CoQ → Cyt b→ Cyt c → Cyt a-a_3 → O_2
(B) FMN→ CoQ → Cyt b → Cyt c → Cyt a-a_3 → O_2

(C) $FAD \rightarrow CoQ \rightarrow Cyt\ c \rightarrow Cyt\ b \rightarrow$
Cyt a-$a_3 \rightarrow O_2$

(D) $FMN \rightarrow CoQ \rightarrow Cyt\ c \rightarrow Cyt\ b \rightarrow$
Cyt a-$a_3 \rightarrow O_2$

(E) $FAD \rightarrow CoQ \rightarrow Cyt\ a$-$a_3 \rightarrow Cyt\ b \rightarrow$
Cyt $c \rightarrow O_2$

10. Which of the following ETC compartments accepts only one electron?

(A) Coenzyme Q
(B) Cytochrome b
(C) FAD
(D) FMN
(E) O_2

11. A 38-year-old woman sees an advertisement for a new weight-loss medication. The ad claims that the drug causes your body to burn calories without having to exercise. In theory, which of the following compounds could make this claim?

(A) Rotenone
(B) Antimycin
(C) Dinitrophenol
(D) Amytal
(E) Atractyloside

12. MELAS is a mitochondrial disorder characterized by mitochondrial encephalopathy, lactic acidosis, and stroke-like episodes. Due to the lack of functional mitochondria, what would be the net ATP that would be produced from 1 molecule of glucose?

(A) 1
(B) 2
(C) 4
(D) 8
(E) 0

13. A 23-year-old college football player sustains a compound fracture on the field. He is taken to surgery, during which the anesthesiologist notes a significantly increased body temperature (102°F). The operation is terminated without completion, as malignant hyperthermia is suspected. Which of the following components of the ETC is likely to be responsible for this phenomenon?

(A) Complex I
(B) Complex II
(C) Complex III
(D) Complex IV
(E) The F_0–F_1 ATPase

14. A 53-year-old, previously successful man recently lost his job and is under investigation for racketeering. His wife returns home to find him slumped over the steering wheel of the idling car in the closed garage. He is nonresponsive and has a cherry color to his lips and cheeks. Which of the following is inhibited by the carbon monoxide in the car's exhaust fumes?

(A) Complex I of the ETC
(B) Cytochrome oxidase
(C) The ATP-ADP antiport
(D) The F_0 component of the F_0–F_1 ATPase
(E) The F_1 component of the F_0-F_1 ATPase

15. A 43-year-old man with a strong family history of Parkinson's disease begins to develop the telltale sign of the disease, a pill-rolling tremor. He visits his neurologist who tells him about the new data that suggests that coenzyme Q may stall the development of the disease. This component of the ETC normally:

(A) receives electrons directly from NADH.
(B) receives electrons from complex IV.
(C) receives electrons from FMN.
(D) transports ATP to the cytoplasm.
(E) contains a heme group.

16. An 8-year-old boy is seen by an ophthalmologist for difficulties in seeing in all visual fields as well as slow eye movements. The ophthalmologist finds ophthalmoplegia and pigmentary retinopathy. She suspects the child has Kearns-Sayre syndrome. Assuming the defect is due to a mutation in complex II of the ETC, electron transfer from which substance would be impaired?

(A) Malate
(B) α-Ketoglutarate
(C) Isocitrate
(D) Succinate
(E) Pyruvate

17. A 6-year-old child has been suffering from muscle weakness that has progressively worsened over the past 6 months. Measurement of oxygen consumption with mitochondria isolated from a muscle biopsy revealed normal rates of succinate oxidation but very poor rates of pyruvate oxidation. Assays conducted on extracts of the mitochondria revealed normal malate dehydrogenase and pyruvate dehydrogenase activities. The patient may have a mutation in a mitochondrial gene encoding a subunit of:

(A) complex I.
(B) complex II.
(C) complex III.
(D) complex IV.
(E) ATP synthase.

18. A 58-year-old man develops progressive lower extremity weakness, confining him to a wheel chair. A neurologist performs a throughout workup, confirming the diagnosis of amyotrophic lateral sclerosis (ALS). The patient recalls that his father had similar symptoms and eventually died of respiratory failure. Some patients with the familial form of ALS have a defect in the enzyme that normally:

(A) catalyzes the conversion of peroxide to water and oxygen.
(B) catalyzes the conversion of superoxide to hydrogen peroxide and water.
(C) converts carbon tetrachloride to CCL_3·.
(D) regenerates oxidized cellular molecules.
(E) converts carbonic acid to carbon dioxide and water.

19. A 53-year-old woman is diagnosed with early-stage breast cancer. She elects to have a lumpectomy followed by radiation therapy because this regimen has been shown to be equivalent to mastectomy in such patients. Radiation works, in part, by:

(A) inhibiting NADH oxidase.
(B) inhibiting the cytochrome b-c_1 complex.
(C) generating reactive oxygen species.
(D) stimulating the production of glutathione.
(E) generating hypochlorous acid.

20. A 3-year-old boy presents with multiple bacterial infections due to catalase-positive organisms (i.e., *Staphylococcus aureus*). Subsequent lab studies show that he has chronic granulomatous disease (CGD). Which of the following characterizes the defect in this patient's neutrophils?

(A) A defect in NADPH oxidase
(B) A dysfunction in the myeloperoxidase-halide system
(C) Deficiency in the ability to produce ATP
(D) A defect in cytochrome oxidase
(E) Mutations in superoxide dismutase

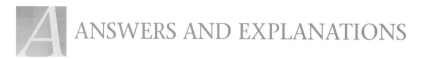

ANSWERS AND EXPLANATIONS

1–D. Cytochrome P450 is in the family of heme proteins termed mono-oxygenases that use O_2 for action on substrates. It is not an oxidase that transfers two electrons to oxygen. Whereas all oxygenases are in the broader class of enzymes that perform reduction-oxidation, it is coupled neither to proton pumping nor electron transport. Antimycin inhibits passage of electrons through the cytochrome b-c_1 complex.

2–D. Oligomycin binds to the stalk of the adenosine triphosphate (ATP) synthase, preventing the re-entry of protons into the mitochondrial matrix. It does not uncouple oxidation from phosphorylation like 2-4-dinitrophenol (DNP); it inhibits synthase, not NADH dehydrogenase (rotenone is an inhibitor); and does not interact with F1 ATPase or stimulate respiration with ADP.

3–E. There is an exchange transporter (not active transport) in the inner mitochondrial membrane (not outer) that imports adenosine diphosphate (ADP) in exchange for an adenosine triphosphate (ATP) exported from the matrix. Atractyloside inhibits ADP/ATP transport, and valinomycin is an ionophore allowing K^+ flow.

4–C. The associated members in the succinate dehydrogenase complex (complex II) are flavin adenine dinucleotides (FAD) (and iron-sulfur [Fe-S] proteins). Cytochromes b and c reside in complex III, with flavin mononucleotide (FMN) in complex I. Coenzyme Q accepts electrons from both FAD and FMN.

5–A. Energetically favorable reactions are "driven" ($\Delta G<0$) and do not require energy input; electrons flow from NADH (or $FADH_2$) toward O_2, and require neither ATP synthesis nor proton translocation. The specific inhibitors act upon parts of the path. Dinitrophenol (DNP), an ionophore, allows protons to circumvent ATP synthase and uncouples oxidation from phosphorylation, and oligomycin binds to the stalk of the ATP synthase, preventing proton re-entry to the mitochondrial matrix.

6–A. Catalase catalyzes hydrogen peroxide, $H_2O_2 \rightarrow H_2O + O_2$. Superoxide dismutase (SOD) catalyzes superoxide anion to $H_2O_2 + O_2$. O_2 is an end product. Dioxygenases do not convert peroxide to water; cytochrome P450 catalyzes electron transfer from NADPH to O_2; and peroxide is not a substrate, but an intermediate.

7–B. Succinate dehydrogenase mediating electron transfer from complex II is not coupled to the synthesis of ATP. The other sites along the ETC listed as choices are coupled to ATP synthesis.

8–E. The term "uncouplers" refers to the dissociation of oxidative phosphorylation (not *reduction*) from ATP synthesis, so respiration is uncontrolled, since there no limit by ADP or organic phosphorus (P_i). The most common uncoupler is 2-4-dinitrophenol (DNP). Atractyloside inhibits ATP/ADP transport, and phosphoenolpyruvate and phosphoglycerate are involved with glycolysis, with phosphoglycerate shuttling reducing equivalents through the mitochondrion.

9–A. See Figure 8-1 concerning the pathway of the ETC and oxidative phosphorylation.

10–B. Cytochrome b is an oxidant that is a one-electron acceptor and donor. All of the other choices are involved with two electrons being donated or accepted.

11–C. Dinitrophenol (DNP) uncouples the ATP synthase from the ETC by carrying protons from the cytosol back into the mitochondrial matrix without going through the ATP synthase pore. Dinitrophenol was actually used by thousands for weight loss until it was discontinued in 1938 after reports of poisoning and deaths. Rotenone inhibits the transfer of electrons from complex I to coenzyme Q. Amytal inhibits complex I of the ETC. Antimycin inhibits complex III, and finally, atractyloside inhibits the ATP-ADP antiport.

12–B. Mitochondria are responsible for both the tricarboxylic acid (TCA) cycle and the ETC. Therefore, diseases that compromise mitochondrial activity will result in energy production solely through glycolysis. This net energy production is 2 ATP and 2 NADH, which are unable to undergo further oxidation via the mitochondrial oxidative phosphorylation.

13–E. Patients with malignant hyperthermia experience uncoupling of oxidative phosphorylation at complex V (the F_0–F_1 ATPase) of the ETC. Rotenone inhibits the transfer of electrons from complex I to coenzyme Q. Complex III is inhibited by antimycin, and complex IV is inhibited by cyanide and carbon monoxide.

14–B. In addition to binding hemoglobin and impairing oxygen transport, carbon monoxide also terminates cellular respiration by inhibiting cytochrome oxidase. Amytal, a barbiturate, inhibits complex I of the ETC. The ATP-ADP antiport is inhibited by the plant toxin atractyloside. The F_0 component of the F_0–F_1 ATPase is inhibited by the drug oligomycin.

15–C. Coenzyme Q receives electrons directly from FMN. FMN receives electrons from NADH. Electrons from complex IV are transferred ultimately to oxygen. ATP is exchanged for ADP by the ATP-ADP antiport. Unlike the cytochromes, coenzyme Q does not contain a heme group.

16–D. Succinate feeds electrons into complex II, which, in this case, would be impaired. The other intermediates of the TCA, including malate, α-ketoglutarate, isocitrate, and pyruvate all feed their electrons via NADH through complex I.

17–A. NADH produced from glycolysis, pyruvate dehydrogenase complex, and the TCA cycle feeds into the ETC at complex I (NADH dehydrogenase) under aerobic conditions. If NADH accumulates due to a defect in the ETC, it will inhibit pyruvate oxidation and divert the substrate to be converted to lactate. The substrate succinate bypasses complex 1 and feeds its energy currency, $FADH_2$, into coenzyme Q.

18–B. Some patients with the familial form of ALS have mutations in the enzyme superoxide dismutase (SOD), which normally catalyzes the conversion of superoxide to hydrogen peroxide and water. Catalase, in turn, converts the hydrogen peroxide to water and oxygen. Carbon tetrachloride (CCl_4), used in the dry cleaning business, is converted to the hepatotoxic free radical CCL_3• by the cytochrome P450 system. Glutathione functions to regenerate oxidized cellular molecules, like hemoglobin. Carbonic anhydrase stimulates the conversion of carbonic acid to carbon dioxide and water.

19–C. Therapeutic radiation works by generating reactive oxygen species (ROS) that damage cellular DNA. Because cancer cells often have impaired abilities to correct such damage, there is a selective effect on such cells. NADH dehydrogenase is inhibited by rotenone. The cytochrome b-c_1 complex is inhibited by antimycin. Glutathione is an intracellular molecule that protects the cell against reactive oxygen species. Hypochlorous acid is produced by the enzyme myeloperoxidase.

20–A. A lab test known as the Nitroblue tetrazolium test is used to diagnose chronic granulomatous disease (CGD) because the neutrophils in such patients cannot produce superoxide anion due to a defect in NADPH oxidase. Immune defects in the myeloperoxidase-halide system are usually less severe. A defect in cytochrome oxidase can be found in some patients with Leigh's disease. Mutations in SODs affect the ability to break down superoxide and are found in familial forms of amyotrophic lateral sclerosis.

chapter 9

Glycogen Metabolism

I. Overview of Glycogen Structure and Metabolism (Figure 9-1)

A. **Glycogen,** the major storage form of carbohydrate in animals, consists of chains of α-1,4–linked D-glucose residues with branches that are attached by α-1,6 linkages (see Figure 9-2).

B. Glycogen is synthesized from glucose.

C. Glycogen degradation produces glucose 1-phosphate as the major product, but free glucose is also formed.

D. Liver glycogen is used to maintain blood glucose during fasting or exercise.

E. Muscle glycogen is used to generate adenosine triphosphate (ATP) for muscle contraction.

II. Glycogen Structure (Figure 9-2)

A. The **linkages** between glucose residues are α-**1,4** except at branch points, where the linkage is α-**1,6.** Branching is more frequent in the interior of the molecule and less frequent at the periphery, the average being an α-1,6 branch every 8 to 10 residues.

B. One glucose unit, located at the reducing end of each glycogen molecule, is attached to the protein **glycogenin.**

C. The glycogen molecule branches like a tree and has **many nonreducing ends** at which addition and release of glucose residues occur during synthesis and degradation, respectively.

III. Glycogen Synthesis

A. **Synthesis of UDP-glucose** (Figure 9-3)

1. Uridine diphosphate glucose (UDP-glucose) is the precursor for glycogen synthesis.
2. Glucose enters cells and is phosphorylated to glucose 6-phosphate by the enzyme **hexokinase** (or by **glucokinase** in the liver). ATP provides the phosphate group.

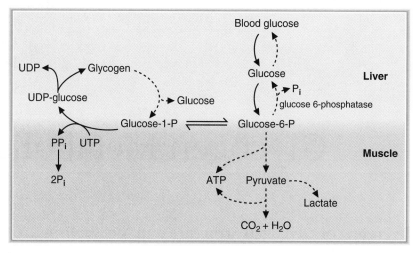

Figure 9-1 Overview of glycogen synthesis and degradation. *Solid arrows* = glycogen synthesis; *broken arrows* = glycogen degradation. ATP = adenosine triphosphate; P = phosphate; P_i = inorganic phosphate; PP_i = inorganic pyrophosphate; UDP = uridine diphosphate; UTP = uridine triphosphate.

3. **Phosphoglucomutase** converts glucose 6-phosphate to glucose 1-phosphate.
4. Glucose 1-phosphate reacts with uridine triphosphate (UTP), forming **UDP-glucose** in a reaction catalyzed by **UDP-glucose pyrophosphorylase.** Inorganic pyrophosphate (PP_i) is released in this reaction.
   a. PP_i is cleaved by a pyrophosphatase to 2 inorganic phosphates (P_i).
   b. This removal of product helps to drive the process in the direction of glycogen synthesis.

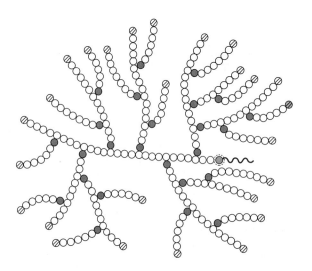

○ Glucose residue linked α-1,4   ◉〰 Reducing end attached to glycogenin

● Glucose residue linked α-1,6   ⊘ Nonreducing ends

Figure 9-2 The structure of glycogen.

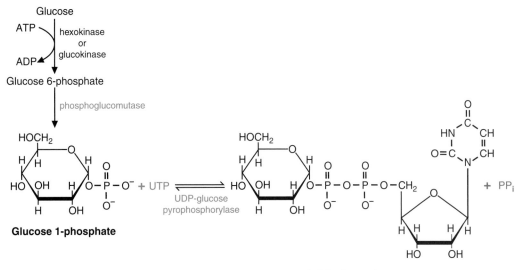

Figure 9-3   Formation of uridine diphosphate glucose (UDP-glucose) from glucose. ADP = adenosine diphosphate; ATP = adenosine triphosphate; PP_i = inorganic pyrophosphate.

B. Action of glycogen synthase (Figure 9-4A)

   1. **Glycogen synthase** is the key regulatory enzyme for glycogen synthesis. It trans-fers glucose residues from UDP-glucose to the nonreducing ends of a glycogen primer.
   2. UDP is released and reconverted to UTP by reaction with ATP.

> *cc* **9.1** Genetic deficiency of **glycogen synthase** is also known as a **type 0** glycogen storage disease (GSD). This inborn error in metabolism results in **fasting hypoglycemia** with **occasional muscle cramping.** It can usually be managed with frequent meals and feeding of uncooked cornstarch to **prevent overnight hypoglycemia.**

   3. The primers, which are attached to glycogenin, are glycogen molecules that were partially degraded in liver during fasting or in muscle and liver during exercise.

C. Formation of branches (see Figure 9-4A)

   1. When a chain contains 11 or more glucose residues, an **oligomer,** 6 to 8 residues in length, is removed from the nonreducing end of the chain. It is **reattached** via an α-1,6 **linkage** to a glucose residue within an α-1,4–linked chain.
   2. These branches are formed by the branching enzyme, a **glucosyl 4:6 transferase** that breaks an α-1,4 bond and forms an α-1,6 bond.
   3. The new branch points are at least 4 residues and an average of 7 to 11 residues from previously existing branch points.

> *cc* **9.2** **Andersen disease,** a **type IV** GSD, results from a genetic **deficiency of this branching enzyme.** Children **fail to thrive.** There is not an increased accumulation of glycogen, but rather, the **glycogen has very long outer branches.** This structural abnormality may trigger an immune response, causing progressive scarring of the liver (**cirrhosis**), which leads to death around age 5.

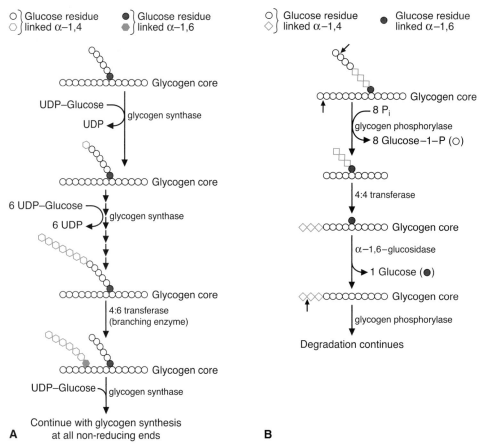

Figure 9-4 Glycogen synthesis (A) and degradation (B). UDP-glucose = uridine diphosphate glucose; P_i = inorganic phosphate.

D. Growth of glycogen chains

1. Glycogen synthase continues to add glucose residues to the **nonreducing ends** of newly formed branches as well as to the ends of the original chains.
2. As the chains continue to grow, additional branches are produced by the branching enzyme.

IV. Glycogen Degradation (see Figure 9-4B)

A. Action of glycogen phosphorylase

1. **Glycogen phosphorylase**—the key regulatory enzyme for glycogen degradation— removes glucose residues, one at a time, from the nonreducing ends of glycogen molecules.

> *cc* **9.3** A genetic deficiency of **liver phosphorylase** results in **Hers disease,** a type VI GSD. Because a complete deficiency of this enzyme would be fatal, patients typically have **partial deficiency of the protein.** As such, the disease can present with **extreme enlargement of the liver,** as a result of glycogen accumulation. However, some patients present with **only mild hypoglycemia** or no symptoms at all.

> *cc 9.4*   **Muscle phosphorylase deficiency, McArdle disease,** is a type V GSD.
> The disorder presents with **exercise-induced cramps and pain secondary
> to rhabdomyolysis.** Most patients live normally, avoiding strenuous exercise; however,
> severe rhabdomyolysis leading to **myoglobinuria** can lead to life-threatening **renal failure.**

2. Phosphorylase uses P_i to cleave α-1,4 bonds, producing **glucose 1-phosphate.**
3. Phosphorylase can act only when it is four glucose units from a branch point.

B. Removal of branches

1. The four units remaining at a branch are removed by the **debranching enzyme,**
   which has both glucosyl 4:4 transferase and α-1,6-glucosidase activity.
2. Three of the four glucose residues that remain at the branch point are removed
   as a trisaccharide and are attached to the nonreducing end of another chain by
   a **4:4 transferase,** which cleaves an α-1,4 bond and forms a new α-1,4 bond.
3. The last glucose unit at the branch point, which is linked α-1,6, is hydrolyzed by
   α-**1,6-glucosidase,** forming free glucose.

> *cc 9.5*   **Cori disease,** a type III GSD, results from a **deficiency of debranching
> enzyme.** Type IIIa is a deficiency of both liver and muscle enzymes and
> manifests with **hepatomegaly, hypoglycemia during fasting,** and **myopathy;** it is
> managed by **small meals** or continuous nasogastric feeding. The rarer type IIIb disease
> is a deficiency of the liver enzyme only, with no muscular involvement.

C. Degradation of glycogen chains

1. The **phosphorylase/debranching process is repeated,** generating glucose
   1-phosphate and free glucose in about a 10:1 ratio that reflects the length of the
   chains in the outer region of the glycogen molecule.

D. Fate of glucosyl units released from glycogen (see Figure 9-1)

1. In the **liver,** glycogen is degraded to **maintain blood glucose.**
   a. Glucose 1-phosphate is converted by **phosphoglucomutase** to glucose
      6-phosphate.
   b. Inorganic phosphate is released by **glucose 6-phosphatase,** and free glucose
      enters the blood. This enzyme also acts in gluconeogenesis.
2. In **muscle,** glycogen is degraded to provide **energy for contraction.**
   a. Phosphoglucomutase converts glucose 1-phosphate to glucose 6-phosphate,
      which enters the pathway of **glycolysis** and is converted either to lactate or
      to CO_2 and H_2O, generating ATP.
   b. Muscle does not contain glucose 6-phosphatase and, therefore, does not
      contribute to the maintenance of blood glucose.

V.   Lysosomal Degradation of Glycogen

A. Glycogen is degraded by an α-**glucosidase** located in lysosomes.

B. Lysosomal degradation is not necessary for maintaining normal blood glucose
levels.

> *cc 9.6* **Pompe disease,** a type II GSD, is a **lysosomal storage disease. Accumulation of glycogen within the lysosome** results in the formation of large lysosomes, which ultimately compromises muscle cellular function. Type IIa is the infantile form that presents with muscle weakness (**floppiness**), **with death by 2 years** secondary to **heart muscle dysfunction.** The milder IIb (juvenile) and IIc (adult) forms have delayed and progressive onset and are dominated by skeletal muscle weakness.

VI. Regulation of Glycogen Degradation (Figure 9-5)

A. **Glucagon,** a peptide hormone, acts on liver cells, and **epinephrine** (adrenaline) acts on both liver and muscle cells to stimulate glycogen degradation.

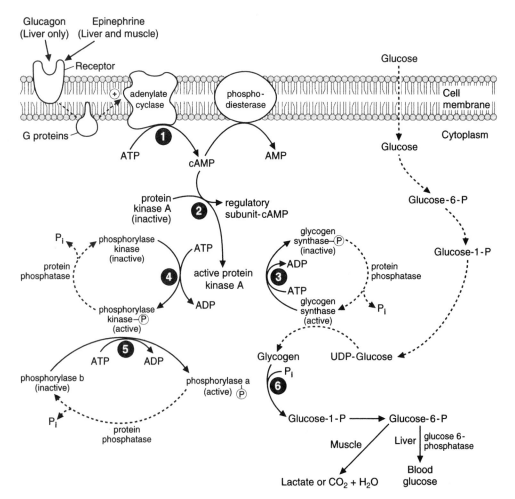

Figure 9-5 Hormonal regulation of glycogen synthesis and degradation. *Solid lines* indicate reactions that predominate when glucagon or epinephrine is elevated. Steps 1 through 6, indicated by *circled numbers,* correspond to VI A-F in the text. *Dashed lines* indicate reactions that predominate when insulin is elevated. Note that protein kinase A phosphorylates both phosphorylase kinase and glycogen synthase. ADP = adenosine diphosphate; ATP = adenosine triphosphate; cAMP = cyclic adenosine monophosphate; P_i = inorganic phosphate.

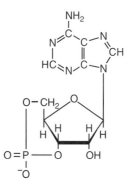

Figure 9-6   Cyclic adenosine monophosphate (cAMP).

    1. These hormones, via G proteins, activate **adenylate cyclase** in the cell membrane, which converts ATP to **3′,5′-cyclic adenosine monophosphate AMP** (cAMP) (Figure 9-6).

    2. Adenylate cyclase is also called adenyl or adenylyl cyclase. (Step 1)

B. cAMP **activates protein kinase A** (see Figure 9-5), which consists of two regulatory and two catalytic subunits. cAMP binds to the regulatory (inhibitory) subunits, releasing the catalytic subunits in an active form. (Step 2)

C. Protein kinase A phosphorylates **glycogen synthase**, causing it to be less active, thus decreasing glycogen synthesis. (Step 3)

D. Protein kinase A phosphorylates **phosphorylase kinase.** (Step 4)

E. Phosphorylase kinase phosphorylates **phosphorylase b**, converting it to its active form, phosphorylase a. (Step 5)

F. Phosphorylase a cleaves glucose residues from the nonreducing ends of glycogen chains, producing glucose 1-phosphate, which is oxidized or, in the liver, converted to blood glucose. (Step 6)

G. The cAMP cascade

    1. The cAMP-activated process is a cascade in which the initial **hormonal signal is amplified** many times.

    2. One hormone molecule, by activating the enzyme adenylate cyclase, produces many molecules of cAMP, which activate protein kinase A.

    3. One active protein kinase A molecule phosphorylates many phosphorylase kinase molecules, which convert many molecules of phosphorylase b to phosphorylase a.

    4. One molecule of phosphorylase a produces many molecules of glucose 1-phosphate from glycogen.

    5. The net result is that one hormone molecule can generate tens of thousands of molecules of glucose 1-phosphate, which form glucose 6-phosphate. Oxidation of glucose 6-phosphate generates hundreds of thousands of molecules of ATP.

H. Additional **regulatory mechanisms in muscle** (Figure 9-7)

    1. In addition to cAMP-mediated regulation, **adenosine monophosphate (AMP)** and **Ca²⁺** stimulate glycogen breakdown in muscle.

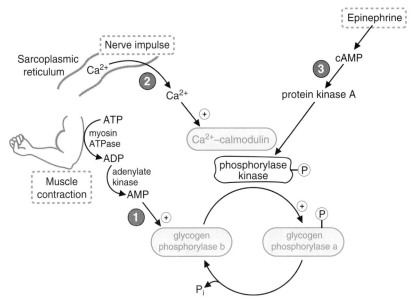

Figure 9-7 Activation of muscle glycogen phosphorylase during exercise. ADP = adenosine diphosphate; AMP = adenosine monophosphate; ATP = adenosine triphosphate; cAMP = cyclic AMP.

2. **Phosphorylase b** is activated by the rise in **AMP,** which occurs during muscle contraction by the following reactions:

contraction
$2\ ATP \rightarrow 2\ ADP + 2\ P_i$
adenylate kinase
(myokinase)
$2\ ADP \rightarrow AMP + ATP$
Sum: $ATP \rightarrow AMP + 2\ P_i$

3. **Phosphorylase kinase** is activated by **Ca²⁺,** which is released from the sarcoplasmic reticulum during muscle contraction.
4. Ca²⁺ binds to **calmodulin,** which serves as a subunit of phosphorylase kinase.

> **cc 9.7** Deficiency of **phosphorylase kinase** is a type IX GSD. It most commonly results in **hepatomegaly, growth retardation, delayed motor development,** and **increased blood lipids.** Phosphorylase kinase is a **complex enzyme,** and several subtypes have been identified. The most common form is the **X-linked form.**

VII. Regulation of Glycogen Synthesis (see Figure 9-5)

A. **Factors that promote glycogen synthesis in the liver**

1. **Insulin,** a pancreatic peptide hormone, is elevated after a meal and stimulates the synthesis of glycogen in liver and muscle.
2. In the **fed state,** glycogen degradation decreases because **glucagon** is **low,** and the cAMP cascade is not activated.
   a. cAMP is converted to AMP by a cell membrane **phosphodiesterase.**

      b. As **cAMP decreases**, the regulatory subunits rejoin the catalytic subunits of **protein kinase** A, and the enzyme is **inactivated**.

      c. **Dephosphorylation** of phosphorylase kinase and phosphorylase a causes these enzymes to be inactivated. **Insulin** causes activation of the **phosphatases** that dephosphorylate these enzymes.

  3. **Glycogen synthesis** is promoted by activation of **glycogen synthase** and by the increased concentration of glucose, which enters liver cells from the hepatic portal vein.

      a. The inactive, phosphorylated form of glycogen synthase is dephosphorylated, causing the enzyme to become active.

      b. **Insulin** causes activation of the **phosphatase** that catalyzes this reaction.

B. **Factors that promote glycogen synthesis in muscle**

  1. After a meal, muscle will have low levels of cAMP, AMP, and Ca^{2+} if it is not contracting and epinephrine is low. Consequently, muscle glycogen degradation will not occur.

  2. **Insulin stimulates glycogen synthesis** by mechanisms similar to those in the liver.

  3. In addition, **insulin stimulates the transport of glucose** into muscle cells, providing increased substrate for glycogen synthesis.

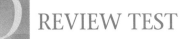

REVIEW TEST

*Directions: Each of the numbered questions or incomplete statements in this section is followed by answers or by completions of the statement. Select the **one** lettered answer or completion that is **best** in each case.*

1. Which enzyme is not present in muscle?

(A) Phosphorylase b
(B) Hexokinase
(C) Glucose 6-phosphatase
(D) Glycogen synthase
(E) Lactate dehydrogenase

2. Glycogenolysis is best described by which of the following statements?

(A) It involves enzymes cleaving β-1,4 and β-1,6 glycosidic bonds.
(B) It requires a dual-action enzyme with an α-1,6-glucosidase and a transferase.
(C) Its inefficiency can be due to Andersen disease.
(D) It requires activation of glycogen synthase.
(E) It uses adenosine triphosphate (ATP) to produce glucose 1-phosphate.

3. Glycogenesis from glucose 1-phosphate requires which of the following?

(A) Phosphoglucomutase
(B) Uridine triphosphate (UTP) glucose
(C) α-1,6-Glucosidase
(D) A glycogen primer
(E) Uridine diphosphate (UDP)

4. In glycogen, glucose residues form a straight chain via which of the following?

(A) α-1,4 linkages
(B) α-1,6 linkages
(C) α-1,4 linkages with glycogenin at the nonreducing end
(D) α-1,6 linkages with UDP-glucose at any end
(E) Straight linkages occur 3 residues apart

5. Finish the following sentence with the correct reaction: In the liver, epinephrine-induced glycogenolysis:

(A) requires UDP-glucose pyrophosphorylase.
(B) requires phosphoglucomutase.

(C) requires phosphorylase a inactivation.
(D) is inhibited by cyclic adenosine monophosphate (cAMP).
(E) acts upon both liver and muscle cells, similar to glucagon.

6. During the breakdown of glycogen, free glucose is formed from which of the following?

(A) Glucose residues in an α-1,4-glycosidic linkage
(B) The reducing end
(C) The nonreducing end
(D) Glucose residues in an α-1,6-glycosidic linkage
(E) Hydrolysis of glucose 1-phosphate

7. Glycogen catabolism is best described by which of the following statements?

(A) In the brain, it yields glucose for skeletal muscle consumption.
(B) It requires a debranching enzyme in mature erythrocytes.
(C) It is not a major pathway in the brain.
(D) It uses phosphorylase a for glucose residue cleavage from the reducing end of glycogen in liver.
(E) It is stimulated by insulin in liver.

8. Which of the following statements explains the synthesis of glycogen *directly* from D-glucose?

(A) It does not use glucose 1-phosphate.
(B) It requires a debranching enzyme.
(C) It occurs in the erythrocyte.
(D) It requires UDP-glucose.
(E) It requires a glucosyl transferase.

9. The degradation of glycogen normally produces which of the following?

(A) More glucose than glucose 1-phosphate
(B) More glucose 1-phosphate than glucose
(C) Equal amounts of glucose and glucose 1-phosphate

(D) Neither glucose nor glucose 1-phosphate

(E) Only glucose 1-phosphate

10. Which of the following statements about liver phosphorylase kinase is most accurate?

(A) It is present in an inactive form when epinephrine is elevated.

(B) It phosphorylates phosphorylase to an inactive form.

(C) It catalyzes a reaction that requires ATP.

(D) It is phosphorylated in response to elevated insulin.

(E) It is not affected by cAMP.

11. A newborn is found to have fasting hypoglycemia. The nursery staff begins overnight feeds by nasogastric tube because they find that the child has consistently low blood sugars. A liver biopsy and molecular studies demonstrate an absence of glycogen synthetase. The normal function of this enzyme is to do which of the following?

(A) Remove glucose residues one at a time from glycogen in the liver

(B) Remove glucose residues one at a time from glycogen in muscles

(C) Transfer UDP-glucose to the nonreducing end of a glycogen primer

(D) Hydrolyze α-1,6 bonds of glycogen

(E) Function as a glucosyl 4:6 transferase

12. A 3-year-old child presents to the pediatrician for failure to thrive. A workup including an ultrasound of his liver shows cirrhosis. A biopsy of the liver demonstrates a deficiency of an enzyme involved in glycogen synthesis. Which of the following is the most likely glycogen storage disease (GSD) that affects this child?

(A) Type I: von Gierke disease

(B) Type II: Pompe disease

(C) Type III: Cori disease

(D) Type IV: Andersen disease

(E) Type V: McArdle disease

13. A newborn is experiencing failure to thrive. On physical exam, organomegaly is appreciated due to accumulation of glycogen in the lysosomes of several organs, including the heart, muscle, and liver. You diagnose the patient with Pompe disease. Which of the following biochemical deficits are seen in this disorder?

(A) Glycogenin deficiency

(B) An α-1,6-glucosidase deficiency

(C) A glucose 6-phosphatase deficiency

(D) A glycogen phosphorylase enzyme deficiency

(E) A lysosomal glucosidase deficiency

14. A second-year medical student decides to do research in a nutrition laboratory that is studying the effects of caffeine on cellular metabolism. Caffeine inhibits cAMP phosphodiesterase. If caffeine is added to cells, which of the following enzymes would be phosphorylated and inactivated in the liver?

(A) Phosphorylase kinase

(B) Pyruvate kinase

(C) Phosphorylase

(D) Protein kinase A

(E) Calmodulin

15. A 28-year-old professional cyclist has been training for an opportunity to race in the Tour de France. His coach strongly suggests the intake of carbohydrates after his workouts to ensure a muscle glycogen storage that can endure the 28-day race. The activity of muscle glycogen synthase in resting muscles is increased by the action of which of the following?

(A) Epinephrine

(B) Glucagon

(C) Insulin

(D) Phosphorylation

(E) Fasting and starvation

16. An infant was brought into the emergency room after her parents witnessed her having a seizure. The child's blood glucose was 28 mmol/L. After a thorough workup, a GSD is suspected, and a muscle biopsy is significant for the accumulation of dextrin, a form of glycogen with branching limited to only a few glucose molecules. Which of the following GSDs is most likely the cause of the hypoglycemia and subsequent seizure?

(A) Type I: von Gierke disease

(B) Type II: Pompe disease

(C) Type III: Cori disease
(D) Type IV: Andersen disease
(E) Type V: McArdle disease

17. A patient had large deposits of liver glycogen, which, after an overnight fast, had shorter than normal branches. This abnormality could be caused by a defective form of:

(A) Glycogen phosphorylase.
(B) Glucagon receptor.
(C) Glycogenin.
(D) Amylo-1,6-glucosidase (α-glucosidase).
(E) Amylo-4,6-transferase (4:6 transferase).

18. A marathon runner is trying to optimize his performance. He has calculated that, even under anaerobic conditions, his glycogen stores will supply him with enough energy to last the race. What would the energy difference be between using glucose from a dietary source versus relying solely on glycogen stores?

(A) Dietary would give 1 more ATP/glucose.
(B) Dietary would give 2 more ATP/glucose.
(C) Dietary would give the same ATP/glucose.
(D) Dietary would give 1 less ATP/glucose.
(E) Dietary would give 2 less ATP/glucose.

19. A 24-year-old student is training for the track and field events at her college. She presents to her physician with complaints of severe muscle cramps and weakness when training. Muscle biopsy demonstrates glycogen accumulation, but liver biopsy is unremarkable. Which of the following is the most likely diagnosis?

(A) Andersen disease
(B) Cori disease
(C) McArdle disease
(D) von Gierke disease
(E) Hers disease

20. A 32-year-old woman receives anesthesia in preparation for a laparoscopic cholecystectomy. The anesthesiologist notices a subtle twitch of the masseter muscle in the jaw, followed by sinus tachycardia and an increase of the end-expiratory CO_2. He immediately recognizes the early signs of malignant hyperthermia and administers dantrolene. Dantrolene is a muscle relaxant that acts specifically on skeletal muscle by interfering with the release of calcium from the sarcoplasmic reticulum. Which of the following enzymes would be affected by this action?

(A) Phosphoglucomutase
(B) Glucokinase
(C) Glycogen synthase
(D) Glycogen phosphorylase kinase
(E) Glucosyl transferase

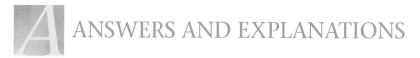

ANSWERS AND EXPLANATIONS

1–C. Glucose 6-phosphatase is not present in muscle and does not contribute to blood glucose. Phosphorylase b and glycogen synthase—part of the degradation cascade—are in muscle. Hexokinase (which converts liver glycogen to blood glucose) and lactate dehydrogenase (which converts pyruvate to lactate) are in muscle.

2–C. Glycogenolysis or glycogen degradation requires debranching enzyme. The last 4 units are removed by a dual-action enzyme with an α-1,6-glycosidase and a transferase. Glycogen synthase is involved in synthesis. Enzymes are required to degrade α-1,4 and α-1,6 bonds, NOT β bonds. Andersen disease (type IV) is a branching enzyme deficiency. Inorganic phosphate (P_i) cleaving α-1,4 bonds produces glucose 1-phosphate.

3–D. Glycogenesis from glucose 1-phosphate requires a primer. Uridine diphosphate (UDP)-glucose is the precursor (neither UDP nor uridine triphosphate [UTP] glucose). Both phosphoglucomutase and α-1,6-glucosidase are involved in glycogen degradation.

4–A. Glucose residues bound by α-1,4 form a straight chain. And α-1,6–bound residues form glycogen branch points with branch points occurring an average of every 8 to 10 residues. A glucose unit, located at the reducing end of each glycogen molecule, is attached to glycogenin. Glucose residues are transferred from UDP-glucose to the nonreducing ends of glycogen.

5–B. In the liver, epinephrine-induced glycogenolysis requires phosphoglucomutase and is activated by cyclic adenosine monophosphate (cAMP) produced from activated adenyl cyclase. UDP-glucose pyrophosphorylase is required for glycogen synthesis, not degradation. Phosphorylase a activation is required. Whereas epinephrine acts on both liver and muscle cells to stimulate glycogen degradation, glucagon has this capacity *only* in liver.

6–A. During glycogenolysis, free glucose is produced by glucose residues in an α-1, 4-glycosidic linkage, not from α-1,6 linkages. Free glucose is not siphoned off of the ends (reducing or nonreducing) of chains. Glucose 1-phosphate is not a source for glucose 1-phosphatase.

7–C. Glycogen catabolism is not a major pathway in the brain (A is incorrect), and it is not a major pathway in erythrocytes (choice B). It is a major pathway in liver and muscle. Phosphorylase a is used for glucose residue cleavage from the nonreducing end of glycogen. Glycogen synthesis is stimulated by insulin in liver and muscle.

8–D. UDP-glucose is the precursor for glycogen synthesis. Glucose is converted to glucose 6-phosphate, then to glucose 1-phosphate, then to UDP-glucose. Erythrocytes do not store glycogen, and debranching and glucosyl transferase enzymes are involved in glycogen branching after a primer is formed and degraded, respectively.

9–B. Phosphorylase produces glucose 1-phosphate from glucose residues linked by α-1,4. Free glucose is produced from α-1,6–linked residues at branch points by an α-1,6-glucosidase. Degradation of glycogen produces glucose 1-phosphate and glucose in about a 10:1 ratio.

10–C. Glucagon in the liver and epinephrine in both the liver and muscle cause cAMP levels to rise, activating protein kinase A. Protein kinase A phosphorylates and activates phosphorylase kinase, which in turn phosphorylates and activates phosphorylase. These phosphorylation reactions require adenosine triphosphate (ATP).

11–C. Glycogen synthase is the first enzyme in the synthesis of glycogen. It transfers UDP-glucose to the nonreducing end of a glycogen primer and adds subsequent residues to the growing chain. The removal of glucose residues during the catabolism of glycogen is mediated by glycogen phosphorylase, a deficiency of which results in Hers disease if in the liver and McArdle disease if in muscle. Debranching enzyme hydrolyzes α-1,6 bonds of glycogen. Finally, deficiency of glucosyl 4:6 transferase results in Andersen disease.

12–D. Andersen disease (type IV glycogen storage disease [GSD]) results from a deficiency of amylo-4,6-glucosidase. This enzyme is responsible for forming branches in glycogen. The other answer choices are all deficiencies in enzymes responsible for the degradation of glycogen: for example, glucose 6-phosphatase deficiency in von Gierke disease; maltase deficiency in Pompe disease; glycogen debrancher deficiency in Cori disease; and as discussed in the previous question, muscle glycogen phosphorylase deficiency in McArdle disease.

13–E. Pompe disease results from a deficiency of α-1,4-glucosidase, halting the release of glucose from its glycogen storage in lysosomes. A very confusing relationship is that McArdle syndrome is caused by the enzyme glycogen phosphorylase, which also cleaves the same α-1,4-glycosidic bond but, instead, presents with muscle symptoms, such as weakness and cramps. Glycogenin initiates glycogen synthesis, and therefore, a deficiency would result in a decrease in glycogen storage. An α-1,6-glucosidase deficiency results in the inability to liberate the 1,6 branch points of glycogen as seen in Cori disease. Glucose 6-phosphatase deficiency, or von Gierke disease, results in hypoglycemia, hepatomegaly, hyperlipidemia, hyperuricemia, gouty arthritis, nephrolithiasis, and chronic renal failure

14–B. Under these conditions, cAMP levels would remain elevated. Phosphorylation of pyruvate kinase causes its inactivation. Phosphorylase kinase and phosphorylase are activated by phosphorylation. Protein kinase A is not regulated by phosphorylation but by dissociation of inhibitory subunits that bind to cAMP. Calmodulin is a calcium-binding protein that serves as a subunit of phosphorylase kinase.

15–C. Glycogen synthesis occurs at times of rest and when the energy needs of the cells are being met. Of the hormones influencing the storage of glucose, insulin promotes the synthesis of energy stores through the dephosporylation and activation of glycogen synthase. In fact, a helpful generalization is that glucagon typically mobilizes energy stores through the activation of enzymes via a direct phosphorylation, while epinephrine and insulin accomplish the contrary.

16–C. Of the GSDs, the presence of limit dextrin is unique to Cori disease. Hypoglycemic seizures may occur in the first decade of life. Long-term morbidity arises from hepatic disease and progressive muscle weakness. von Gierke disease, a deficiency of glucose 6-phosphatase, and Pompe disease, a deficiency of acid α-glucosidase, both result in excessive glycogen with normal structure and cardiomyopathy. McArdle disease also results in excessive glycogen with normal structure, but the deficient muscle phosphorylase results in symptoms of muscle cramps and myoglobinuria. Andersen disease results from the deficiency of the branching enzyme, transglucosidase, which is found in all tissue.

Due to abnormal glycogen, hepatic deposition may occur and result in severe cirrhosis, hepatic failure, or neuromuscular failure. It also can present as abnormal liver function tests in its mildest presentation.

17–D. If, after fasting, the branches were shorter than normal, phosphorylase must be functional and capable of being activated by glucagon. The branching enzyme (the 4:6 transferase) must be normal because branches are present. The protein glycogenin must be present in order for large amounts of glycogen to be synthesized and deposited. The defect has to be in the debranching enzyme (which contains an α-1,6-glucosidase). If the debrancher is defective, phosphorylase would break the glycogen down to the branch points, but complete degradation would not occur. Therefore, short branches would be present in the glycogen. If the short branches contain only one glucose unit, the defect is in the α-1,6-glucosidase activity of the debrancher. If they contain four glucose units, the defect is in the 4:4 transferase activity of the debrancher.

18–C. There are two points that must be taken into account for this question: energy of absorption and the energy cost for the degradation of glycogen. Under a condition such as drinking a high-energy drink, the glucose will be absorbed via facilitated diffusion at no energy cost. The degradation of glycogen, however, requires that the terminal glucose be converted to glucose 1-phosphate at the cost of 1 ATP/glucose.

19–C. McArdle disease (type V GSD) is due to a defect specific to muscle phosphorylase, with normal liver phosphorylase. A presentation involving muscle failure during demands such as exercise is typical. Many affected individuals also experience myoglobinuria due to rhabdomyolysis. A rhabdomyolysis with spillage of myoglobin into the bloodstream can result in serious renal damage. The diagnosis can be made by observing gross blood in the urine, but lacking red blood cells on microscopic examination. Andersen disease primarily affects the liver and skeletal muscle. Cori disease is a deficiency of debranching enzyme. Lastly, von Gierke and Hers diseases primarily target the liver.

20–D. Glycogen regulation in skeletal muscle versus the liver is matched well to the functions of the muscle and liver. Muscle glycogen functions as a storage for mechanical energy needs, whereas liver glycogen functions to maintain blood glucose levels. With regard to regulation, when a motor neuron stimulates the release of calcium from the sarcoplasmic reticulum, the calcium binds to calmodulin and activates phosphorylase kinase, which in turn activates glycogen phosphorylase. Glucokinase (in the liver) converts glucose to glucose 6-phosphate. Phosphoglucomutase converts glucose 6-phosphate to glucose 1-phosphate. Glycogen synthase is activated via phosphorylation. Finally, glucosyl transferase is a debranching enzyme that removes the branches of glycogen to allow glycogen synthase to elongate the newly formed branch.

CHAPTER 10

Gluconeogenesis and the Maintenance of Blood Glucose Levels

I.   Overview (Figure 10-1)

A.   Gluconeogenesis, which **occurs mainly in the liver** and to a small degree in the kidney, is the synthesis of glucose from compounds that are not carbohydrates.

B.   The major precursors for gluconeogenesis are **lactate, amino acids** (which form pyruvate or tricarboxylic acid [TCA] cycle intermediates), and **glycerol** (which forms dihydroxyacetone phosphate [DHAP]). Even-chain fatty acids do not produce any net glucose.

C.   Gluconeogenesis involves several enzymatic steps that do not occur in glycolysis; thus, glucose is **not generated by a simple reversal of glycolysis.**

D.   The synthesis of 1 mole of glucose from 2 moles of pyruvate requires the energy equivalent of about 6 moles of adenosine triphosphate (ATP).

E.   Blood glucose levels are maintained within a very narrow range, even though the nature of a person's diet may vary widely and the normal person eats periodically during the day and fasts between meals and at night. Even under circumstances when a person does not eat for extended periods of time, blood glucose levels decrease only slowly.

F.   The major hormones that regulate blood glucose are **insulin** and **glucagon.**

G.   After a meal, blood glucose is supplied by dietary carbohydrate. However, during fasting, the liver maintains blood glucose levels by the processes of glycogenolysis and gluconeogenesis.

H.   All cells use glucose for energy; however, the production of glucose during fasting is particularly important for tissues such as the brain and red blood cells.

I.   During exercise, blood glucose is also maintained by liver glycogenolysis and gluco-neogenesis.

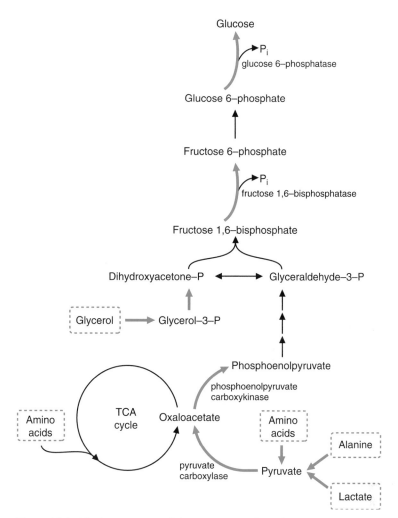

Figure 10-1 The key reactions of gluconeogenesis from the precursors alanine, lactate, and glycerol. *Heavy arrows* indicate steps that differ from those of glycolysis. *Broken arrows* are reactions that are inhibited under conditions in which gluconeogenesis is occurring. P_i = inorganic phosphate.

II. Reactions of Gluconeogenesis

A. Conversion of pyruvate to phosphoenolpyruvate (Figure 10-2)

1. In the liver, pyruvate is converted to phosphoenolpyruvate (PEP).
2. **Pyruvate** (produced from lactate, alanine, and other amino acids) (Step 1) is first converted to oxaloacetate (OAA) (Step 2) by **pyruvate carboxylase**, a mitochondrial enzyme that requires biotin and ATP.
    a. OAA cannot directly cross the inner mitochondrial membrane.
    b. Therefore, it is converted to malate (Step 3) or to aspartate, which can cross the mitochondrial membrane and be reconverted to OAA in the cytosol.
3. **OAA** is decarboxylated by **phosphoenolpyruvate carboxykinase (PEPCK)** to form PEP. (Step 4) This reaction requires guanosine triphosphate (GTP).
4. **PEP** is converted to fructose 1,6-bisphosphate by reversal of the glycolytic reactions (see Figure 10-3).

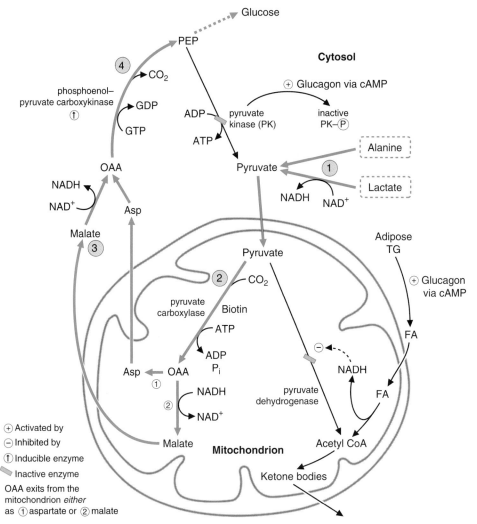

Figure 10-2 The conversion of pyruvate to phosphoenolpyruvate (PEP). Follow the diagram by starting with the precursors alanine and lactate (on the right). Asp = aspartate; ATP = adenosine triphosphate; cAMP = cyclic adenosine monophosphate; FA = fatty acid; GDP = guanosine diphosphate; GTP = guanosine triphosphate; OAA = oxaloacetate; P_i = inorganic phosphate; TG = triacylglycerol.

B. Conversion of fructose 1,6-bisphosphate to fructose 6-phosphate (Figure 10-3)

1. **Fructose 1,6-bisphosphate** is converted to fructose 6-phosphate in a reaction that releases inorganic phosphate and is catalyzed by **fructose 1,6-bisphosphatase**.
2. Fructose 6-phosphate is converted to glucose 6-phosphate by the same isomerase used in glycolysis.

C. Conversion of glucose 6-phosphate to glucose

1. **Glucose 6-phosphate** releases inorganic phosphate (P_i), which produces free glucose that enters the blood. The enzyme is **glucose 6-phosphatase**.
2. **Glucose 6-phosphatase** is involved both in **gluconeogenesis and glycogenolysis** (see Figure 9-5).

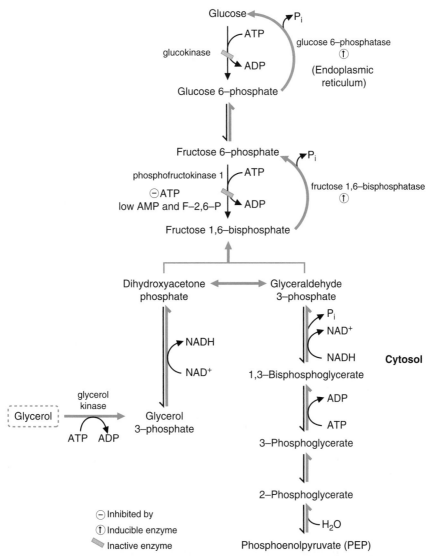

Figure 10-3   The conversion of phosphoenolpyruvate and glycerol to glucose. *Heavy arrows* indicate the pathway. F-2,6-P = fructose 2,6-bisphosphate.; ADP = adenosine diphosphate; AMP = adenosine monophosphate; ATP = adenosine triphosphate; P_i = inorganic phosphate.

> *cc* **10.1**   Deficiency of **glucose 6-phosphatase, von Gierke disease,** is a type I glycogen storage disease (GSD). Failure to convert glucose 6-phosphate to glucose results in intracellular accumulation of glucose 6-phosphate and **severe hypoglycemia** that can cause **lethargy, seizures,** and **brain damage.** Patients often have **hepatomegaly,** increased bleeding (due to platelet dysfunction), and **growth retardation. Frequent meals** and nighttime nasogastric feedings help control the disease.

D. **Regulatory enzymes of gluconeogenesis**

1. Under fasting conditions, **glucagon** is elevated and stimulates gluconeogenesis.
   a. Because of changes in the activity of certain enzymes, futile cycles are prevented from occurring, and the overall flow of carbon is from pyruvate to glucose (see Figures 10-2 and 10-3).

   b. A futile cycle is the continuous recycling of substrates and products with the net consumption of energy and no useful result.
2. *Pyruvate dehydrogenase (PDH)* (see Figure 10-2)
   a. Decreased insulin and increased glucagon stimulate the **release of fatty acids** from adipose tissue.
   b. **Fatty acids** travel to the liver and **are oxidized**, producing acetyl coenzyme A (CoA), NADH, and ATP, which cause inactivation of PDH.
   c. Because **PDH** is relatively **inactive**, pyruvate is converted to OAA, not to acetyl CoA.
   d. See the Clinical Correlation on pyruvate dehydrogenase complex deficiency in Chapter 7 (cc 7.3).
3. *Pyruvate carboxylase*
   a. Pyruvate carboxylase, which converts pyruvate to OAA, is **activated by acetyl CoA.**
   b. Note that pyruvate carboxylase is active in both the fed and fasting states.
   c. See the Clinical Correlation on pyruvate carboxylase deficiency in Chapter 7 (cc 7.6).
4. *Phosphoenolpyruvate carboxykinase (PEPCK)*
   a. PEPCK is an **inducible** enzyme.
   b. **Transcription** of the gene encoding PEPCK is stimulated by binding of proteins that are phosphorylated in response to cyclic adenosine monophosphate (cAMP) and by binding of glucocorticoid–protein complexes to regulatory elements in the gene.
   c. Increased production of PEPCK messenger RNA (mRNA) leads to increased translation, resulting in higher PEPCK levels in the cell.

> *cc 10.2* **PEPCK deficiency** is a rare but severe metabolic defect. Absence of the cytosolic form of the enzyme results in severe **cerebral atrophy,** optic atrophy, **fatty infiltration** of the liver and kidney, and **intractable hypoglycemia.**

5. *Pyruvate kinase (PK)*
   a. **Glucagon**, via cAMP and protein kinase A, causes PK to be phosphorylated and **inactivated.**
   b. Because PK is relatively inactive, PEP formed from OAA is not reconverted to pyruvate but, in a series of steps, forms fructose 1,6-bisphosphate, which is converted to fructose 6-phosphate.
   c. See the Clinical Correlation on PK deficiency in Chapter 6 (cc 6.9).
6. *Phosphofructokinase 1* (see Figure 10-3)
   a. Phosphofructokinase 1 is relatively **inactive** because the concentrations of its activators, adenosine monophosphate (AMP) and fructose 2,6-bisphosphate, are low and its inhibitor, ATP, is relatively high.
   b. See Clinical Correlation for phosphofructokinase deficiency in Chapter 6 (cc 6.8).
7. *Fructose 1,6-bisphosphatase (F-1,6-BP)*
   a. The level of **fructose 2,6-bisphosphate**, an inhibitor of F-1,6-BP, is **low** during fasting. Therefore, F-1,6-BP is **more active.**
   b. F-1,6-BP is also **induced** in the fasting state.

> *cc 10.3* **Deficiency of F-1,6-BP** commonly presents as **neonatal hypoglycemia,** along with **acidosis,** irritability, tachycardia, dyspnea, **hypotonia,** and **moderate hepatomegaly.** This deficiency is typically only of the liver enzyme, and the **muscular F-1,6-BP activity is normal.**

8. *Glucokinase*
   a. **Glucokinase** is relatively **inactive** because it has a **high K_m** for glucose, and under conditions that favor gluconeogenesis, the glucose concentration is low. Therefore, free glucose is not reconverted to glucose 6-phosphate.
   b. See the Clinical Correlation on maturity-onset diabetes of the young (MODY) in Chapter 6 (cc 6.7).

E. Precursors for gluconeogenesis

1. Lactate, amino acids, and glycerol are the major precursors for gluconeogenesis in humans.
2. **Lactate** is oxidized by NAD^+ in a reaction catalyzed by **lactate dehydrogenase** to form pyruvate, which can be converted to glucose (see Figure 10-2). Sources of lactate include red blood cells and exercising muscle.

> *cc* **10.4** Genetic **deficiency of lactate dehydrogenase** has been described. These patients present with **muscle cramping** and **myoglobinuria after intense exercise.**

3. **Amino acids** for gluconeogenesis come from degradation of muscle protein.
   a. Amino acids are released directly into the blood from muscle, or carbons from amino acids are converted to alanine and glutamine and released.
      (1) **Alanine** is also formed by transamination of pyruvate that is derived by oxidation of glucose.
      (2) **Glutamine** is converted to alanine by tissues such as gut and kidney.
   b. Amino acids travel to the liver and provide carbon for gluconeogenesis. Quantitatively, **alanine is the major gluconeogenic amino acid.**
   c. Amino acid **nitrogen** is converted to **urea.**
4. **Glycerol,** which is derived from **adipose** triacylglycerols, reacts with ATP to form glycerol-3-phosphate, which is oxidized to DHAP and converted to glucose (see Figure 10-3).

F. Role of fatty acids in gluconeogenesis

1. *Even-chain fatty acids*
   a. Fatty acids are oxidized to acetyl CoA, which enter the TCA cycle.
   b. For every 2 carbons of acetyl CoA that enter the TCA cycle, 2 carbons are released as CO_2. Therefore, there is **no net synthesis of glucose from acetyl CoA.**
   c. The **PDH** reaction is irreversible, thus acetyl CoA cannot be converted to pyruvate.
   d. Although even-chain fatty acids do not provide carbons for gluconeogenesis, β-oxidation of fatty acids provides **ATP** that drives gluconeogenesis.
2. *Odd-chain fatty acids*
   a. The three carbons at the ω-end of an odd-chain fatty acid are converted to propionate.
   b. **Propionate** enters the TCA cycle as succinyl CoA, which forms **malate,** an intermediate in glucose formation (see Figure 10-2).

G. Energy requirements for gluconeogenesis

1. *From pyruvate* (see Figures 10-2 and 10-3)
   a. Conversion of pyruvate to OAA by **pyruvate carboxylase** requires 1 ATP.
   b. Conversion of OAA to PEP by phosphoenolpyruvate carboxykinase requires 1 GTP (the equivalent of 1 ATP).

      c. Conversion of 3-phosphoglycerate to 1,3-bisphosphoglycerate by **phosphoglycerate kinase** requires 1 ATP.

      d. Since 2 moles of pyruvate are required to form 1 mole of glucose, **6 moles of high-energy phosphate are required for synthesis of 1 mole of glucose.**

  2. *From glycerol*

      a. Glycerol enters the gluconeogenic pathway at the DHAP level.

      b. Conversion of glycerol to glycerol-3-phosphate, which is oxidized to DHAP, requires 1 ATP.

      c. Because 2 moles of glycerol are required to form 1 mole of glucose, 2 moles of high-energy phosphate are required for synthesis of 1 mole of glucose.

III.   Maintenance of Blood Glucose Levels

A. Blood glucose levels in the fed state

  1. *Changes in insulin and glucagon levels* (Figure 10-4)

      a. Blood insulin levels increase as a meal is digested, following the rise in blood glucose.

> *cc 10.5*   **Decreased production of insulin,** which is usually caused by autoimmune destruction of pancreatic β-cells, results in **type 1** (formerly called insulin-dependent) diabetes mellitus. Type 1 diabetes is characterized by **hyperglycemia,** the result of decreased uptake of glucose by cells and increased output of glucose by the liver (due to low insulin and high glucagon levels in the blood). These patients are dependent on exogenous insulin to survive.

> *cc 10.6*   **Decreased release of insulin** from the pancreas or **decreased sensitivity** of tissues to insulin (insulin resistance) results in **type 2** (formerly called non–insulin-dependent) **diabetes mellitus.** This condition also is characterized by **hyperglycemia.**

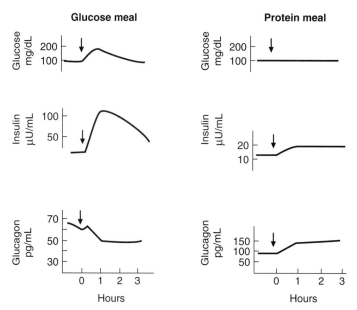

Figure 10-4   Changes in blood glucose, insulin, and glucagon levels in response to a glucose or protein meal.

(1) Glucose enters the **pancreatic β-cells** via the insulin-independent glucose transporter, GLUT-2, which stimulates release of preformed insulin and promotes the synthesis of new insulin.

(2) Additionally, amino acids (particularly **arginine** and **leucine**) cause the release of preformed insulin from β-cells of the pancreas.

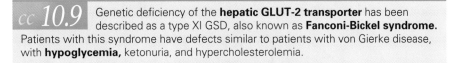

cc **10.7** One group of drugs used in the **management of type 2 diabetes mellitus** is known as the **sulfonylureas.** These drugs **stimulate the release of preformed insulin** from the pancreatic islets cells to decrease serum glucose concentrations, thereby preventing hyperglycemia.

b. Blood glucagon levels change depending on the content of the meal.
  (1) **A high-carbohydrate meal causes glucagon levels to decrease.**
  (2) **A high-protein meal causes glucagon to increase** (see Figure 10-4).
  (3) On a normal mixed diet, glucagon will remain relatively constant after a meal, while insulin increases.

cc **10.8** Tumors of the α-cells of the pancreas, the source of glucagons, are known as **glucagonomas.** As a result of increased levels of circulating glucagons, patients present with mild diabetes, characteristic skin lesions, and anemia.

2. *Fate of dietary glucose in the liver*
  a. Glucose enters the hepatocyte via the insulin-independent **GLUT-2 transporter.**

cc **10.9** Genetic deficiency of the **hepatic GLUT-2 transporter** has been described as a type XI GSD, also known as **Fanconi-Bickel syndrome.** Patients with this syndrome have defects similar to patients with von Gierke disease, with **hypoglycemia,** ketonuria, and hypercholesterolemia.

  b. Glucose is **oxidized** for energy. Excess glucose is converted to **glycogen** and to the **triacylglycerols** of **very low–density lipoprotein (VLDL).**
  c. The enzyme **glucokinase** has a **high K_m** for glucose (about 6 mM), thus its velocity increases after a meal when glucose levels are elevated. On a high-carbohydrate diet, glucokinase is **induced.**
  d. Glycogen synthesis is promoted by insulin, which stimulates the phosphatase that dephosphorylates and activates glycogen synthase.
  e. Synthesis of triacylglycerols is also stimulated. The triacylglycerols are converted to VLDLs and released into the blood.
3. *Fate of dietary glucose in peripheral tissues*
  a. All cells oxidize glucose for energy.
  b. Insulin stimulates the **transport** of glucose into **adipose** and **muscle** cells.

cc **10.10** Another class of agents used in the **treatment of type 2 diabetes** is known as the **thiazolidinediones,** of which rosiglitazone and pioglitazone are examples. These drugs induce genes that **increase the cells' responsiveness to circulating insulin.**

  c. In **muscle,** insulin stimulates the synthesis of **glycogen.**
  d. Adipose cells convert glucose to the **glycerol** moiety for synthesis of triacylglycerols.
4. *Return of blood glucose to fasting levels*
  a. The **uptake of dietary glucose** by tissues (particularly liver, adipose, and muscle) causes blood glucose to decrease.

b. **By 2 hours after a meal**, blood glucose has returned to the fasting level of 5 mM or 80 to 100 mg/dL.

> cc *10.11* The **oral glucose tolerance test** is one test used to diagnose diabetes. Patients drink a liquid containing 75 g of glucose dissolved in water. **After 2 hours,** the serum glucose is measured. A blood glucose of **<139 mg/dL is normal,** whereas a level of **140 to 199 mg/dL represents "pre-diabetes"** or impaired glucose tolerance. A serum level of **>200 mg/dL is indicative of diabetes.**

B. **Blood glucose levels in the fasting state** (Figure 10-5)

1. *Changes in insulin and glucagon levels*
    a. During fasting, insulin levels decrease, and glucagon levels increase.
    b. These hormonal changes promote **glycogenolysis** and **gluconeogenesis** in the liver so that blood glucose levels are maintained.

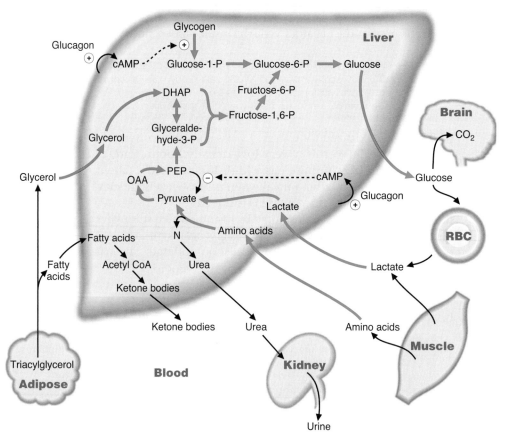

Figure 10-5 Tissue inter-relationships in glucose production during fasting. Trace the precursors lactate, amino acids, and glycerol to blood glucose. cAMP = cyclic adenosine monophosphate; CoA = coenzyme A; DHAP = dihydroxyacetone phosphate; OAA = oxaloacetate; P = phosphate; PEP = phosphoenolpyruvate; RBC = red blood cell.

cc 10.12 Diabetes is more often diagnosed based on **fasting plasma glucose tests.** Patients are required to **fast for at least 8 hours,** and the tests are most reliable in the morning. Normally, the serum glucose should be <100 mg/dL; a blood glucose, on **at least two separate occasion,** of **>126 mg/dL indicate diabetes,** whereas a value **100 to 125 mg/dL** indicates **impaired glucose tolerance** (prediabetes).

2. *Stimulation of glycogenolysis*
   a. Within a few hours after a meal, **glucagon** levels increase.
   b. As a result, **glycogenolysis** is stimulated and begins to supply glucose to the blood (see Figure 9-5).

3. *Stimulation of gluconeogenesis*
   a. **By 4 hours after a meal,** the liver is supplying glucose to the blood via gluconeogenesis and glycogenolysis (Figure 10-6).
   b. Regulatory mechanisms prevent futile cycles from occurring and promote the conversion of gluconeogenic precursors to glucose (see Figures 10-2 and 10-3).

4. *Stimulation of lipolysis* (see Figure 10-5)
   a. During fasting, the **breakdown of adipose triacylglycerols** is stimulated, and fatty acids and glycerol are released into the blood.
   b. **Fatty acids** are **oxidized** by certain tissues and converted to **ketone bodies** by the liver. The ATP and NADH produced by β-oxidation of fatty acids promotes gluconeogenesis.
   c. **Glycerol** is a source of carbon for gluconeogenesis in the liver.

5. *Relative roles of glycogenolysis and gluconeogenesis in maintaining blood glucose* (see Figure 10-6)
   a. **Glycogenolysis** is stimulated as blood glucose falls to the fasting level after a meal. It is the main source of blood glucose for the next 8 to 12 hours.
   b. **Gluconeogenesis** is stimulated within a few hours (4) after a meal and supplies an increasingly larger share of blood glucose as the fasting state persists.
   c. By 16 hours of fasting, **gluconeogenesis and glycogenolysis** are approximately **equal** as sources of blood glucose.
   d. As liver glycogen stores become depleted, **gluconeogenesis predominates.**
   e. By about 30 hours of fasting, liver glycogen is depleted, and thereafter, **gluconeogenesis** is the **only source** of blood glucose.

Figure 10-6 Sources of blood glucose in fed, fasting, and starved states. Note that the scale changes from hours to days. (Modified from Hanson RW and Mehlman MA (eds): *Gluconeogenesis: Its Regulation in Mammalian Species.* p 518. Copyright © 1976 by John Wiley & Sons, Inc. Reprinted with permission from John Wiley & Sons, Inc.)

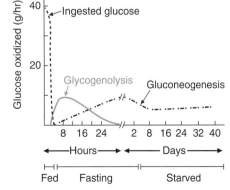

> **cc 10.13** The class of drugs known as **biguanides,** of which **metformin** is an example, is important in the management of **type 2 diabetes mellitus.** Although the mechanism is not completely clear, these drugs work primarily by **inhibiting hepatic gluconeogenesis** because an "average" person with type 2 diabetes has three times the normal rate of gluconeogenesis. The effect of this drug is to **decrease circulate glucose concentrations** in the post-absorptive state.

C. **Blood glucose levels during prolonged fasting (starvation)**

1. Even after 5 to 6 weeks of starvation, blood glucose levels are still in the range of 65 mg/dL.
2. Changes in fuel utilization by various tissues prevent blood glucose levels from decreasing abruptly during prolonged fasting.
3. The levels of ketone bodies rise in the blood, and the **brain uses ketone bodies** for energy, decreasing its utilization of blood glucose.
4. The rate of **gluconeogenesis** and, therefore, of **urea** production by the liver **decreases.**
5. **Muscle protein is spared.** Less muscle protein is used to provide amino acids for gluconeogenesis.

D. **Blood glucose levels during exercise**

1. During exercise, blood glucose is maintained by essentially the same mechanisms that are used during fasting.
2. *Use of endogenous fuels*
   a. As the exercising muscle contracts, **ATP** is used.
   b. ATP is regenerated initially from **creatine phosphate.**
   c. **Muscle glycogen** is oxidized to produce ATP. AMP activates phosphorylase b, and Ca^{2+}-calmodulin activates phosphorylase kinase. The hormone epinephrine causes the production of cAMP, which stimulates glycogen breakdown (see Figure 9-5).
3. *Use of fuels from the blood*
   a. As blood flow to the exercising muscle increases, blood glucose and fatty acids are taken up and oxidized by muscle.
   b. As blood glucose levels begin to decrease, the **liver,** by the processes of **glycogenolysis** and **gluconeogenesis,** acts to maintain blood glucose levels.

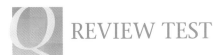

REVIEW TEST

Directions: Each of the numbered questions or incomplete statements in this section is followed by answers or by completions of the statement. Select the **one** lettered answer or completion that is **best** in each case.

1. Regulation of the activity of the pyruvate dehydrogenase (PDH) complex is best described by which of the following statements?

(A) It occurs by phosphorylation to a more active form.
(B) It is directly stimulated by cyclic adenosine monophosphate (cAMP).
(C) The active form synthesizes oxaloacetate (OAA).
(D) Activity is stimulated by adenosine triphosphate (ATP), NADH, and acetyl coenzyme A (CoA).
(E) It is inactivated by oxidation of fatty acids in the liver.

2. Which of the following statements best describes phosphoglycerate kinase?

(A) It is NAD+ dependent.
(B) It yields ATP by oxidative phosphorylation in mitochondria.
(C) It can be used for gluconeogenesis and glycolysis.
(D) It consumes ATP during glycolysis.
(E) It uses 2-phosphoglycerate as substrate.

3. Which of the following is a major precursor for gluconeogenesis?

(A) Glycogen
(B) Glycerol
(C) Glucagon
(D) Galactose
(E) Glucose 1-phosphate

4. Following the binding of epinephrine to its receptor sites on liver cells, a series of events occur, including which of the following?

(A) Decreased intracellular levels of cAMP
(B) Activation of phosphorylase
(C) Inhibition of the active form of glycogen synthase
(D) Inhibition of adenylate cyclase
(E) Inhibition of protein kinase

5. A high ratio of insulin to glucagon can:

(A) promote gluconeogenesis.
(B) promote glycogenolysis.
(C) promote triacylglyceride storage.
(D) occur in type 1 diabetes.
(E) occur in the fasting state.

6. The conversion of pyruvate to fructose 1,6-bisphosphate by the glucogenic pathway involves which of the following?

(A) Requires lactate dehydrogenase
(B) Requires hexokinase
(C) Produces 2 ATP + 2 guanosine triphosphates (GTP)
(D) Requires 4 ATP + 2 GTP
(E) Acetyl CoA is not required to activate the pathway

7. Which of the following glycolytic enzymes is used in gluconeogenesis?

(A) Glucokinase
(B) Phosphofructokinase 1
(C) Pyruvate kinase
(D) Aldolase B
(E) Phosphoglycerate kinase

8. In the conversion of pyruvate to glucose during gluconeogenesis:

(A) biotin is required.
(B) CO_2, added in one reaction, appears in the final product.
(C) energy is used only in the form of GTP.
(D) all of the reactions occur in the cytosol.
(E) PDH is the allosteric enzyme used.

9. Which of the following is a common intermediate in the conversion of glycerol and lactate to glucose?

(A) Pyruvate
(B) Oxaloacetate
(C) Malate
(D) Glucose 6-phosphate
(E) Phosphoenolpyruvate

10. In an individual at rest, who has fasted for 12 hours, which of the following occurs?

(A) Gluconeogenesis is the major process by which blood glucose is maintained.
(B) Adenylate cyclase is inactivated in liver.
(C) Liver glycogen stores are depleted.
(D) Phosphorylase, pyruvate kinase, and glycogen synthetase are phosphorylated in liver.
(E) Glycogen synthase is activated in liver.

11. A 32-year-old bodybuilder has decided to go on a diet consisting of only egg whites to ensure optimal protein for muscle growth. After a few weeks, he notices decreased energy and is found to be hypoglycemic. A nutritionist tells the patient that he most likely has a deficiency in the vitamin biotin. Which of the following enzymes is unable to catalyze its step in synthesizing glucose from pyruvate?

(A) Pyruvate carboxylase
(B) Phosphoenolpyruvate carboxykinase (PEPCK)
(C) Fructose 1,6-bisphosphatase
(D) Glucose 6-phosphase
(E) Phosphoglycerate kinase

12. An 8-year-old boy presents with frequent episodes of weakness, accompanied by sweating and feelings of dizziness. Physical exam is remarkable for palpably enlarged liver and kidneys. Labs revealed hypoglycemia and an elevated lactic acidemia. The patient is diagnosed with an enzyme deficiency of glucose 6-phospatase, which is normally only expressed in:

(A) liver and muscle.
(B) liver and brain.
(C) liver and kidney.
(D) erythrocytes.
(E) liver and adipose tissue.

13. A 14-year-old high school girl who is extremely conscious about her appearance has gone a full day without eating. She hopes to fit into a dress she intentionally bought a size too small by the day of her school dance. Which of the following organs contributes to the glucose that is being synthesized through gluconeogenesis?

(A) Spleen
(B) Red blood cells
(C) Skeletal muscle
(D) Liver
(E) Brain

14. A newborn infant is found to have persistent hypoglycemia, despite decreased feeding intervals. The child is also irritable with a moderate degree of hepatomegaly. He is found to have normal levels of muscular fructose 1,6-bisphophatase but decreased levels of the hepatic isoform. Which of the following statements is true of fructose 1,6-bisphophatase?

(A) It is induced by adenosine monophosphate (AMP).
(B) It is induced by insulin.
(C) It is inhibited by fructose 2,6-bisphosphate.
(D) It is induced in the fed state.
(E) It is inhibited during fasting.

15. A 6-year-old boy begins playing soccer in a community league. After his first game of the year, he is brought to see his pediatrician because of severe muscle cramps and what appears to be blood in his urine. He is subsequently found to have a deficiency of lactate dehydrogenase. This enzyme is important in which of the following conversions?

(A) Pyruvate to acetyl CoA
(B) Pyruvate to alanine
(C) Pyruvate to oxaloacetate
(D) Pyruvate to lactate
(E) Pyruvate to phosphoenolpyruvate

16. A 33-year-old, obese man with an impressive family history of type 2 diabetes is concerned he may develop the disease as well. During a health maintenance exam, his family physician orders several lab tests to evaluate the patient. Which of the following results would lead to a diagnosis of diabetes?

(A) A single random glucose level of 190 mg/dL

(B) The presence of a reducing sugar in his urine

(C) A single fasting blood glucose level of 160 mg/dL

(D) A 2-hour oral glucose tolerance test with a blood glucose level of 210 mg/dL

(E) A single fasting blood glucose level of 110 mg/dL

17. A 56-year-old, newly diagnosed type 2 diabetic fails an initial attempt at controlling her diabetes with dietary measures alone. She follows up with her family physician, who starts her on a sulfonylurea. This drug works by doing which of the following?

(A) Stimulating the production of GLUT-2

(B) Stimulating the synthesis of new insulin

(C) Antagonizing the effects of arginine on pancreatic β-cells

(D) Inhibiting the release of glucagon

(E) Stimulating the release of preformed insulin

18. A 62-year-old, obese man complains of polydipsia (increased drinking), polyuria (increased urination), and fatigue. A glucose tolerance test confirms the diagnosis of diabetes. He is placed on metformin, which works by which of the following the mechanisms?

(A) Inhibiting hepatic gluconeogenesis

(B) Increasing glucagon levels

(C) Increasing cellular responsiveness to circulating insulin

(D) Stimulating the release of preformed insulin

(E) Replacing the need for endogenous insulin

19. A 34-year-old woman presents with central obesity, relatively thin extremities, and purple stria on her abdomen. Further workup reveals an excessive serum cortisol level and a blood sugar level of 258 mg/dL. Which of the following is the most likely cause of her hyperglycemia?

(A) A pancreatic adenoma secreting adrenocorticotropic hormone (ACTH) and glucagons

(B) Glucocorticoid-enhanced translation of PEPCK

(C) Increased gluconeogenesis substrates through excess fatty acid degradation

(D) Cortisol inhibition of insulin secretion

(E) Excess consumption of processed carbohydrates

20. A 4-month-old boy is being evaluated for seizures, psychomotor retardation, and hypotonia. Workup reveals elevated serum levels of lactate, alanine, pyruvate, and ketoacids. Based on the clinical presentation, pyruvate carboxylase activity is measured using fibroblasts from a skin biopsy and is found to be markedly decreased. This enzyme is normally used to directly synthesize which of the following molecules?

(A) Pyruvate

(B) Oxaloacetate

(C) Malate

(D) Acetyl CoA

(E) α-Ketoglutarate

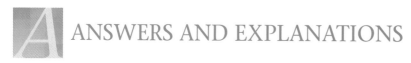

ANSWERS AND EXPLANATIONS

1–E. One of the modes of regulation of pyruvate dehydrogenase (PDH) activity is by fatty acids being oxidized in the liver, producing acetyl coenzyme A (CoA), NADH, and adenosine triphosphate (ATP) and inactivating the complex (choice D). The active form produces acetyl CoA; oxaloacetate (OAA) is produced by pyruvate carboxylase. Phosphorylation inactivates PDH as well as cyclic adenosine monophosphate (cAMP).

2–C. Phosphoglycerate kinase is one of the enzymes used for both gluconeogenesis and glycolysis. The reaction is not a dehydrogenation, and it does not yield an ATP (it requires 1 ATP in gluconeogenesis). The substrate is 3-phosphoglycerate.

3–B. One of the major precursors for gluconeogenesis is glycerol, which forms dihydroxyacetone phosphate (DHAP). Glycogen is for glucose storage and is not a precursor for gluconeogenesis. Glucagon is a hormone-regulating glucose concentration. Neither the disaccharide galactose nor glucose 1-phosphate is a major precursor for gluconeogenesis.

4–B. The hormone epinephrine activates phosphorylase and causes an increase in the production of cAMP. Epinephrine stimulates glycogen breakdown by inhibiting glycogen synthase, and activates adenyl cyclase and protein kinase.

5–C. A high ratio of insulin to glucagon indicates synthesis of triacylglycerols. Gluconeogenesis and glycogenolysis, as well as the fasting state, cause insulin to decrease and glucagons to increase. Type 1 diabetes results in decreased uptake of glucose by cells (due to low insulin and high glucagon in blood).

6–D. Because 2 moles of pyruvate are required to form 1 mole of fructose 1,6-bisphosphate, 6 moles of high-energy phosphate are required for synthesis in the form of 4 ATP and 2 guanosine triphosphates (GTP). The glucogenic pathway requires neither hexokinase nor lactate dehydrogenase, but it does require acetyl CoA.

7–D. During gluconeogenesis, glucokinase, phosphofructokinase 1, and pyruvate kinase are not active, and thus, futile cycles do not occur. Aldolase B, the liver isozyme, is used both in glycolysis and gluconeogenesis. Phosphoglycerate kinase is present only in gluconeogenesis.

8–A. In the mitochondria, CO_2 is added to pyruvate to form OAA. The enzyme is pyruvate carboxylase, which requires biotin and ATP. OAA leaves the mitochondrion as malate or aspartate and is regenerated in the cytosol. OAA is converted to phosphoenolpyruvate by a reaction that uses GTP and releases the same CO_2 that was added in the mitochondrion. The remainder of the reactions occur in the cytosol. PDH is inactive; pyruvate is not converted to acetyl CoA.

9–D. The only intermediate included among the choices that glycerol has in common with lactate is glucose 6-phosphate. Glycerol enters gluconeogenesis as dihydroxyacetone phosphate (DHAP). Therefore, it bypasses the other compounds.

10–D. After 12 hours of fasting, liver glycogen stores are still substantial. Glycogenolysis is stimulated by glucagon, which activates adenylate cyclase. cAMP activates protein kinase A, which phosphorylates phosphorylase kinase, pyruvate kinase, and glycogen synthase. As a result, phosphorylase is activated, whereas glycogen synthase and pyruvate kinase are inactivated. Gluconeogenesis does not become the major process for maintaining blood glucose until 18 to 20 hours of fasting. After about 30 hours, liver glycogen is depleted.

11–A. Pyruvate carboxylase requires the cofactor biotin to catalyze the irreversible carboxylation of pyruvate to OAA. Although the conversion of OAA to phosphoenolpyruvate is also irreversible and requires energy in the form of GTP, the enzyme catalyzing this step, phosphoenolpyruvate carboxykinase (PEPCK), does not require a cofactor. As with pyruvate carboxylase and PEPCK, fructose 1,6-bisphosphatase and glucose 6-phosphatase are used to bypass the irreversible steps of glycolysis. Phosphoglycerate kinase is the only enzyme, in addition to the first two in the gluconeogenesis pathway, that uses ATP.

12–C. Type 1 glycogen storage disease, von Gierke disease, results from the deficiency of glucose 6-phosphatase. The deficiency blocks the release of glucose from glycogen stores and also obstructs glucose synthesis in the last step of gluconeogenesis. Thus, glucose is only available from the diet, resulting in severe hypoglycemia when fasting. Although muscle is a major storage area for glycogen, the glucose 6-phosphate is converted to glucose **in the liver** before it can be used by muscle as an energy source. Brain and erythrocytes depend on glucose in the serum for their energy source, whereas adipose tissue uses fatty acids entering the Kreb's cycle as their main source of energy.

13–D. The two organs that translate the enzymes necessary for gluconeogenesis are the liver and kidneys. Although the kidneys only supply 10% of the newly formed glucose, their participation takes on a major role in starvation. Mature red blood cells lack a nucleus and, therefore, are unable to transcribe the messenger RNA (mRNA) needed to translate and synthesize the needed enzymes for gluconeogenesis. Skeletal muscle and brain tissue also lack the ability to transcribe and translate the enzymes for gluconeogenesis and must rely on the blood glucose supplied by the diet, gluconeogenesis, and glycogenolysis for their needed energy requirements.

14–C. Fructose 1,6-bisphophatase is an important regulator step in gluconeogenesis. It is inhibited by fructose 2,6-bisphosphate. It is also inhibited by adenosine monophosphate (AMP). In addition, it is induced during the fasting state but not in the fed state. Insulin has no direct effect on this critical regulatory enzyme.

15–D. Lactate is formed from pyruvate via the enzyme lactate dehydrogenase. Pyruvate plays a critical role in metabolism because it is at the crossroads of several pathways. Pyruvate can be converted to acetyl CoA for entry into lipid metabolism. The conversion of pyruvate to alanine by alanine aminotransferase merges glucose and amino acid metabolism. Conversion of pyruvate to OAA by pyruvate carboxylase allows interconversion between glucose metabolism and the tricarboxylic acid (TCA) cycle. Finally, the conversion of pyruvate to PEP for gluconeogenesis requires two steps: the above reaction to produce OAA and an additional step to convert OAA to PEP, mediated by PEPCK.

16–D. Of all the test values, the one that renders a diagnosis of diabetes in a single episode is a 2-hour oral glucose tolerance test yielding a blood glucose level of 200 mg/dL. A single random glucose level of >200 mg/dL with symptoms of diabetes would confirm the diagnosis. Concerning fasting glucose levels, there must be blood glucose levels of >126 mg/dL on at least two occasions. Two fasting blood glucose levels between 100 and 125 mg/dL indicate impaired glucose tolerance or so called prediabetes. The presence of a reducing sugar in the urine is not sufficient because patients with benign fructosuria would be positive and not necessarily diabetic.

17–E. Sulfonylureas stimulate the release of preformed insulin from pancreatic islets and have been important drugs in the management of diabetes. Sulfonylureas have the same action as in response to arginine, in that preformed insulin is released. Neither sulfonylureas nor arginine are capable of stimulating the production of new insulin. No agent listed directly inhibits glucagon. The production of GLUT-2 is insulin independent and would not be altered with sulfonylurea treatment.

18–A. Metformin, a biguanide, is beneficial in the treatment of type 2 diabetes because it inhibits hepatic gluconeogenesis, which is often increased in patients with type 2 diabetes. No known agent to treat diabetes directly affects glucagon. Thiazolidinediones are used in the treatment of diabetes because they increase cellular responsiveness to insulin. Sulfonylureas stimulate the release of preformed insulin. None of these agents completely replaces the need for exogenous insulin in patients with insulin-dependent diabetes.

19–B. Cushing syndrome results in increased circulating glucocorticoids, primarily cortisol. Glucocorticoids bind to cytosolic receptor proteins that traverse the nuclear envelope and bind to specific sequences in the PEPCK gene and cause an increase in PEPCK gene expression. PEPCK RNA is translated into PEPCK protein in the cytosol. The increased PEPCK protein concentration then catalyzes the formation of PEP from OAA, which is an initiating step prior to gluconeogenesis; this results in hyperglycemia. Tumors of the pancreas more commonly produce insulin or glucagon. There are documented cases of pancreatic tumors secreting ACTH, but this is much less likely than another form of Cushing syndrome, as described by the patient's signs and symptoms. Fatty acid degradation produces primarily 2 carbon units, which bypass gluconeogenesis and enter the TCA cycle. Cortisol actually stimulates insulin secretion, although, paradoxically, it decreases the tissues' sensitivity to the hormone. Excess consumption of carbohydrates would cause hypoglycemia, not hyperglycemia.

20–B. Pyruvate carboxylase converts pyruvate to OAA, which can then either enter the Kreb's cycle (or TCA cycle) or enter the gluconeogenesis pathway, depending on energy needs. In a fed state, gluconeogenesis is active in the liver, and OAA is diverted to form glucose (via PEP). When energy needs are high, acetyl CoA is produced, for instance, from the β-oxidation of fatty acids. In this condition, OAA condenses with the acetyl CoA to enter the Kreb's cycle and subsequent oxidative phosphorylation. Both α-ketoglutarate and malate will eventually be synthesized, if pyruvate is catalyzed by pyruvate dehydrogenase to form acetyl CoA (which enters the TCA cycle).

Miscellaneous Carbohydrate Metabolism

I.   Fructose and Galactose Metabolism

A.   Metabolism of fructose

 The major dietary source of fructose is the disaccharide sucrose in table sugar and fruit, but it is also present as the monosaccharide in corn syrup, which is used as a sweetener.

1. *Conversion of fructose to glycolytic intermediates* (Figure 11-1)

   a. Fructose is metabolized mainly in the **liver**, where it is converted to pyruvate or, under fasting conditions, to glucose.

   (1) Fructose is phosphorylated by adenosine triphosphate (ATP) to form fructose 1-phosphate. The enzyme is **fructokinase.**

> *cc 11.2* Deficiency of **fructokinase** is also known as **benign fructosuria.** It is an autosomal recessive disorder usually **diagnosed incidentally,** as fructose accumulates in the urine and is **detected as a reducing sugar** that may give falsely high glucose readings.

   (2) Fructose 1-phosphate is cleaved by **aldolase B** to form dihydroxyacetone phosphate (DHAP) and glyceraldehyde, which is phosphorylated by ATP to form glyceraldehyde 3-phosphate. DHAP and glyceraldehyde 3-phosphate are intermediates of glycolysis. (Aldolase B is the same liver enzyme that cleaves fructose 1,6-bisphosphate in glycolysis.)

   (3) See Chapter 6 for clinical correlation on absence of the A isoform of aldolase (cc 6.3).

   b. In tissues other than liver, the major fate of fructose is phosphorylation by hexokinase to form fructose 6-phosphate, which enters glycolysis. Hexokinase has an affinity for fructose about one-twentieth of that for glucose.

2. *Production of fructose from glucose*

   a. Glucose is reduced to sorbitol by **aldose reductase**, which reduces the aldehyde group to an alcohol (Figure 11-2).

   b. Sorbitol is then reoxidized at carbon 2 by **sorbitol dehydrogenase** to form fructose.

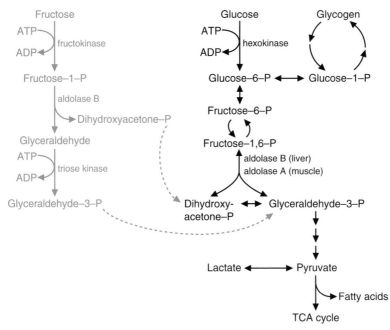

Figure 11-1 Conversion of fructose to intermediates of glycolysis. ADP = adenosine diphosphate; ATP = adenosine triphosphate; P = phosphate; TCA = tricarboxylic acid.

> *cc* **11.3** **Fructose,** derived from glucose in **seminal vesicles,** is the major energy source for sperm cells. During an **infertility workup,** semen fructose concentrations may be analyzed.

B. Metabolism of galactose

> *cc* **11.4** The disaccharide **lactose,** found in milk or milk products, is the major dietary source of galactose. It is also found in many artificial sweeteners and as "filler" in some medications.

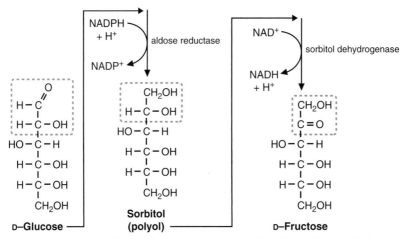

Figure 11-2 Reduced forms of sugars. Sorbitol is produced by reduction of glucose and can be reoxidized at carbon 2 to form fructose. Galactitol is produced by reduction of galactose.

1. *Conversion of galactose to intermediates of glucose pathways* (Figure 11-3)
   a. **Galactose** is phosphorylated by ATP to galactose 1-phosphate. The enzyme is **galactokinase.**

   > *cc* **11.5**   **Galactokinase deficiency** results in increased levels of galactose in the blood (galactosemia) and urine (galactosuria). This results in the development of **cataracts** in infants without appropriate dietary restriction; however, these patients are **otherwise asymptomatic,** unlike the more severe classic galactosemia.

   b. **Galactose 1-phosphate** reacts with uridine diphosphate glucose (UDP-glucose) and forms glucose 1-phosphate and UDP-galactose. The enzyme is **galactose 1-phosphate uridyltransferase.**

   > *cc* **11.6**   **Classic galactosemia** is a serious disorder that results from a deficiency of **galactose 1-phosphate uridyltransferase.** The disorder typically presents with **hepatomegaly,** jaundice, **hypoglycemia, convulsions,** and **lethargy.** The infant may hay have difficulties feeding, with poor weight gain and the development of **cataracts.** Infants are at increased risk for **neonatal sepsis** due to *Escherichia coli.* **Neonatal screening** tests typically detect the disorder early, allowing for the elimination of all dietary galactose and preventing the development of more serious complications including **mental retardation** and cirrhosis.

   c. **UDP-galactose** is epimerized to UDP-glucose in a reaction that is readily reversible. The enzyme is **UDP-glucose epimerase.**

   > *cc* **11.7**   **Deficiency of UDP-glucose epimerase** occurs in two distinct forms. The first is a benign condition, in which there is a deficiency in only leukocytes and erythrocytes. The second is more serious, as it involves all tissues, with symptoms similar to classic galactosemia with the addition of hypotonia and nerve deafness. Again, the management requires the elimination of dietary galactose.

   d. Repetition of reactions described above (in a–c) results in conversion of galactose to **UDP-glucose** and **glucose 1-phosphate.**
      (1) In the **liver,** these glucose derivatives are converted to blood glucose during fasting or to glycogen after a meal.

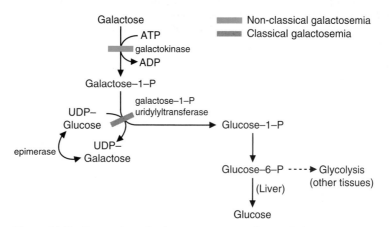

Figure 11-3   Conversion of galactose to intermediates of glucose metabolism. Galactose 1-phosphate uridyltransferase is deficient in classic galactosemia. ADP = adenosine diphosphate; ATP = adenosine triphosphate; P = phosphate.

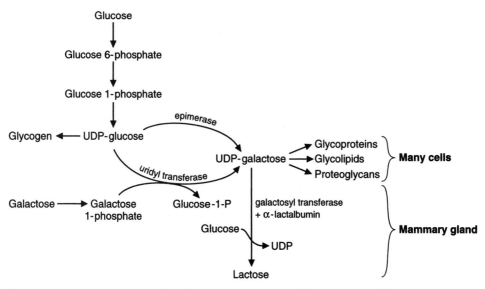

Figure 11-4 Metabolism of uridine diphosphate galactose (UDP-galactose). UDP-galactose can be produced from dietary glucose or galactose.

      (2) In various tissues, the glucose 1-phosphate forms glucose 6-phosphate and feeds into glycolysis.

  2. *Other fates of UDP-galactose* (Figure 11-4)

    a. UDP-galactose can be produced either from galactose or from glucose via UDP-glucose and an epimerase.

    b. UDP-galactose supplies galactose moieties for the synthesis of **glycoproteins, glycolipids,** and **proteoglycans.** The enzyme that adds galactose units to growing polysaccharide chains is **galactosyl transferase.**

    c. UDP-galactose reacts with glucose in the **lactating mammary gland** to produce the milk sugar **lactose.** The modifier protein, α-**lactalbumin,** reacts with galactosyl transferase, lowering its K_m for glucose so that glucose adds to galactose (from UDP-galactose), forming lactose.

> *cc* **11.8** The synthesis of α-**lactalbumin** in the **mammary gland** is stimulated by the hormone **prolactin.** Lactose and milk proteins are only produced in the presence of prolactin. (Prolactin is released from the **anterior pituitary.**)

  3. Conversion of galactose to galactitol. Aldose reductase reduces the aldehyde of galactose to an alcohol, forming galactitol (see Figure 11-2).

> *cc* **11.9** **Galactitol,** like **sorbitol (see cc 1.11),** accumulates in cells, increasing their osmotic pressure and **promoting cell swelling.** It is this swelling that ultimately leads to **damage of nerves, lens of the eye,** and **liver cells** in the defects in galactose metabolism described earlier.

II.   Pentose Phosphate Pathway

A. Reactions of the pentose phosphate pathway (Figure 11-5)

  1. *The oxidative reactions* (Figure 11-6)

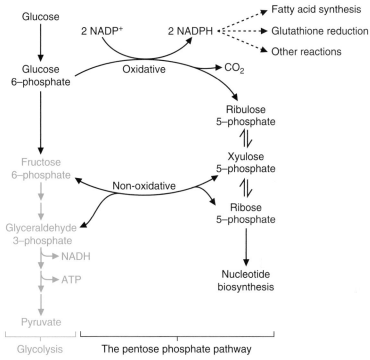

Figure 11-5 Overview of the pentose phosphate pathway. ATP = adenosine triphosphate.

a. **Glucose 6-phosphate** is converted, via the enzyme **glucose 6-phosphate dehydrogenase**, to 6-phosphogluconolactone, and $NADP^+$ is reduced to $NADPH + H^+$.

> **cc 11.10** A deficiency of **glucose 6-phosphate dehydrogenase** causes **insufficient amounts of NADPH** to be produced under certain conditions (e.g., when antimalarial **drugs** are being used). As a result, glutathione is not adequately reduced and, in turn, is not available to reduce compounds that are produced by the metabolism of these drugs. Red blood cells lyse, and a **hemolytic anemia** can occur.

b. **6-Phosphogluconolactone is hydrolyzed to 6-phosphogluconate,** with the help of the enzyme **gluconolactonase.**
c. **6-Phosphogluconate** is oxidatively decarboxylated. The enzyme involved is **6-phosphogluconate dehydrogenase.**
  (1) CO_2 is released, and a second $NADPH + H^+$ is generated from $NADP^+$.
  (2) The remaining carbons form ribulose 5-phosphate.
2. *The nonoxidative reactions* (see Figure 11-5)
  a. **Ribulose 5-phosphate** is isomerized to ribose 5-phosphate or epimerized to xylulose 5-phosphate.
  b. **Ribose 5-phosphate** and **xylulose 5-phosphate** undergo reactions, catalyzed by **transketolase** and **transaldolase,** that transfer carbon units, ultimately forming fructose 6-phosphate and glyceraldehyde 3-phosphate.
    (1) **Transketolase,** which requires **thiamine pyrophosphate,** transfers two-carbon units (Figure 11-7).
    (2) **Transaldolase** transfers three-carbon units.

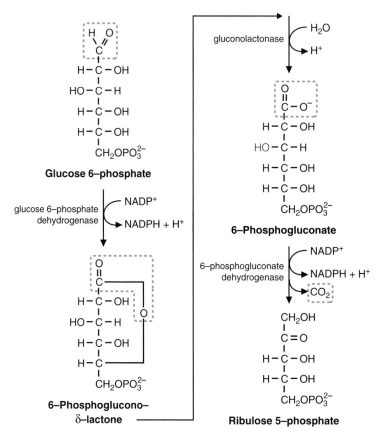

Figure 11-6 The oxidative reactions of the pentose phosphate pathway. These reactions are irreversible. Deficiency of glucose 6-phosphate dehydrogenase can result in hemolytic anemia.

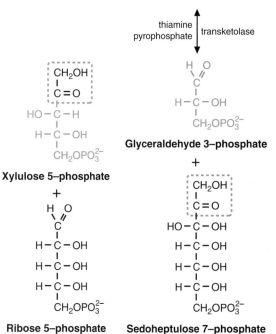

Figure 11-7 A two-carbon unit transferred by transketolase. Thiamine pyrophosphate is a cofactor for this enzyme.

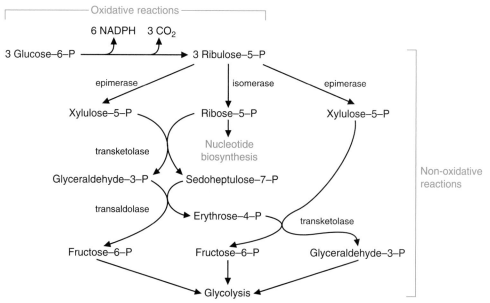

Figure 11-8 The reactions of the pentose phosphate pathway.

3. *Overall reactions of the pentose phosphate pathway* (Figure 11-8)

$$3 \text{ glucose-6-P} + 6 \text{ NADP}^+ \rightarrow 3 \text{ ribulose-5-P} + 3 \text{ CO}_2 + 6 \text{ NADPH}$$

$$3 \text{ ribulose-5-P} \rightarrow 2 \text{ xylulose-5-P} + \text{ribose-5-P}$$

$$2 \text{ xylulose-5-P} + \text{ribose-5-P} \rightarrow 2 \text{ fructose-6-P} + \text{glyceraldehyde-3-P}$$

B. **Functions of NADPH** (see Figure 11-5)

1. The pentose phosphate pathway produces NADPH for **fatty acid synthesis.** Under these conditions, the fructose 6-phosphate and glyceraldehyde 3-phosphate generated in the pathway re-enter glycolysis.
2. NADPH is also used to **reduce glutathione** (γ-glutamylcysteinylglycine).
   a. Glutathione helps to prevent oxidative damage to cells by reducing hydrogen peroxide (H_2O_2).
   b. Glutathione is also used to transport amino acids across the membranes of certain cells by the γ-glutamyl cycle.

C. **Generation of ribose 5-phosphate** (see Figure 11-5)

1. When **NADPH levels are low,** the oxidative reactions of the pathway can be used to generate ribose 5-phosphate for nucleotide biosynthesis.
2. When **NADPH levels are high,** the reversible nonoxidative portion of the pathway can be used to generate ribose 5-phosphate for nucleotide biosynthesis from fructose 6-phosphate and glyceraldehyde 3-phosphate.

III. Proteoglycans, Glycoproteins, and Glycolipids

A. Proteoglycans

1. *Synthesis of proteoglycans*
   a. The **protein** is synthesized on the endoplasmic reticulum (ER).

b. **Glycosaminoglycans** are produced by the addition of sugars to serine or threonine residues of the protein. UDP-sugars serve as the precursors.

c. In the ER and the Golgi, the glycosaminoglycan chains grow by sequential addition of sugars to the nonreducing end.

   (1) **Sulfate groups,** donated by 3'-phosphoadenosine 5'-phosphosulfate (PAPS), are added after the hexosamine is incorporated into the chain.

   (2) Because of the uronic acid and sulfate groups, the glycosaminoglycans are **negatively charged,** causing the chains to be heavily hydrated.

---

cc 11.11 **Glycosaminoglycans** are important **components of the fluid in joints (synovial fluid)** and the vitreous humor of the eye. These solutions are mucous and **highly compressible** as water can be "squeezed out" from between the chains. Patients with **osteoarthritis** have a relative **deficiency** of these important "cushioning" molecules, resulting in damage to the joint.

---

d. **Proteoglycans** are **secreted** from the cell.

e. Proteoglycans can associate noncovalently with **hyaluronic acid** (a glycosaminoglycan), forming large aggregates, which act as molecular sieves that can be penetrated by small, but not by large, molecules.

2. *Degradation of proteoglycans by lysosomal enzymes*

   a. Because proteoglycans are located outside the cell, they are taken up by **endocytosis.** The endocytic vesicles fuse with lysosomes.

   b. **Lysosomal enzymes** specific for each monosaccharide remove the sugars, one at a time, from the nonreducing end of the chain.

   c. **Sulfatases** remove the sulfate groups before the sugar residue is hydrolyzed.

   d. Several rare diseases known as **mucopolysaccharidoses, result from deficiencies of these lysosomal enzymes,** with subsequent accumulation of substrate. Tissues become engorged with these "residual bodies," and their function is impaired. **(See Table 11-1.)**

TABLE 11-1	*Mucopolysaccharidoses (MPS)*			
	Disease	Enzyme Deficiency	Accumulated Products	Clinical Consequence
cc 11.12	Hurler syndrome (MPS I)	α-L-Iduronidase	Heparin sulfate, dermatan sulfate	**Deficiency** of this enzyme results in **mental retardation, micrognathia, coarsening of facial features** with **macroglossia** (enlarged tongue), retinal degeneration, **corneal clouding,** and **cardiomyopathy.**

TABLE 11-1	*Mucopolysaccharidoses (MPS) (Continued)*			
	Disease	**Enzyme Deficiency**	**Accumulated Products**	**Clinical Consequence**
cc 11.13	**Hunter syndrome** (MPS II)	Iduronate sulfatase	Heparin sulfate, dermatan sulfate	This **X-linked deficiency** is generally milder than Hurler syndrome, **without corneal clouding.** However, it is associated with **variable mental retardation.**
cc 11.14	**Sanfilippo syndrome A** **Sanfilippo syndrome B** **Sanfilippo syndrome C** (MPS IIIA-C)	Heparan sulfamidase *N*-acetylgluco-saminidase *N*-acetylgluco-samine 6-sulfatase	Heparin sulfate Heparin sulfate Heparin sulfate	This biochemically heterogenous syndrome results in **developmental delay, severe hyperactivity, spasticity, and progressive loss of motor skills** with death by the second decade.
cc 11.15	**Morquio syndrome** (MPS IV)	Galactose 6-sulfatase	Keratan sulfate, chondroitin 6-sulfate	Unlike other MPS syndromes, Morquio syndrome **is not associated with CNS involvement.** The disease is predominated by **severe skeletal dysplasia** and short stature. Motor involvement results from spinal cord impingement on motor neurons.
cc 11.16	**Sly syndrome** (MPS VII)	β-Glucuronidase	Heparan sulfate, dermatan sulfate, Chondroitin 4-,6-sulfate	Results in **hepatomegaly, skeletal deformity** with short stature, corneal clouding, and **developmental delay.** Although rare, much work has been accomplished in terms of **gene therapy** and **bone marrow transplantation** as a cure for this MPS.

CNS = central nervous system.

B. Glycoproteins

1. *Synthesis of glycoproteins*

a. The protein is synthesized on the ER. In the ER and the Golgi, the **carbohydrate chain** is produced by the sequential addition of monosaccharide units to the nonreducing end. UDP-sugars, guanosine diphosphate (GDP)-mannose, GDP-L-fucose, and cytisine monophosphate-N-acetylneuraminic acid (CMP-NANA) act as precursors.

b. For O-linked glycoproteins, the initial sugar is added to a **serine or threonine** residue in the protein, and the carbohydrate chain is then elongated.

---

cc **11.17** Blood group antigens are **O-linked glycoproteins** and lipid ceramides. Most individuals produce a **fructose linked to a galactose at the nonreducing end** of the blood group antigen, the so called **H substance**. Individuals with **A blood group** produce an N-acetylgalactosamine transferase, which transfers an **N-acetylgalactosamine moiety to the H substance.** Individuals with **B blood group** produce a galactosyltransferase that adds **galactose to the H substance.** Individuals with **AB blood group produce both transferases,** whereas individuals with **O blood type produce neither** and, therefore, have only the H substance at the nonreducing end (**Figure 11-9**).

---

c. **Dolichol phosphate** is involved in the synthesis of N-linked glycoproteins in which the carbohydrate moiety is attached to the amide N of asparagine.

---

cc **11.18** A heterogenous group of diseases, known as **congenital disorders of glycosylation (CDG),** result from defects in the various enzymes involved in **N-linked oligosaccharide synthesis.** A spectrum of clinical symptoms has been described, with most presenting with **severe motor involvement, mental retardation,** and **coagulopathy** resulting in abnormal bleeding and **stroke-like episodes.**

Blood Type

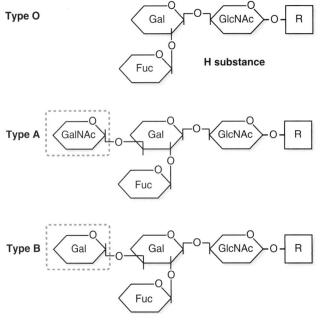

Figure 11-9 Structures of blood group substances. Note that these structures are the same except that type A has N-acetylgalactosamine (GalNAc) at the nonreducing end, type B has galactose (Gal), and type O has neither. R is either a protein or the lipid ceramide.

(1) Dolichol phosphate, a long-chain alcohol containing about 20 five-carbon isoprene units, can be synthesized from acetyl coenzyme A (CoA).
(2) Sugars are added sequentially to dolichol phosphate, which is associated with the membrane of the ER.
(3) The branched polysaccharide chain is transferred to an amide N of an asparagine residue in the protein.
(4) In the ER and the Golgi, sugars are removed from the chain and other sugars are added.

d. **Glycoproteins** are **segregated** into lysosomes within the cell, **attached** to the cell membrane, or **secreted** by the cell.

(1) **Lysosomal enzymes** are glycoproteins. A mannose phosphate residue targets these glycoproteins to lysosomes.

> *cc* **11.19** **I-cell disease** results form a defect in the addition of **mannose 6-phosphate** tag on enzymes destined for the **lysosome.** As such, these **hydrolytic enzymes** end up being secreted from the cell. **Substrates within lysosomes accumulate, resulting in large inclusion bodies,** hence I-cells. Patients have **skeletal abnormalities, joint impairment, coarse facial features,** and **psychomotor impairment** culminating in death by the age of 8 years.

(2) When a glycoprotein is attached to the **cell membrane**, the carbohydrate portion extends into the extracellular space and a hydrophobic segment of the protein is anchored in the membrane.

2. *Degradation of glycoproteins*

- **Lysosomal enzymes** specific for each monosaccharide remove sugars sequentially from the nonreducing ends of the chains.

> *cc* **11.20** Analogous to the mucopolysaccharidoses (MPS), there are a heterogeneous group of disorders known as **glycoproteinoses.** They are associated with deficiencies in numerous **lysosomal enzymes** important in the **catabolism of glycoproteins.** Glycoproteinoses (i.e., α-mannosidase deficiency, α-fucosidase deficiency, and aspartyl glucosaminidase deficiency) typically present with **recurrent respiratory infections** secondary to **impaired immune function, developmental delay, neurodegeneration, and facial coarsening.**

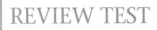

REVIEW TEST

Directions: Each of the numbered questions or incomplete statements in this section is followed by answers or by completions of the statement. Select the **one** lettered answer or completion that is **best** in each case.

1. The reactions of the pentose phosphate pathway using glucose 6-phosphate as the initial substrate are best described by which of the following statements?

(A) They produce 2 moles of NADPH for each mole of CO2 released.
(B) They generate 2 moles of adenosine triphosphate (ATP) per mole of glucose 6-phosphate metabolized to ribulose 6-phosphate.
(C) They occur in the matrix of mitochondria.
(D) They are not required for the production of NADPH in the mature red blood cell.
(E) They are required for the metabolism of glucose in muscle.

2. Concerning fructose, which of the following statements is correct?

(A) Fructose uses hexokinase in the liver to enter glycolysis.
(B) Fructose is converted to fructose 6-phosphate by fructokinase and ATP.
(C) Fructose 1-phosphate is cleaned by aldolase to form DHAP and glyceraldehyde.
(D) Deficiency of fructose 1-phosphate aldolase leads to fructosuria.
(E) Fructosuria is a disease with severe medical consequences.

3. In the pentose phosphate pathway, the major products are which of the following?

(A) Ribulose or xylulose and ATP
(B) Ribulose or xylulose and NADP⁺
(C) Ribose and NADH
(D) Ribose and NADPH
(E) Ribose and NADP⁺

4. Which of the following statements is true about UDP derivatives of monosaccharides?

(A) They are sometimes formed during glucose metabolism.

(B) Uridine diphosphate (UDP) glucose is used by glycogen synthetase in the liver.
(C) One is formed when uridine triphosphate (UTP) reacts with glucose 6-phosphate.
(D) They are required during the conversion of pyruvate to glucose in the liver.
(E) UDP-galactose is epimerized to UDP-glucose via UDP-galactose epimerase.

5. For *O*-linked glycosylation of secreted or membrane proteins, which of the following statements best describes the process?

(A) A complex oligosaccharide is synthesized on dolichol phosphate and then transferred to the protein.
(B) Sugars are linked to the side chain of asparagine.
(C) Sugars are linked to the side chain of tyrosine.
(D) Sugars are added to the carbohydrate chain one at a time in the Golgi.
(E) Defects are known as congenital disorders of glycosylation (CDG).

6. Which of the following statements best describes glycosaminoglycans?

(A) They contain repeating disaccharides.
(B) They are usually positively charged.
(C) They contain short oligosaccharide chains.
(D) They rarely contain sulfate groups.
(E) They contain branches of *N*-acetylneuraminic acid.

7. Which of the following statements concerning lactose synthesis is correct?

(A) The reactions occur in most tissues.
(B) α-Lactalbumin acts as a modifier of galactosyl transferase.
(C) UDP-glucose reacts with galactose.
(D) UDP-galactose requires dietary galactose for its synthesis.
(E) Lactase is present in the mammary gland.

178

8. Dietary fructose is phosphorylated in the liver and cleaved to form which of the following choices?

(A) 2 molecules of dihydroxyacetone phosphate
(B) 1 molecule each of dihydroxyacetone phosphate and glyceraldehyde
(C) 1 molecule each of dihydroxyacetone phosphate and glyceraldehyde 3-phosphate
(D) 1 molecule each of dihydroxyacetone and glyceraldehyde 3-phosphate
(E) 2 molecules of glyceraldehyde 3-phosphate

9. Glycoproteins are best described by which of these statements?

(A) They are usually positively charged.
(B) They never contain branched oligosaccharide chains.
(C) They contain oligosaccharides that are synthesized on dolichol phosphate and transferred to serine residues.
(D) They are degraded by lysosomal enzymes.
(E) They are all secreted into the blood.

10. A 14-day-old neonate fails to gain weight during infancy despite breast feeding. Although concerned, the mother continues to breast feed and wait. The infant subsequently develops cataracts, an enlarged liver, and mental retardation. Urinalysis is significant for high levels of galactose in the urine, as well as galactosemia. What food product in the baby's diet is leading to her symptoms?

(A) Fructose
(B) Lactose
(C) Phenylalanine
(D) Glucose
(E) Sorbitol

11. A 19-year-old, African-American male military recruit is about to be sent to Iraq on his assignment. In preparation for his tour of duty, he is given a prophylactic dose of primaquine to prevent malaria. Several days after he begins taking the drug, he develops fatigue and hemolytic anemia.

Which of the following proteins is likely deficient?

(A) Fructokinase
(B) Aldolase B
(C) Glucose 6-phosphate dehydrogenase
(D) Galactokinase
(E) Galactosyl transferase

12. A 3-year-old girl presents with developmental delay and growth failure. Physical exam is remarkable for coarse facial features, craniofacial abnormalities, gingival hyperplasia, prominent epicanthal fold, and macroglossia. The patient was diagnosed with I-cell disease resulting from the enzyme responsible for attaching mannose 6-phosphate residues on lysosomal hydrolase glycoproteins. Rather than being targeted for the cell's lysosomes, I-cell disease results in the proteins being:

(A) accumulated in the endoplasmic reticulum (ER).
(B) degraded in the lysosome.
(C) targeted for the mitochondria.
(D) exported from the cell.
(E) accumulated in the cytoplasm.

13. A 65-year-old man with a long history of diabetes presents to his physician after failing the driver's license renewal eye exam. Patients with diabetes have abnormally high blood glucose levels. Glucose can enter the lens of the eye, where it can be converted to sorbitol. Which of the following converts glucose to sorbitol?

(A) Hexokinase
(B) Aldose reductase
(C) Aldose mutase
(D) Sorbitol dehydrogenase
(E) Aldose oxidase

14. A 23-year-old woman gives birth to a healthy baby. She plans on breast feeding the infant. Prolactin is an important hormone for the synthesis of milk in the breast because it stimulates the synthesis of α-lactalbumin. The function of this protein is to do which of the following?

(A) Convert galactose to galactitol
(B) Lower the K_m of galactosyl transferase for glucose

(C) Add galactose for the glycosylation of proteins
(D) Reduce oxidized glutathione
(E) Form fructose from sorbitol

15. A 5-year-old child presents with Hurler syndrome, which is characterized by dwarfism, hunchback, coarse facies, mental retardation, clouding of the cornea, and sensorineural deafness. The patient also has organomegaly due to the accumulation of which of the following?

(A) Glucocerebroside
(B) Sphingolipids
(C) Heparin sulfate and dermatan sulfate
(D) Glycogen
(E) Galactose 1-phosphate

16. A newborn undergoes a physical exam relevant for hepatomegaly, inguinal hernia, and deformed chest (pectus carinatum). A family history of mucopolysaccharidosis (MPS) leads you to check enzyme activities from a sample including fibroblasts. The findings were significant for decreased activity in β-glucuronidase, which is indicative of which of the following syndromes?

(A) MPS type IH–Hurler syndrome
(B) MPS type IS–Scheie syndrome
(C) MPS type II–Hunter syndrome
(D) MPS type III–Sanfilippo syndrome
(E) MPS type VII–Sly syndrome

17. A 58-year-old man with a 30-year history of heavy drinking presents with confusion, unstable gait, and nystagmus. On mini-mental exam, he scores 21/30. A running diagnosis of Wernicke-Korsakoff syndrome is made. Which of the patient's enzymes of the pentose phosphate pathway is inhibited due to the vitamin deficiency in this case?

(A) Transaldolase
(B) Phosphopentose isomerase
(C) Transketolase
(D) Phosphopentose epimerase
(E) Glucose 6-phosphate dehydrogenase

18. A 24-year-old man comes in with multiple gunshot wounds. A type and cross give his blood type as type B⁻. He is taken immediately to the operating room because his blood pressure is dropping rapidly. Which of the following carbohydrate units will be found on the reducing end of his red blood cell surface protein?

(A) *N*-acetylgalactosamine
(B) *N*-acetylglucosamine
(C) Galactose
(D) Glucose
(E) Fructose

19. A 2-year-old child is brought for evaluation for developmental delay, mental retardation, and abnormal bleeding. After a thorough workup by a pediatric geneticist, the child is found to have a congenital disorder of *N*-linked oligosaccharides. Which of the following substances is involved in the synthesis of *N*-linked glycoproteins?

(A) α-Mannosidase
(B) α-Lactalbumin
(C) Thiamine pyrophosphate
(D) α-Fucosidase
(E) Dolichol phosphate

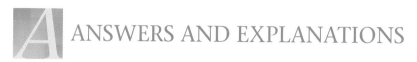

ANSWERS AND EXPLANATIONS

1–A. Starting from glucose 6-phosphate via the pentose phosphate pathway (occurring in the cytosol), 2 moles of NADPH are produced for each mole of CO_2 released. **No** adenosine triphosphate (ATP) is generated to ribulose 6-phosphate. Production of NADPH is the mainstay of the pathway and is present in red blood cells. In muscle, glycolysis is the major route of glucose metabolism, producing ATP.

2–C. Fructose 1-phosphate is cleaved by aldolase B (not fructokinase) to form dihydroxyacetone phosphate (DHAP) and glyceraldehydes. Hexokinase is used in other organs (**not the liver**) for entering glycolysis. Fructokinase produces fructose 1-phosphate. Deficiency of fructokinase leads to benign fructosuria, which is diagnosed incidentally.

3–D. The major products from the pentose phosphate pathway are ribose and NADPH. Ribulose 5-phosphate is isomerized to ribose 5-phosphate or epimerized to xylulose 5-phosphate, and the pathway does not produce ATP. $NADP^+$ is a hydrogen acceptor, and NADH is a hydrogen donor in glycolysis.

4–D. UDP derivatives of monosaccharides occur during the conversion of pyruvate to glucose in the liver. They are never formed for glucose metabolism. Galactose 1-phosphate + UDP-glucose → glucose 1-phosphate + UDP-galactose. The conversion of UDP-galactose to UDP-glucose occurs via UDP-glucose epimerase.

5–D. For *O*-linked glycoproteins, the initial sugar is added to a serine or threonine, and the sugars are added sequentially in the Golgi and the ER. Dolichol phosphate, sugar linkage to asparagines, and congenital disorders of glycosylation (CDG) refer to *N*-linked glycoproteins. No sugars are linked to tyrosine.

6–A. Glycosaminoglycans are long, linear carbohydrate chains that contain repeating disaccharide units, which usually contain a hexosamine and a uronic acid. They often contain sulfate groups. The uronic acid and sulfate residues cause them to be negatively charged. They are unbranched and do not contain *N*-acetylneuraminic acid.

7–B. UDP-galactose reacts with glucose to form lactose only in the mammary gland. α-Lactalbumin acts as a modifier of the enzyme galactosyl transferase, lowering its K_m for glucose. Glucose can be converted to UDP-glucose and epimerized to form the UDP-galactose used in lactose synthesis; therefore, dietary galactose is not required. Lactase is involved in lactose degradation.

8–B. Fructose 1-phosphate is cleaved by the action of aldolase B to form the products dihydroxyacetone phosphate and glyceraldehyde.

9–D. Glycoproteins contain branched oligosaccharide chains. These chains may be synthesized by addition of sugars to serine or threonine residues of the protein, or they may be synthesized on dolichol phosphate and transferred to asparagine residues on the protein. They are not positively charged. They are synthesized in the rough endoplasmic reticulum (RER) and Golgi and may be secreted from cells, anchored in the cell membrane, or segregated into lysosomes. They are internalized by endocytosis and degraded by lysosomal enzymes.

10–B. This patient has classic galactosemia, resulting from the inability to process galactose once the lactose in the breast milk is cleaved to its monomers, galactose and glucose. This disease results from an autosomal recessively inherited mutation in galactose 1-phosphate uridyltransferase. Logically, treatment is removal of lactose and galactose from the diet.

11–C. Drugs that cause oxidative stress, like primaquine and sulfa-containing drugs, result in hemolytic disease in patients with glucose 6-phosphate dehydrogenase (G6PD) deficiency. Deficiency of fructokinase is a benign disorder. Deficiency of aldolase B leads to hereditary fructose intolerance. Galactokinase deficiency leads to galactosemia, a slightly milder form then seen with galactose 1-phosphate uridyltransferase deficiency. Galactosyl transferase is important in the glycosylation of proteins as well as the metabolism of substances like bilirubin.

12–D. The cell delivers proteins based on the post-translational addition of carbohydrates, similar to putting an address on an envelope and dropping it at the post office. In I-cell disease the enzyme responsible for addressing the lysosomal hydrolase glycoprotein is deficient. Although the child's physical abnormalities are similar to other storage diseases, gingival hyperplasia is a unique clinical feature to I-cell disease.

13-B. Glucose enters tissues such as nerves, kidney, and the lens of the eye without the need of insulin being present. In these tissues, glucose is reduced to sorbitol by aldose reductase. The damage to these tissues is believed to be due to an osmotic effect because the sorbitol is unable to escape these tissues readily.

14–B. Prolactin, released from the anterior pituitary, stimulates the synthesis of α-lactalbumin, which lowers the K_m of galactosyl transferase for the substrate glucose. Glucose is then joined to galactose, thereby forming lactose. The same enzyme, galactosyl transferase, is also responsible for the glycosylation of proteins. Aldose reductase converts galactose to galactitol. NADPH is required to reduce glutathione. Sorbitol is converted to fructose by the action of sorbitol dehydrogenase.

15–C. Hurler syndrome results from a deficiency of α-L-iduronidase. Children with this illness have progressive mental retardation and have an average life span of 10 years. Death is usually due to accumulation of the glycosaminoglycans, such as heparin sulfate and dermatan sulfate, in the arteries, leading to arterial damage and ischemia.

16–E. Sly syndrome is one of the few lysosomal storage disorders with clinical manifestations in utero or at birth. The signs of coarse facial feature (gargoyle facies), mental developmental problems, and short stature can be seen in Sly syndrome as well as all the mucopolysaccharidoses.

17–C. Wernicke-Korsakoff syndrome results from a deficiency of thiamine due to any condition resulting in a poor nutritional intake. Heavy, long-term alcohol use is the most common association with Wernicke-Korsakoff syndrome. Thiamine is converted to thiamine pyrophosphate, which serves as a cofactor for several enzymes that function in glucose utilization. These enzymes include transketolase, pyruvate dehydrogenase, and α-ketoglutarate.

18–C. The human ABO blood types arise from differences in oligosaccharides glycoproteins and glycolipids on blood cell. Differences in a single sugar on the nonreducing end result in blood A, B, or O. In all three blood types, a generic oligosaccharide consisting of N-acetylglucosamine is attached to the red blood cell surface proteins. In the absence of an additional sugar, the result is type O. When galactose or *N*-acetylgalactose is covalently bound to the galactose, the type is considered B and A, respectively.

19–E. Dolichol phosphate is a long-chain alcohol associated with the ER that transfers branched polysaccharide chains to proteins during the synthesis of *N*-linked glycoproteins. Both α-mannosidase and α-fucosidase are enzymes involved in the lysosomal degradation of glycoproteins. α-Lactalbumin is involved in the synthesis of lactose. Thiamine pyrophosphate is a cofactor for transketolase in the pentose phosphate pathway.

CHAPTER 12

Fatty Acid and Triacylglycerol Synthesis

I. Fatty Acid and Triacylglycerol Synthesis

A. **Conversion of glucose to acetyl CoA for fatty acid synthesis** (Figure 12-1)

   1. **Glucose** enters liver cells and is converted via glycolysis to pyruvate, which enters mitochondria.
   2. **Pyruvate** is converted to acetyl coenzyme A (CoA) by pyruvate dehydrogenase and to **oxaloacetate** (OAA) by pyruvate carboxylase.
   3. Because acetyl CoA cannot directly cross the mitochondrial membrane and enter the cytosol to be used for the process of fatty acid synthesis, acetyl CoA and OAA condense to form **citrate**, which can cross the mitochondrial membrane.
   4. In the cytosol, **citrate is cleaved** to OAA and acetyl CoA by citrate lyase, an enzyme that requires adenosine triphosphate (ATP) and is induced by insulin.
      a. **OAA** from the citrate lyase reaction is reduced in the cytosol by NADH, producing NAD^+ and **malate.** The enzyme is cytosolic malate dehydrogenase.
      b. In a subsequent reaction, **malate** is converted to pyruvate, NADPH is produced, and CO_2 is released. The enzyme is the **malic enzyme** (also known as decarboxylating malate dehydrogenase or $NADP^+$-dependent malate dehydrogenase).
         (1) **Pyruvate** re-enters the mitochondrion and is reutilized.
         (2) **NADPH** supplies reducing equivalents for reactions that occur on the fatty acid synthase complex.
         (3) **NADPH** is produced not only by the **malic enzyme** but also by the **pentose phosphate pathway.**
   5. **Acetyl CoA** (from the citrate lyase reaction or from other sources) supplies carbons for fatty acid synthesis in the cytosol.

B. **Synthesis of fatty acids by the fatty acid synthase complex** (Figure 12-2)

   1. *Fatty acid synthase* is a multienzyme complex located in the cytosol. It has two identical subunits with seven catalytic activities.
      a. This enzyme contains a **phosphopantetheine residue,** derived from the vitamin pantothenic acid, and a **cysteine residue;** both contain sulfhydryl groups that can form thioesters with acyl groups.
      b. The growing fatty acyl chain moves from one to the other of these sulfhydryl residues as it is elongated.

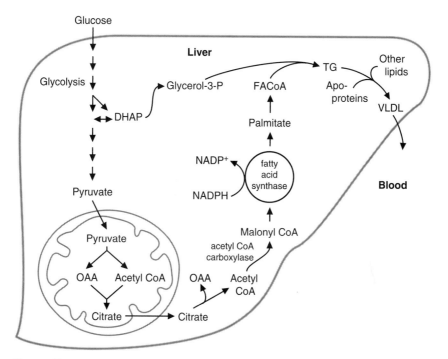

Figure 12-1   Lipogenesis, the synthesis of fatty acids (FA) and triacylglycerols (TG) from glucose, occurs mainly in the liver. CoA = coenzyme A; DHAP = dihydroxyacetone phosphate; OAA = oxaloacetate; VLDL = very low–density lipoprotein.

2. *Addition of two-carbon units*
   a. Initially, **acetyl CoA** reacts with the phosphopantetheinyl residue, and then the acetyl group is transferred to the cysteinyl residue. This acetyl group provides the ω-**carbon** of the fatty acid produced by the fatty acid synthase complex.
   b. A malonyl group from **malonyl CoA** forms a **thioester** with the phospho-pantetheinyl sulfhydryl group.
      (1) **Malonyl CoA** is formed from acetyl CoA by a carboxylation reaction that requires **biotin** and ATP.
      (2) The enzyme is **acetyl CoA carboxylase**, a regulatory enzyme that is inhibited by phosphorylation, activated by dephosphorylation and by citrate, and induced by insulin.
   c. The **acetyl group** on the fatty acid synthase complex condenses with the malonyl group; the CO_2 that was added to the malonyl group by acetyl CoA carboxylase is released; and a β-**ketoacyl group**, containing four carbons, is produced.
3. *Reduction of the β-ketoacyl group*
   a. The β-keto group is **reduced** by NADPH to a β-hydroxy group.
   b. Then **dehydration** occurs, producing an **enoyl group** with the double bond between carbons 2 and 3.
   c. Finally, the double bond is reduced by NADPH, and a **four-carbon acyl group** is generated.
   d. The **NADPH** for these reactions is produced by the **pentose phosphate pathway** and by the **malic enzyme**.

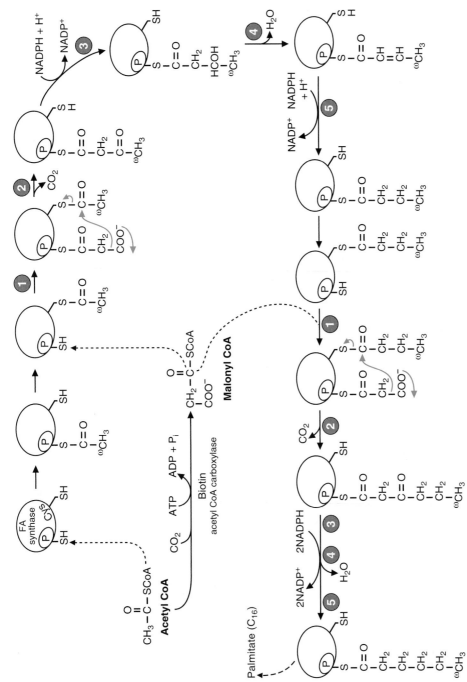

Figure 12-2 Fatty acid (FA) synthesis (palmitate). Malonyl coenzyme A (CoA) provides the 2-carbon units that are added to the growing fatty acyl chain. The addition and reduction steps (1–5) are repeated until palmitic acid is produced. ADP = adenosine diphosphate; ATP = adenosine triphosphate; Cys-SH = a cysteinyl residue; P = a phosphopantetheinyl group attached to the FA synthase complex; P_i = inorganic phosphate.

4. *Elongation of the growing fatty acyl chain*
   a. The acyl group is transferred to the cysteinyl sulfhydryl group, and **malonyl CoA** reacts with the phosphopantetheinyl group. Condensation of the acyl and malonyl groups occurs with the release of CO_2, followed by the three reactions that reduce the β-keto group. The chain thus grows longer by two carbons.
   b. This sequence of reactions repeats until the growing chain is 16 carbons in length.
   c. **Palmitate**, a 16-carbon saturated fatty acid, is the final product released by hydrolysis from the fatty acid synthase complex.

C. Elongation and desaturation of fatty acids

   1. *Palmitate* can be elongated and desaturated to form a **series of fatty acids.**
   2. *Elongation of long-chain fatty acids* occurs on the endoplasmic reticulum by reactions similar but not identical to those that occur on the fatty acid synthase complex.
      a. **Malonyl CoA** provides the two-carbon units that add to palmitoyl CoA or to longer-chain fatty acyl CoAs.
      b. Malonyl CoA condenses with the carbonyl group of the fatty acyl residue, and CO_2 is released.
      c. The β-keto group is reduced by NADPH to a β-hydroxy group; dehydration occurs; and a double bond is formed, which is reduced by NADPH.
   3. *Desaturation of fatty acids* is a complex process that requires O_2, NADPH, and cytochrome b_5.
      a. In humans, desaturases may add double bonds at the 9–10 position of a fatty acyl CoA and at intervals between carbon 9 and the carboxyl group.
      b. Plants can introduce double bonds between carbon 9 and the ω-carbon, but animals cannot. Therefore, certain unsaturated fatty acids from plants are required in the human diet.
      c. **Linoleate** (18:2, $\Delta^{9,12}$) and α-**linolenate** (18:3, $\Delta^{9,12,15}$) are the major sources of the essential fatty acids required in the human diet. They are used for synthesis of **arachidonic acid** and other polyunsaturated fatty acids from which eicosanoids (e.g., prostaglandins) are produced.

> *cc 12.1* **Total parenteral nutrition (TPN)** is an **intravenous** form of nutrition containing **essential fatty acids required in the diet.** TPN can be administered in cases of stress from chronic illness, infection, trauma, burn patients, postsurgery recovery, starvation, kidney failure, or liver failure. TPN allows intake of nutritional requirements **without using the gastrointestinal tract.**

> *cc 12.2* **Olestra** (Olean) is a **fat replacement** that has a sucrose polyester backbone with 6 to 8 fatty acid side chains, making it **too bulky to be digested and absorbed** in intestinal cells. Olestra passes through the gastrointestinal tract without being absorbed, leading to side effects, such as **flatulence, bloating,** and **diarrhea.**

D. Synthesis of triacylglycerols (Figure 12-3)

   1. **In intestinal epithelial** cells, triacylglycerol synthesis occurs by a different pathway than in other tissues. This triacylglycerol becomes a component of chylomicrons. Ultimately, the fatty acyl groups are stored in adipose triacylglycerols.
   2. **In the liver and adipose tissue,** glycerol 3-phosphate provides the glycerol moiety that reacts with two fatty acyl CoAs to form **phosphatidic acid.** The phosphate

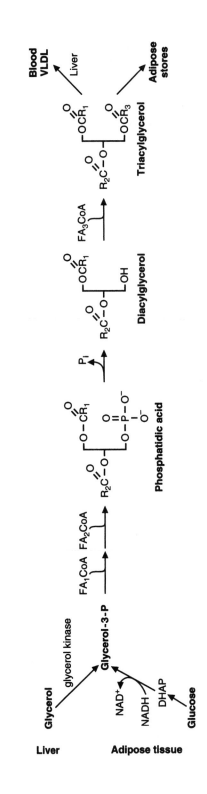

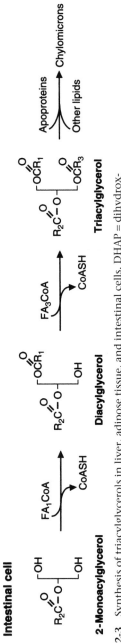

Figure 12-3 Synthesis of triacylglycerols in liver, adipose tissue, and intestinal cells. DHAP = dihydroxyacetone phosphate; glycerol-3-P = glycerol 3-phosphate; R = aliphatic chain of a fatty acid; P_i = inorganic phosphate; VLDL = very low-density lipoprotein.

group is cleaved to form a diacylglycerol, which reacts with another fatty acyl CoA to form a triacylglycerol.

> *cc* **12.3** Elevation of the **serum triglyceride (triacylglycerol) level above 1000 mg/dL** can cause **pancreatitis,** an inflammation of the pancreas that causes severe abdominal pain.

a. **The liver** can use glycerol to produce glycerol 3-phosphate by a reaction that requires ATP and is catalyzed by glycerol kinase.
b. **Adipose tissue,** which **lacks glycerol kinase,** cannot generate glycerol 3-phosphate from glycerol.

> *cc* **12.4** **Alcoholic fatty liver** occurs due to excessive consumption of ethanol. The liver changes from a normal red, dense appearance to a yellow, oily, fatty appearance due to excessive fat globule deposition.

c. **Both liver and adipose tissue** can convert glucose, through glycolysis, to **dihydroxyacetone phosphate (DHAP),** which is reduced by NADH to glycerol 3-phosphate.
d. **Triacylglycerol** is **stored in adipose tissue.**
e. In the **liver,** triacylglycerol is incorporated into **very low–density lipoprotein (VLDL),** which enters the blood. Ultimately, the fatty acyl groups are stored in adipose triacylglycerols.

> *cc* **12.5** **Chylous ascites** is the **extravasation of milky chyle** (lymphatic fluid) with a triglyceride (triacylglycerol) level > 200 mg/dL **into the peritoneal cavity of the abdomen.** (Fluid collection in the peritoneal cavity is called ascites.) Chylous ascites occurs in conditions such as **abdominal surgery, abdominal trauma,** and **cancers** such as lymphomas and in conditions causing obstruction or disruption of the lymphatic system.

E. **Regulation of triacylglycerol synthesis from carbohydrate**

1. Synthesis of triacylglycerols from carbohydrate occurs in the liver in the **fed state.**
2. **Key regulatory enzymes** in the pathway are activated, and a high-carbohydrate diet causes their induction.
   a. The glycolytic enzymes **glucokinase, phosphofructokinase 1,** and **pyruvate kinase** are active.
   b. **Pyruvate dehydrogenase** is dephosphorylated and active.
   c. **Pyruvate carboxylase** is activated by acetyl CoA.
   d. **Citrate lyase** is inducible.
   e. **Acetyl CoA carboxylase** is induced, activated by citrate, and converted to its active, dephosphorylated state by a phosphatase that is stimulated by insulin.
   f. The **fatty acid synthase complex** is inducible.
3. **NADPH,** which provides the reducing equivalents for fatty acid synthesis, is produced by the inducible **malic enzyme** and by the inducible enzymes of the pentose phosphate pathway: **glucose 6-phosphate dehydrogenase** and **6-phosphogluconate dehydrogenase.**
4. **Malonyl CoA,** the product of acetyl CoA carboxylase, **inhibits carnitine acyltransferase I** (carnitine palmitoyl transferase I), thus preventing newly synthesized fatty acids from entering mitochondria and undergoing β-oxidation. (Figure 12-4)

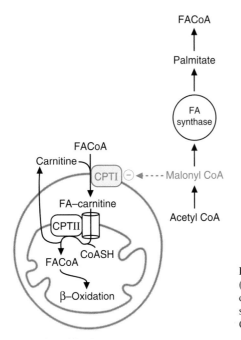

Figure 12-4 Inhibition of carnitine acyltransferase I (carnitine palmitoyl transferase I [CPTI]) by malonyl coenzyme A (CoA). This mechanism prevents newly synthesized fatty acids from immediately oxidizing. CoASH = ; FA = fatty acyl group.

II. Formation of Triacylglycerol Stores in Adipose Tissue

A. **Hydrolysis of triacylglycerols of chylomicrons and VLDL** (Figure 12-5)

1. The triacylglycerols of chylomicrons and VLDL are hydrolyzed to **fatty acids** and **glycerol** by lipoprotein lipase, which is attached to membranes of cells in the walls of capillaries in adipose tissue.

2. **Lipoprotein lipase** is synthesized in adipose cells and is secreted by a process stimulated by insulin, which is elevated after a meal. **Apoprotein C$_{II}$,** which is transferred from high-density lipoprotein (HDL) to chylomicrons and VLDL, is an activator of lipoprotein lipase.

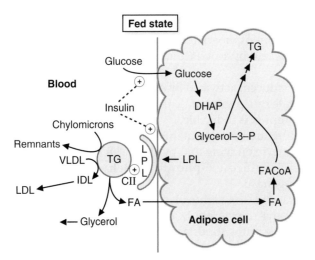

Figure 12-5 Formation of triacylglycerol (TG) stores in adipose tissue in the fed state. CII = apoprotein C$_{II}$; CoA = coenzyme A; DHAP = dihydroxyacetone phosphate; FA = fatty acid; IDL = intermediate-density lipoprotein; LPL = lipoprotein lipase; ⊕ = stimulated by; circled TG = triacylglycerol of chylomicrons and very low–density lipoprotein (VLDL).

Obesity is associated with **genetics, overeating,** and sedentary life habits. This condition is more common in industrialized countries.

B. **Synthesis of triacylglycerols in adipose tissue**

1. **Fatty acids** released from chylomicrons and VLDL by lipoprotein lipase are taken up by adipose cells and converted to triacylglycerols, but glycerol is not used because adipose tissue lacks glycerol kinase (see Figure 12-3).
   a. The **transport of glucose** into adipose cells is **stimulated by insulin**, which is elevated after a meal.
   b. Glucose is converted to **DHAP**, which is reduced by NADH to form **glycerol 3-phosphate**, which is used to produce the glycerol moiety.
2. The triacylglycerols are stored in large fat globules in adipose cells.

cc 12.7 **Hyperlipidemias (types I, IIa, IIb, III, IV, and V) are defined as triglyceride (triacylglycerol) levels >200 mg/dL.** All hyperlipidemias, except type IIa, cause elevations in serum triglyceride level. Clinical manifestations include **pancreatitis** (when triacylglycerol level is >1000 mg/dL), **xanthomas** (yellow fat papules on the skin), lipemia retinalis (pale pink or milky appearance of retinal blood vessels), and **hepatomegaly.**

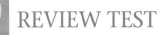 REVIEW TEST

*Directions: Each of the numbered questions or incomplete statements in this section is followed by answers or by completions of the statement. Select the **one** lettered answer or completion that is **best** in each case.*

1. Which of the following is a correct step in the conversion of glucose to acetyl CoA for fatty acid synthesis?

(A) Glucose enters the mitochondria and then undergoes glycolysis.
(B) Pyruvate is converted to acetyl coenzyme A (CoA) and oxaloacetate.
(C) Acetyl CoA crosses the mitochondrial membrane to be used as carbons for fatty acid synthesis.
(D) Two acetyl CoA molecules condense to form citrate.
(E) Citrate is cleaved to form malonyl CoA.

2. Which of the following supplies the two-carbon units that are added to the elongating fatty acid chain?

(A) Glucose
(B) Acetyl CoA
(C) Malonyl CoA
(D) β-Ketoacyl group
(E) NADPH

3. In the synthesis of fatty acids from glucose, which of the following is the complex that forms the growing fatty acyl chain?

(A) Pyruvate dehydrogenase
(B) Pyruvate carboxylase
(C) Citrate lyase
(D) Malate dehydrogenase
(E) Fatty acid synthase

4. Fatty acids are stored in adipose tissue as which of the following?

(A) Chylomicrons
(B) Very low–density lipoprotein (VLDL)
(C) Glycerol
(D) Triacylglycerols
(E) Acetyl CoA

5. The conversion of acetyl CoA to malonyl CoA requires which of the following?

(A) Biotin
(B) Adenosine diphosphate (ADP) + inorganic phosphorus (P_i)

(C) NAD^+
(D) NADPH
(E) H_2O

6. NADPH is synthesized via the action of which of the following enzymes?

(A) Glucose 6-phosphate dehydrogenase
(B) Pyruvate dehydrogenase
(C) Acetyl CoA carboxylase
(D) Glycerol kinase
(E) Lipoprotein lipase

7. Which of the following hydrolyzes triacylglycerols from chylomicrons and VLDL to fatty acids and glycerol?

(A) Glucokinase
(B) Pyruvate carboxylase
(C) Lipoprotein lipase
(D) Citrate lyase
(E) Fatty acid synthase complex

8. Which of the following is the initial step of fatty acid synthesis?

(A) Glucose is converted to pyruvate.
(B) Oxaloacetate and acetyl CoA form citrate.
(C) Citrate is cleaved to form oxaloacetate.
(D) Oxaloacetate is reduced to form malate.
(E) Malate is converted to pyruvate.

9. Insulin promotes which of the following?

(A) Transport of glucose into cells
(B) Triacylglycerol conversion to diacylglycerol
(C) Fatty acid oxidation
(D) Inactivity of lipoprotein lipase
(E) Increased blood glucose level

10. Glucose can be converted to glycerol 3-phosphate through which of the following intermediates?

(A) Glycerol
(B) Dihydroxyacetone phosphate (DHAP)

(C) Acetyl CoA
(D) Pyruvate
(E) Malate

11. A 35-year-old man presents with yellow xanthomas on his skin and hepatomegaly (enlarged liver). His triglyceride (triacylglycerol) level is 1500 mg/dL (normal: 150–199 mg/dL). He is diagnosed with type V hyperlipidemia. Triacylglycerols are primarily synthesized in which of the following tissues?

(A) Skeletal muscle
(B) Heart muscle
(C) Liver
(D) Spleen
(E) Blood cells

12. A 45-year-old woman presents with severe upper abdominal pain, nausea, and vomiting. She is diagnosed with pancreatitis (an inflammation of the pancreas). Her serum triacylglycerol level is found to be 5000 mg/dL and is deemed as the cause of her pancreatitis. To form triacylglycerol, which of the following is added to diacylglycerol?

(A) Glycerol
(B) Glycerol 3-phosphate
(C) Fatty acyl CoA
(D) Acetyl CoA
(E) Malonyl CoA

13. An 18-year-old woman presents with xanthomas on her eyelids. She is found to have a rare genetic deficiency of lipoprotein lipase and is diagnosed with type I hyperlipidemia. In this disorder, chylomicrons are abnormally elevated in the serum. In what type of cell are triacylglycerols packaged into chylomicrons?

(A) Intestinal epithelial cell
(B) Liver cell
(C) Muscle cell
(D) Heart cell
(E) Adipose cell

14. A 30-year-old pregnant woman has a sugar craving and consumes a hot fudge sundae. Her serum glucose level increases, which induces production of insulin. Insulin induces the action of acetyl CoA carboxylase in fatty acid synthesis. Which of the following statements best describes this regulatory enzyme?

(A) It is activated by carboxylation.
(B) It is inhibited by phosphorylation.
(C) It converts malonyl CoA to acetyl CoA.
(D) It catalyzes a reaction that requires biotin and ATP.
(E) It catalyzes a reaction that condenses an acetyl group with a malonyl group.

15. A 70-year-old man with a history of lymphoma (a blood cell cancer that causes swollen lymph nodes) presents with abdominal distension from fluid collection (ascites). This fluid is collected from his abdomen, revealing chylous ascites, which is fluid with an abnormally high triacylglycerol content. In the synthesis of triacylglycerols from fatty acids, how many carbons are in the product released from the fatty acid synthase complex?

(A) 14
(B) 16
(C) 18
(D) 20
(E) 22

16. An 18-year-old woman is diagnosed as obese. She maintains a sedentary lifestyle and eats a high-fat, high-sugar diet. Maintenance of this diet and lifestyle has led to lipogenesis and obesity. Which aspect of lipogenesis affects fatty acids?

(A) The primary source of carbons for fatty acid synthesis is from glycerol.
(B) Fatty acids are synthesized from acetyl CoA in the mitochondria.
(C) Fatty acid synthesis and esterification to glycerol to form triacylglycerols occur mainly in muscle cells.
(D) The fatty acyl chain on the fatty acid synthase complex is elongated two carbons at a time.
(E) $NADP^+$, which is important for fatty acid synthesis, is produced by the pentose phosphate pathway.

17. A 50-year-old, alcoholic male presents with a ruddy face, distended abdomen, and an enlarged, fatty liver. Fatty acids react with glycerol 3-phosphate to form triacylglycerols, which accumulate and cause fatty liver. The liver has glycerol kinase, while adipose tissue lacks glycerol kinase. As a result, in adipose tissue, which of the following occurs?

(A) Glucose cannot be converted to DHAP.
(B) Glycerol cannot be converted to glycerol 3-phosphate.
(C) DHAP cannot be converted to glycerol 3-phosphate.
(D) Diacylglycerol cannot be converted to triacylglycerol.
(E) Triacylglycerols cannot be stored.

18. A 25-year-old man is brought to the emergency room after a motor vehicle accident. He has a dislocated hip, rib fractures, and a facial laceration. Toxicology screen shows a high level of ethanol in his blood. Oxidation of ethanol produces acetaldehyde and NADH. A high level of NADH relative to NAD slows the tricarboxylic acid (TCA) cycle and promotes the conversion of dihydroxyacetone phosphate to glycerol 3-phosphate. In the liver and adipose tissue, glycerol 3-phosphate combines with two fatty acyl CoAs to form which of the following?

(A) Phosphatidic acid
(B) 2-Monoacylglycerol

(C) Diacylglycerol
(D) Triacylglycerol
(E) VLDL

19. A 45-year-old man presents with multiple gunshot wounds to the abdomen. He undergoes emergent surgery, during which a part of his intestines is resected. After surgery, he is placed on total parenteral nutrition (TPN), an intravenous form of nutrition. TPN supplies an essential fatty acid required in the human diet. Which of the following is this essential fatty acid?

(A) Palmitate
(B) Linoleate
(C) Phosphatidic acid
(D) Glycerol
(E) Glucose

20. A 35-year-old woman presents with flatulence, bloating, and steatorrhea (fat in the stool). She has been eating large amounts of potato chips that were made using Olestra, a fat substitute. Normally, dietary triacylglycerols are hydrolyzed into components that are reconstructed into triacylglycerols that become a component of chylomicrons. In the intestinal cell, the initial precursor for triacylglycerol synthesis is which of the following?

(A) Glycerol
(B) Glycerol 3-phosphate
(C) 2-Monoacylglycerol
(D) Phosphatidic acid
(E) Acetyl CoA

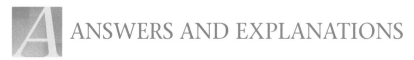

1–B. Glucose enters the cytosol and undergoes glycolysis to be converted to pyruvate. Pyruvate enters the mitochondria and is subsequently converted to acetyl coenzyme A (CoA) and oxaloacetate. Since acetyl CoA cannot cross the mitochondrial membrane, acetyl CoA and oxaloacetate condense to form citrate, which crosses back into the cytosol. In the cytosol, citrate is cleaved back to acetyl CoA and oxaloacetate. Oxaloacetate is reduced by NADH, producing NAD^+ and malate.

2–C. The three-carbon compound, malonyl CoA, is decarboxylated to provide a two-carbon unit for fatty acid synthesis. With each two-carbon addition, the β-ketoacyl group on the growing chain is reduced by NADPH. Glucose is the precursor and source of carbons for fatty acid synthesis.

3–E. Fatty acid synthase is a multienzyme complex that initially reacts with acetyl CoA, and eventually elongates to form a fatty acid. Pyruvate dehydrogenase, pyruvate carboxylase, citrate lyase, and malate dehydrogenase are involved in the conversion of glucose to acetyl CoA, which then binds to the fatty acid synthase complex.

4–D. Fatty acids are stored in adipose tissue as triacylglycerols. Triacylglycerols are packaged into very low–density lipoproteins (VLDLs) in the liver and released into the blood. Triacylglycerols are secreted in chylomicrons via the lymph into the blood.

5–A. The conversion of acetyl CoA to malonyl CoA requires biotin and adenosine triphosphate (ATP). NADPH supplies reducing equivalents for reactions that occur on the fatty acid synthase complex.

6–A. NADPH is produced by the inducible malic enzyme and by the inducible enzymes of the pentose phosphate pathway: glucose 6-phosphate dehydrogenase and 6-phosphogluconate dehydrogenase. Pyruvate dehydrogenase and acetyl CoA carboxylase are involved in fatty acid synthesis from carbohydrate. Glycerol kinase is involved in triacylglycerol synthesis in the liver. Lipoprotein lipase is involved in the hydrolysis of triacylglycerols.

7–C. Lipoprotein lipase hydrolyzes triacylglycerols from chylomicrons and VLDL to fatty acids and glycerol. Glucokinase, pyruvate carboxylase, citrate lyase, and the fatty acid synthase complex are enzymes involved in fatty acid synthesis.

8–A. In the initial step of fatty acid synthesis, glucose enters liver cells and is converted via glycolysis to form pyruvate. Pyruvate undergoes subsequent reactions to form oxaloacetate, malate, and acetyl CoA. Acetyl CoA and oxaloacetate condense to form citrate.

9–A. Insulin promotes transport of glucose into cells for triacylglycerol synthesis, resulting in a decreased blood glucose level. Triacylglycerols are formed from diacylglycerol and a fatty acyl CoA. Fatty acid synthesis is promoted. Lipoprotein lipase is activated.

10–B. Through glycolysis, glucose can be converted to dihydroxyacetone phosphate (DHAP), which is reduced by NADH to glycerol 3-phosphate (G-3-P). Glycerol is converted to G-3-P by glycerol kinase. Through glycolysis, glucose is converted to pyruvate, which is converted to acetyl CoA by pyruvate dehydrogenase. Malate is converted to pyruvate by the malic enzyme.

11–C. Triacylglycerols are formed primarily in the liver, but they can also be generated in adipose tissue and intestinal cells. In the liver, they are packaged in VLDL and are secreted into the blood. Triacylglycerols are stored in adipose tissue.

12–C. A triacylglycerol is formed when a diacylglycerol reacts with a fatty acyl CoA. Glycerol and glycerol 3-phosphate form the backbone of the triacylglycerol. Acetyl CoA and malonyl CoA are involved in fatty acid synthesis.

13–A. In intestinal epithelial cells, triacylglycerols are bound to apoproteins and other lipids to form chylomicrons. In the liver, triacylglycerols are incorporated into VLDL, which enter the blood. Triacylglycerols are stored in adipose tissue.

14–B. Acetyl CoA carboxylase is a regulatory enzyme that is inhibited by phosphorylation, activated by dephosphorylation, and induced by insulin. Acetyl CoA carboxylase catalyzes a carboxylation reaction requiring biotin and ATP, in which acetyl CoA is converted to malonyl CoA.

15–B. Palmitate, a 16-carbon fatty acid, is the product released by hydrolysis from the fatty acid synthase complex. It can be elongated by 2 carbons to form stearate. Arachidonic acid can be synthesized from the essential fatty acid linoleate, but it cannot be produced from palmitate. Fatty acids synthesized in the liver are converted to triacylglycerols.

16–D. The primary source of carbons for fatty acid synthesis is from dietary carbohydrate. Fatty acids are synthesized from acetyl CoA in the cytosol, and esterification to glycerol to form triacylglycerols occurs primarily in the liver. The fatty acyl chain on the fatty acid synthase complex is elongated 2 carbons at a time. With each 2-carbon addition to the elongating chain, the β-keto group is reduced in a reaction that requires NADPH. NADPH is a reducing equivalent produced by the pentose phosphate pathway and the malic enzyme.

17–B. The liver can use glycerol to produce glycerol 3-phosphate (G-3-P) by a reaction that requires ATP and is catalyzed by glycerol kinase. The liver can also produce G-3-P by converting glucose through glycolysis to DHAP, which is reduced to G-3-P. Adipose tissue lacks glycerol kinase and thus cannot generate G-3-P from glycerol; therefore, it must convert glucose to DHAP, which is then reduced to G-3-P.

18–A. Glycerol 3-phosphate and two fatty acyl CoAs combine to form phosphatidic acid. Diacylglycerol, triacylglycerol, and VLDL are then formed from phosphatidic acid in the liver. 2-Monoacylglycerol is the precursor of triacylglycerol synthesis in the intestinal cell.

19–B. Linoleate and α-linolenate are the major sources of the essential fatty acids required in the human diet. Palmitate is the fatty acid released from the fatty acid synthase complex. Phosphatidic acid is an intermediate in triacylglycerol synthesis, which is formed using glycerol as a precursor in the liver and using glucose as a precursor in adipose tissue.

20–C. The precursors for triacylglycerol synthesis in the intestinal cell are fatty acids and 2-monoacylglycerol. Glycerol is converted to glycerol 3-phosphate as the precursors for triacylglycerol synthesis, in which phosphatidic acid serves as an intermediate. Acetyl CoA provides the carbons for fatty acid synthesis.

Fatty Acid Oxidation

I. Fatty Acid Oxidation

A. Activation of fatty acids

1. In the cytosol of the cell, long-chain fatty acids are activated by **adenosine triphosphate (ATP)** and **coenzyme A (CoA)**, and **fatty acyl CoA** is formed (Figure 13-1). Short-chain fatty acids are activated in mitochondria.

2. The **ATP** is converted to **adenosine monophosphate (AMP) and pyrophosphate (PP$_i$)**, which is cleaved by pyrophosphatase to two inorganic phosphates (2 P$_i$). Because two high-energy phosphate bonds are cleaved, the equivalent of 2 molecules of ATP is used for fatty acid activation.

> *cc 13.1* **Anorexia nervosa** is a disease of intentional **starvation** or **bingeing/ purging** resulting in weight loss of 25% below expected weight. Food restriction results in increased fatty acid oxidation for ATP generation.

B. Transport of fatty acyl CoA from the cytosol into mitochondria (Figure 13-2)

1. **Fatty acyl CoA** from the cytosol reacts with **carnitine** in the outer mitochondrial membrane, forming fatty acyl carnitine. The enzyme is **carnitine acyl transferase I (CATI)**, which is also called carnitine palmitoyl transferase I (CPTI). **Fatty acyl carnitine** passes to the inner membrane, where it **re-forms fatty acyl CoA**, which enters the matrix. The second enzyme is carnitine acyl transferase II (CAT II).

> *cc 13.2* **Primary carnitine deficiency** is caused by a deficiency in the plasma membrane carnitine transporter, leading to **urinary wasting of carnitine.** Subsequent depletion of intracellular carnitine impairs transport of long-chain fatty acids into mitochondria. Thus, long-chain fatty acids are not available for oxidation and energy production.

> *cc 13.3* **Jamaican vomiting syndrome** manifests as sudden onset of **vomiting, abdominal discomfort,** and **hypoglycemia** (low serum glucose level) and is caused by ingestion of unripe ackee fruit, which contains high levels of hypoglycin. Hypoglycin is metabolized to **form nonmetabolizable carnitine** and CoA esters.

2. **CATI,** which catalyzes the transfer of acyl groups from coenzyme A to carnitine, is **inhibited by malonyl CoA**, an intermediate in fatty acid synthesis. Therefore, when fatty acids are being synthesized in the cytosol, malonyl CoA inhibits their

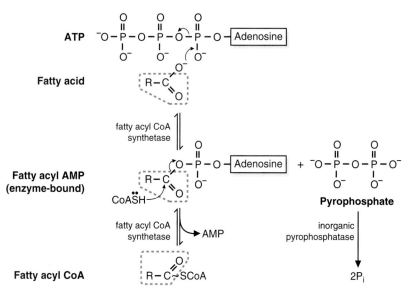

Figure 13-1 Activation of a fatty acid by coenzyme A (CoA) synthetase. AMP = adenosine monophosphate; ATP = adenosine triphosphate; P_i = inorganic phosphate.

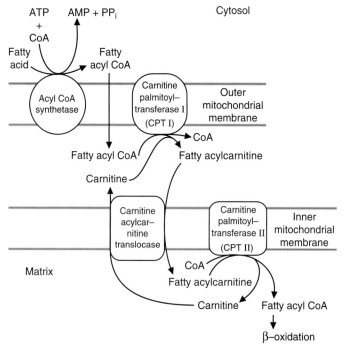

Figure 13-2 Transport of long-chain fatty acids into the mitochondria. AMP = adenosine diphosphate; ATP = adenosine triphosphate; CoA = coenzyme A; PP_i = inorganic pyrophosphate.

transport into mitochondria and thus prevents a futile cycle (synthesis followed by immediate degradation).

> cc *13.4* **CATI deficiency** results in intermittent **ataxia, oculomotor palsy** (cranial nerve [CN] III), hypotonia, **mental confusion,** and disturbance of consciousness.

3. Inside the mitochondrion, fatty acyl CoA undergoes β-**oxidation.**

C. β-**Oxidation of even-chain fatty acids**

1. β-**Oxidation** (in which all reactions involve the β-carbon of a fatty acyl CoA) is a spiral consisting of four sequential steps.
   a. The first three steps are similar to those in the tricarboxylic acid (TCA) cycle between succinate and oxaloacetate.
   b. These steps are repeated until all the carbons of an even-chain fatty acyl CoA are converted to acetyl CoA (Figure 13-3). (Step 1)

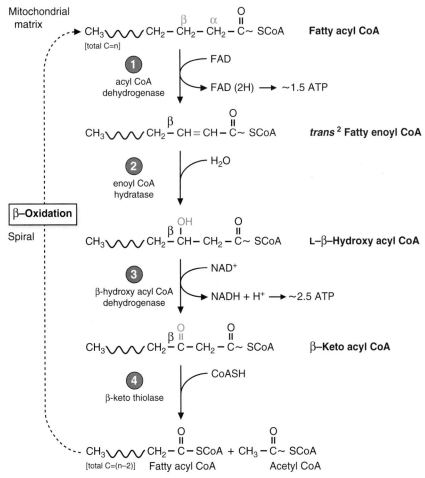

Figure 13-3 Steps of β-oxidation. The four steps are repeated until the even-chain fatty acid is completely converted to acetyl coenzyme A (CoA). ATP = adenosine triphosphate.

2. **Flavin adenine dinucleotide (FAD) accepts hydrogens** from a fatty acyl CoA in the first step.
   a. A double bond is produced between the α-and β-carbons, and an enoyl CoA is formed.
   b. The $FADH_2$ that is produced interacts with the electron transport chain, generating ATP.
   c. Enzyme: **acyl CoA dehydrogenase**

> cc **13.5** **Medium-chain acyl CoA dehydrogenase (MCAD) deficiency** is a **deficiency of acyl CoA dehydrogenase,** an enzyme required in the first step of the β-oxidation cycle. In patients with this deficiency, when serum glucose levels are low (**hypoglycemia**) due to fasting, infection, or increased amount of time between feedings, **fatty acids cannot be oxidized** as an alternate form of energy.

3. **H_2O adds across the double bond,** via the enzyme **enoyl CoA hydratase,** and a β-hydroxyacyl CoA is formed. (Step 2)
4. **β-Hydroxyacyl CoA is oxidized** by NAD^+ to a γ-ketoacyl CoA.
   a. The NADH that is produced interacts with the electron transport chain, generating ATP.
   b. The enzyme: L-3-hydroxyacyl CoA dehydrogenase (which is specific for the L-isomer of the β-hydroxyacyl CoA) (Step 3)
5. The **bond between the α- and β-carbons** of the β-ketoacyl CoA is cleaved by a **thiolase** that requires coenzyme A.
   a. Acetyl CoA is produced from the 2 carbons at the carboxyl end of the original fatty acyl CoA, and the remaining carbons form a fatty acyl CoA that is 2 carbons shorter than the original.
   b. Enzyme: **β-keto thiolase** (Step 4)
6. The shortened **fatty acyl CoA repeats** these four steps. Repetitions continue until all the carbons of the original fatty acyl CoA are converted to acetyl CoA.
   a. The 16-carbon palmitoyl CoA undergoes seven repetitions.
   b. In the last repetition, a 4-carbon fatty acyl CoA (butyryl CoA) is cleaved to 2 acetyl CoAs.
7. **Energy is generated** from the products of β-oxidation.
   a. When 1 palmitoyl CoA is oxidized, 7 $FADH_2$, 7 NADH, and 8 acetyl CoA are formed.
      (1) The 7 $FADH_2$ each generate approximately 2 ATP, for a total of about 14 ATP.
      (2) The 7 NADH each generate about 3 ATP, for a total of about 21 ATP.
      (3) The 8 acetyl CoA can enter the TCA cycle, each producing about 12 ATP, for a total of about 96 ATP.
      (4) From the oxidation of palmitoyl CoA to CO_2 and H_2O, a total of about 131 ATP are produced.
   b. The **net ATP** produced from palmitate that enters the cell from the blood is about 129 because palmitate must undergo activation (a process that requires the equivalent of 2 ATP) before it can be oxidized (131 ATP–2 ATP = 129 ATP).
   c. **Oxidation of other fatty acids** will yield different amounts of ATP.

> cc **13.6** **Short bowel syndrome** is a disorder defined by functional or anatomic loss of the small intestine, causing **diarrhea** and **fat malabsorption** and leading to **increased β-oxidation to generate energy.**

> cc *13.7* **Gastric bypass surgery** can be performed in cases of morbid obesity to induce permanent weight loss by **increased β-oxidation to generate energy.** The stomach is made smaller using **staples or banding,** and the stomach is then connected to the jejunum, bypassing the proximal portion of the small intestines.

D. **Oxidation of odd-chain and unsaturated fatty acids**

1. **Odd-chain fatty acids** produce acetyl CoA and propionyl CoA.
   a. These fatty acids repeat the four steps of the β-oxidation spiral, producing **acetyl CoA** until the last cleavage when the 3 remaining carbons are released as propionyl CoA.
   b. **Propionyl CoA,** but not acetyl CoA, can be converted to glucose.
2. **Unsaturated fatty acids,** which comprise about half the fatty acid residues in human lipids, require enzymes in addition to the four enzymes that catalyze the repetitive steps of the β-oxidation spiral.
   a. **β-Oxidation** occurs until a double bond of the unsaturated fatty acid is near the carboxyl end of the fatty acyl chain.
   b. If the double bond is not between the α- and β-carbons in a trans-configuration, it is moved so that it is α–β trans. The normal steps of β-oxidation can then proceed.

E. **ω-Oxidation of fatty acids** (Figure 13-4)

1. The ω (omega)-**carbon** (the methyl carbon) of fatty acids is oxidized to a carboxyl group in the endoplasmic reticulum.
2. β-Oxidation can then occur in mitochondria at this end of the fatty acid as well as from the original carboxyl end. **Dicarboxylic acids** are produced.

F. **Oxidation of very long–chain fatty acids in peroxisomes** (Figure 13-5)

1. The process differs from β-oxidation in that **molecular O_2 is used, hydrogen peroxide** (H_2O_2) is formed, and **no ATP** is generated.
2. The shorter chain fatty acids that are produced travel to mitochondria, where they undergo β-oxidation, generating ATP.

> cc *13.8* **Zellweger syndrome** is a peroxisomal disorder resulting in **accumulation of very long–chain fatty acids** because the **peroxisome is not properly formed.** Clinical manifestations include congenital craniofacial dysmorphism, psychomotor retardation, and seizures. Death results in the first year of life.

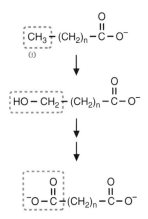

Figure 13-4 ω-Oxidation of fatty acids converts them to dicarboxylic acid.

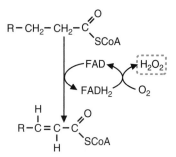

Figure 13-5 Oxidation of fatty acids in peroxisomes. The first step of β-oxidation is catalyzed by a flavin adenine dinucleotide (FAD)–containing oxidase.

> *cc 13.9* **Adrenoleukodystrophy** is the rare metabolic disorder depicted in the 1993 film "Lorenzo's Oil." **Very long–chain fatty acids (VLCFA) accumulate** in the brain (causing demyelination) and in the adrenal cortex (causing degeneration) because of an **inability to transport VLCFA into peroxisomes.** Clinical manifestations include psychomotor retardation and seizures.

G. **α-Oxidation of fatty acids**

1. **VLCFA** are oxidized at the α-carbon (mainly in brain and other nervous tissue), and the carboxyl carbon is released as CO_2.
2. The fatty acid is thus degraded 1 carbon at a time.

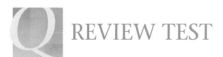

*Directions: Each of the numbered questions or incomplete statements in this section is followed by answers or by completions of the statement. Select the **one** lettered answer or completion that is **best** in each case.*

1. Newly synthesized fatty acids are not immediately degraded because of which of the following reasons?

(A) Fatty acid synthesis occurs in tissues that do not contain the enzymes that degrade fatty acids.

(B) High NAD^+ levels inhibit fatty acid breakdown.

(C) Transport of fatty acids into mitochondria is inhibited under fatty acid synthesis.

(D) Fatty acid synthesis occurs in the mitochondria, while fatty acid β-oxidation occurs in the cytosol.

(E) Newly synthesized fatty acids cannot be converted to their coenzyme A (CoA) derivatives.

2. Odd-chain long fatty acid breakdown produces which of the following?

(A) Acetyl CoA only

(B) Acetyl CoA and propionyl CoA

(C) Butyryl CoA

(D) Decanoyl CoA

(E) Palmitoyl CoA

3. The activation of long-chain fatty acids requires which of the following?

(A) 2 adenosine triphosphates (ATP)

(B) 2 ATP and CoA

(C) 2 ATP, CoA, and fatty acyl CoA

(D) Fatty acyl carnitine

(E) Carnitine acyltransferase I and II

4. Which of the following statements describes β-oxidation of fatty acids?

(A) One acetyl CoA molecule is produced in each turn of the β-oxidation spiral.

(B) β-oxidation is the synthesis of a fatty acyl CoA.

(C) Energy is consumed during β-oxidation of fatty acids.

(D) β-oxidation of all fatty acids yields the same amount of ATP.

(E) Carnitine is produced.

5. Which of the following statements about fatty acids is accurate?

(A) Fatty acids are very insoluble in water and are transported in the blood by albumin.

(B) When fatty acids are activated in the cytosol, ATP is converted to adenosine diphosphate (ADP).

(C) Fatty acids can be oxidized to CO_2 and H_2O in the mitochondria of red blood cells.

(D) In α-oxidation, dicarboxylic acids are produced.

(E) In ω-oxidation, the carboxyl carbon is released as CO_2; thus the fatty acid is degraded 1 carbon at a time.

6. In one turn of the β-oxidation spiral, how many carbons are removed from fatty acyl CoA?

(A) 1

(B) 2

(C) 3

(D) 4

(E) 6

7. β-Oxidation of long-chain fatty acids occurs primarily in which of the following locations?

(A) Cytosol

(B) Peroxisome

(C) Mitochondria

(D) Endoplasmic reticulum

(E) Golgi apparatus

8. Abundance of which of the following promotes β-oxidation of fatty acids?

(A) ATP

(B) NAD^+

(C) FADH$_2$
(D) Acetyl CoA
(E) Propionyl CoA

9. What is the role of the thiolase in the last step of β-oxidation?

(A) Cleaves off CoA
(B) Cleaves the bond between the α- and β-carbons
(C) Adds H$_2$O across the double bond
(D) Generates NADH
(E) Generates FADH$_2$

10. In α-oxidation, which of the following products is released?

(A) CoA
(B) CO$_2$
(C) H$_2$O
(D) Acetyl CoA
(E) Hydrogen peroxide (H$_2$O$_2$)

11. A 16-year-old girl presents with extreme slenderness, with a body weight that is 35% below expected. She feels as though she is obese and severely restricts her food intake. She is diagnosed with anorexia nervosa. In this patient, breakdown of fatty acids is required to provide energy. In fatty acid oxidation, when fatty acids are activated in the cytosol before β-oxidation, which of the following is formed?

(A) ATP
(B) CoA
(C) Fatty acyl CoA
(D) Carnitine
(E) Malonyl CoA

12. A 5-year-old boy presents with altered mental status, heart failure, and muscle weakness. His serum levels of ketones and glucose are abnormally low. He is diagnosed with primary carnitine deficiency. In which of the following is carnitine directly involved?

(A) Activation of fatty acids
(B) Transport of fatty acyl CoA
(C) β-Oxidation
(D) ω-Oxidation
(E) α-Oxidation

13. A 10-year-old girl presents with difficulty walking, muscle weakness, and altered mental status. She is diagnosed with carnitine acetyltransferase deficiency. Carnitine acyl transferase I (CATI) catalyzes a reaction that produces which of the following?

(A) Fatty acyl CoA
(B) Fatty acyl carnitine
(C) Fatty enoyl CoA
(D) β-Hydroxyacyl CoA
(E) β-Ketoacyl CoA

14. After surgical resection of part of her small intestines, a 40-year-old woman presents with chronic foul-smelling diarrhea and weight loss. She is diagnosed with short bowel syndrome. Since fat cannot be properly absorbed, long-chain fatty acids are mobilized and undergo oxidation. β-Oxidation starts with what product?

(A) Long-chain fatty acid
(B) Fatty acyl carnitine
(C) Fatty acyl CoA
(D) β-Hydroxyacyl CoA
(E) Acetyl CoA

15. An infant is born with a high forehead, abnormal eye folds, and deformed ear lobes. He shows little muscle tone and movement. After multiple tests, he is diagnosed with Zellweger syndrome, a disorder caused by malformation of the peroxisome. What type of fatty acid is oxidized in the peroxisome?

(A) Short-chain fatty acids
(B) Acetyl CoA
(C) Dicarboxylic acids
(D) Long-chain fatty acids
(E) Very long–chain fatty acids (VLCFA)

16. An obese, 40-year-old woman, who recently underwent gastric bypass surgery, presents with severe vomiting due to rapid intake of large quantities of food, which must be avoided after gastric bypass surgery. She had successfully lost 10 lb over the last month after the surgery due to mobilization of fat stores to provide acetyl CoA and energy. When palmitoyl CoA is oxidized, how many acetyl CoA are formed?

(A) 1
(B) 2
(C) 6
(D) 8
(E) 10

17. A 16-year-old marathon runner trains by running 15 miles every morning, requiring a constant supply of ATP. Approximately how many ATP are produced when palmitoyl CoA is oxidized to CO_2 and H_2O?

(A) 100
(B) 130
(C) 160
(D) 190
(E) 210

18. A 4-month-old infant presents with a seizure. His mother reports that her infant has been irritable and lethargic over the past several days. The infant is found to have a profoundly low serum glucose level (hypoglycemia) and a profoundly low ketone body level. The infant is diagnosed with medium-chain acyl CoA dehydrogenase (MCAD) deficiency. What is the etiology of this patient's symptoms?

(A) β-oxidation of fatty acids is blocked.
(B) He is consuming a diet that is too low in protein.
(C) Triacylglycerols are being stored in adipose tissue.
(D) Glucose is being used up for fatty acid synthesis.
(E) Fatty acyl CoA cannot be transported into mitochondria.

19. A 12-year-old Jamaican boy presents with intractable vomiting, abdominal pain, and lethargy. He is profoundly hypoglycemic (low blood glucose level). His symptoms are caused by Jamaican vomiting syndrome, a sickness caused by ingestion of hypoglycin, which is present in unripe ackee fruit. Hypoglycin is metabolized to a form of nonmetabolizable carnitine that cannot be used. Carnitine does which of the following?

(A) Activates long-chain fatty acids in the cytosol
(B) Binds to fatty acyl CoA
(C) Is converted to enoyl CoA
(D) Is converted to β-hydroxyacyl CoA
(E) Is involved in breakdown of even-chain, but not odd-chain, fatty acids

20. A 5-year-old boy presents with impaired hearing, poor coordination, and seizures. Two years later, he goes into a vegetative state and dies. He was diagnosed with adrenoleukodystrophy, a disorder in which very long–chain fatty acids (VLCFA) are not properly degraded and accumulate in the brain. How does oxidation of VLCFA differ from oxidation of long-chain fatty acids?

(A) Molecular oxygen is used, and the shorter chain fatty acids produced travel to the mitochondria, generating ATP.
(B) VLCFA cannot be broken down and used for energy.
(C) VLCFA are oxidized in the mitochondria and not in peroxisomes like long-chain fatty acids.
(D) VLCFA are broken down by β-oxidation.
(E) VLCFA undergo ω-oxidation.

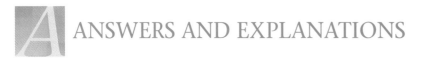
ANSWERS AND EXPLANATIONS

1–C. Fatty acid synthesis occurs primarily in the cytosol, while fatty acid β-oxidation occurs primarily in mitochondria. During fatty acid synthesis, malonyl coenzyme A (CoA) is produced from acetyl CoA as the product of acetyl CoA carboxylase. Malonyl CoA inhibits carnitine acyltransferase I (CATI), an enzyme involved in transport of fatty acids into mitochondria where β-oxidation occurs. NAD$^+$ is important in β-oxidation of fatty acids.

2–B. Odd-chain long fatty acid oxidation produces acetyl CoA and propionyl CoA. β-Oxidation involves the β-carbon of a fatty acyl CoA to sequentially produce acetyl CoA until the last 3 carbons remain as propionyl CoA. Because long-chain fatty acids are broken down at the β-carbon, the remaining carbon chain will always be odd, and thus, butyryl CoA, decanoyl CoA, and palmitoyl CoA will not be created.

3–B. When long-chain fatty acids are activated by 2 adenosine triphosphates (ATP) and CoA in the cytosol, fatty acyl CoA is formed. Fatty acyl CoA reacts with carnitine in the outer mitochondrial membrane, forming fatty acyl carnitine. This reaction is catalyzed by carnitine acyltransferase I (CATI). Fatty acyl carnitine passes through the inner mitochondrial membrane, where it re-forms fatty acyl CoA, catalyzed by carnitine acyltransferase II (CATII).

4–A. β-oxidation is the process by which a fatty acyl CoA is broken down to acetyl CoA. One acetyl CoA is produced from the carboxyl end of a fatty acyl CoA, in each turn of the β-oxidation spiral. ATP is generated during β-oxidation of fatty acids, and different amounts of ATP are generated from different fatty acids. Carnitine is used in the transport of a fatty acyl CoA from the cytosol into mitochondria.

5–A. Fatty acids are very insoluble in water and are carried by serum albumin in the blood. They cross the plasma membrane of a cell and are converted to fatty acyl CoA by CoASH and ATP. Thus, when fatty acids are activated in the cytosol, ATP is converted to adenosine monophosphate (AMP), using the equivalent of 2 ATP. Fatty acids can be oxidized to CO_2 and H_2O in mitochondria of skeletal and heart muscle cells, but red blood cells do not have mitochondria. In α-oxidation, the carboxyl carbon is released as CO_2; thus the fatty acid is degraded 1 carbon at a time. In ω-oxidation, dicarboxylic acids are produced.

6–B. In one turn of the β-oxidation spiral, 2 carbons are removed from fatty acyl CoA as acetyl CoA.

7–C. β-Oxidation of long-chain fatty acids occurs in the mitochondria. Activation of fatty acids occurs in the cytosol. Oxidation of very long–chain fatty acids (VLCFA) occurs in the peroxisome. ω-Oxidation of VLCFA occurs in the endoplasmic reticulum, not in the Golgi apparatus.

8–B. NAD$^+$ is reduced to NADH and FAD is reduced to $FADH_2$ in β-oxidation. β-Oxidation is regulated by the demand for ATP. Acetyl CoA and propionyl CoA are the products of β-oxidation.

9–B. In the last step of β-oxidation, the thiolase cleaves the bond between the α- and β-carbons of the β-ketoacyl CoA in a reaction that requires CoA. Acetyl CoA is produced from the 2 carbons that are cleaved off at the carboxyl end of the fatty acyl CoA. A hydratase is responsible for adding water across the double bond of the fatty enoyl CoA. Dehydrogenases promote generation of NADH and $FADH_2$ during β-oxidation.

10–B. In α-oxidation, VLCFA are oxidized 1 carbon at a time, and the carboxyl carbon is released as CO_2. Acetyl CoA is released during one turn of the β-oxidation spiral. Hydrogen peroxide is formed when VLCFA are oxidized in peroxisomes.

11–C. Long-chain fatty acids are activated by ATP and CoA, forming fatty acyl CoA. Carnitine reacts with fatty acyl CoA, forming fatty acyl carnitine. Malonyl CoA is an intermediate in fatty acid synthesis.

12–B. Fatty acyl CoA reacts with carnitine in the outer mitochondrial membrane, forming fatty acyl carnitine, which passes to the inner mitochondrial membrane. Activation, β-oxidation, ω-oxidation, and α-oxidation do not directly involve carnitine.

13–B. CATI catalyzes the transfer of acyl groups from fatty acyl CoA to carnitine, resulting in fatty acyl carnitine. Fatty enoyl CoA, β-hydroxyacyl CoA, and β-ketoacyl CoA are products in β-oxidation.

14–C. Fatty acyl CoA undergoes β-oxidation in a spiral involving four steps. Long-chain fatty acids are released from adipose cells and must be activated and transported into mitochondria for oxidation. Fatty acyl CoA reacts with carnitine, forming fatty acyl carnitine, which then re-forms fatty acyl CoA, which enters the mitochondrial matrix. β-Hydroxyacyl CoA is one of the products in the β-oxidation spiral. Acetyl CoA is the final product of one β-oxidation spiral.

15–E. VLCFA are oxidized in peroxisomes to hydrogen peroxide. Short-chain and long-chain fatty acids are β-oxidized in mitochondria to acetyl CoA. ω-Oxidation of short-chain and long-chain fatty acids in the endoplasmic reticulum, and subsequent β-oxidation produces dicarboxylic acids.

16–D. When one 16-carbon palmitoyl CoA is oxidized, 8 acetyl CoA molecules are formed.

17–B. 129 ATP are produced when palmitoyl CoA is oxidized to CO_2 and H_2O.

18–A. Medium-chain acyl CoA dehydrogenase (MCAD) deficiency is a deficiency of acyl CoA dehydrogenase, an enzyme required in the first step of the β-oxidation cycle. In patients with MCAD, when serum glucose levels are low (hypoglycemia) due to fasting, infection, or increased amount of time between feedings, fatty acids cannot be broken down as an alternate form of energy.

19–B. In the outer mitochondrial membrane, carnitine reacts with fatty acyl CoA (even- or odd-chain), forming fatty acyl carnitine, which can then pass to the inner mitochondrial membrane. Therefore, carnitine is important for transport of fatty acyl

CoA from the cytosol to the mitochondria, where β-oxidation occurs. Carnitine is not involved in activation of fatty acids or β-oxidation itself. As a note of interest, hypoglycin also causes decreased production of NADH and acetyl CoA. Since NADH is a cofactor for 3-phosphoglyceraldehyde phosphate dehydrogenase and since acetyl CoA is an activator of pyruvate carboxylase, decreased levels of NADH and acetyl CoA lead to inhibition of gluconeogenesis. Profound hypoglycemia (low blood glucose level) results, which is how hypoglycin was named.

20–A. The breakdown of VLCFA differs from long-chain fatty acids, in that molecular oxygen is used and no ATP is generated until the shorter chain fatty acids that are produced travel to the mitochondria and undergo β-oxidation. VLCFA undergo α-oxidation in peroxisomes, while long chain fatty acids undergo β-oxidation in mitochondria.

chapter 14

Cholesterol Metabolism and Blood Lipoproteins

I. Cholesterol and Bile Salt Metabolism

A. Cholesterol is synthesized from **cytosolic acetyl coenzyme A (CoA)** by a sequence of reactions. (Figure 14-1)

1. **Glucose** is a major source of carbon for acetyl CoA. Acetyl CoA is produced from glucose by the same sequence of reactions used to produce cytosolic acetyl CoA for fatty acid biosynthesis (Figure 14-2).
2. **Cytosolic acetyl CoA** forms acetoacetyl CoA, which condenses with another acetyl CoA to form hydroxymethylglutaryl CoA (HMG-CoA) (see Figure 14-1). Acetyl CoA undergoes similar reactions in the mitochondrion, where HMG-CoA is used for ketone body synthesis.
3. **Cytosolic HMG-CoA,** a key intermediate in cholesterol biosynthesis, is reduced in the endoplasmic reticulum to mevalonic acid by the regulatory enzyme HMG-CoA reductase.
    a. **HMG-CoA reductase** is inhibited by cholesterol.
    b. In the liver, it is also inhibited by bile salts and is induced when blood insulin levels are elevated.

> *cc* *14.1* **Statins** are medications that function as **competitive inhibitors of HMG-CoA reductase,** thus **reducing the serum level of cholesterol.** Statins have shown benefit in reducing incidence of heart disease and stroke.

4. **Mevalonic acid** is phosphorylated and decarboxylated to form the 5-carbon (C-5) isoprenoid, isopentenyl pyrophosphate (see Figure 14-1).
5. Two **isopentenyl pyrophosphate** units condense, forming a C-10 compound, geranyl pyrophosphate, which reacts with another C-5 unit to form a C-15 compound, farnesyl pyrophosphate (see Figure 14-1).
6. **Squalene** is formed from two C-15 units and then oxidized and cyclized, forming lanosterol (see Figure 14-1).
7. **Lanosterol** is converted to **cholesterol** in a series of steps (see Figure 14-1).
8. The **ring structure** of cholesterol **cannot be degraded** in the body. The bile salts in the feces are the major form in which the steroid nucleus is excreted.

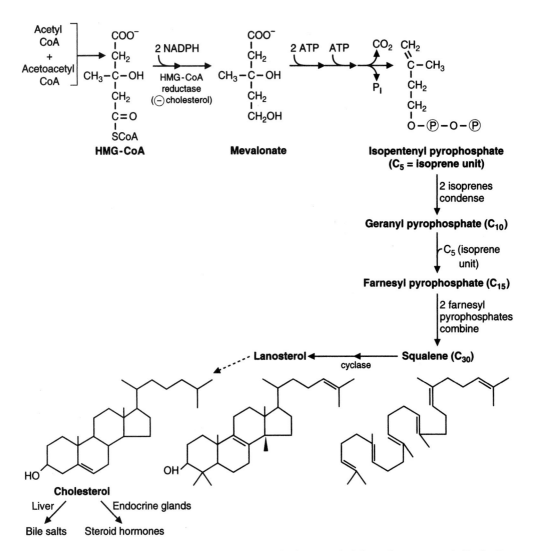

Figure 14-1 Cholesterol biosynthesis. HMG-CoA = hydroxymethylglutaryl coenzyme A (CoA); ⊝ = inhibited by; circled P = phosphate.

---

cc 14.2 **Gallstones** can be made of cholesterol. **Ursodeoxycholate** is a medication used to inhibit the formation of cholesterol gallstones. This medication is a hydrophilic bile salt that **decreases the content of cholesterol in bile.**

---

cc 14.3 **Atherosclerosis** is the **buildup of lipid-rich plaques** in the intima layer of **arteries.** Blood clots can form on these lipid-rich plaques, or part of the plaque may suddenly break loose, occluding a coronary or cerebral artery. **Occlusion of a coronary artery** can cause a **myocardial infarct** (heart attack), and **occlusion of a cerebral artery** can cause an ischemic cerebrovascular accident (**stroke**).

B. **Bile salts** are synthesized in the liver from cholesterol (Figure 14-3)

1. An **α-hydroxyl group** is added to carbon 7 of cholesterol. A **7α-hydroxylase,** which is inhibited by bile salts, catalyzes this rate-limiting step.

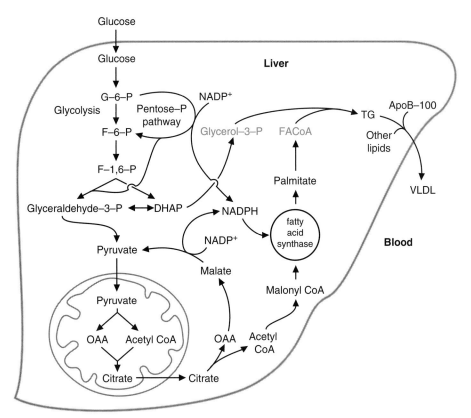

Figure 14-2 Synthesis of fatty acids and triaglycerols from glucose. DHAP = dihydroxyacetone phosphate; F-6-P = fructose 6-phosphate; F-1,6-P = fructose-1,6-biphosphate; G-6-P = glucose 6-phosphate; OAA = oxaloacetate; VLDL = very low–density lipoprotein.

2. The **double bond** is **reduced,** and **further hydroxylations** occur, resulting in two compounds. One has α-hydroxyl groups at positions 3 and 7; and the other has α-hydroxyl groups at positions 3, 7, and 12.
3. The **side chain is oxidized** and converted to a branched, 5-carbon chain, containing a carboxylic acid at the end.
   a. The bile acid with hydroxyl groups at positions 3 and 7 is **chenocholic acid.** The bile acid with hydroxyl groups at positions 3, 7, and 12 is **cholic acid.**
   b. These bile acids each have a **pK** of about 6.
      (1) Above pH 6, the molecules are salts (i.e., they ionize and carry a negative charge).
      (2) At pH 6 (the pH in the intestinal lumen), half of the molecules are ionized and carry a negative charge.
      (3) Below pH 6, the molecules become protonated, and their charge decreases as the pH is lowered.
4. *Conjugation of the bile salts* (see Figure 14-3, *middle*)
   a. The bile salts are activated by adenosine triphosphate (ATP) and coenzyme A, forming their CoA derivatives, which can form conjugates with either **glycine** or **taurine.**
   b. **Glycine,** an amino acid, forms an amide with the carboxyl group of a bile salt, forming **glycocholic acid or glycochenocholic acid.**
      (1) These bile salts each have a **pK** of about **4.**

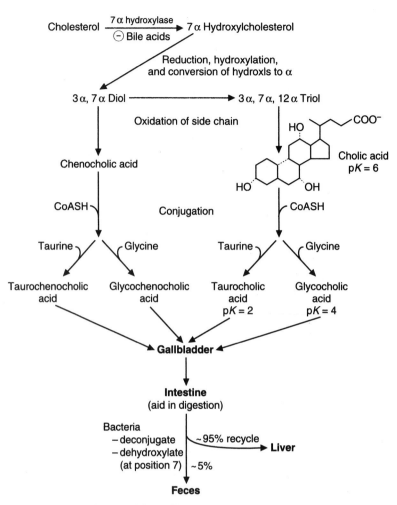

Figure 14-3 Synthesis and fate of bile salts.

  (2) This pK is lower than the unconjugated bile salts, so they are more completely ionized at pH 6 in the gut lumen and serve as better detergents.
  c. **Taurine,** which is derived from the amino acid cysteine, forms an amide with the carboxyl group of a bile salt.
   (1) Because of the sulfite group on the taurine moiety, the **taurocholic** and **taurochenocholic acids** have a **pK of about 2.**
   (2) They ionize very readily in the gut and are the best detergents among the bile salts.
 5. *Fate of the bile salts* (see Figure 14-3, *bottom*)
  a. Cholic acid, chenocholic acid, and their conjugates are known as the **primary bile salts.** They are made in the liver and secreted via the **bile** through the **gallbladder** into the **intestine,** where, because they are amphipathic (contain both hydrophobic and hydrophilic regions), they aid in **lipid digestion.**
  b. In the intestine, bile salts can be **deconjugated** and **dehydroxylated** (at position 7) **by intestinal bacteria.**

c. Bile salts are **resorbed** in the ileum and return to the liver, where they can be reconjugated with glycine or taurine. However, they are not rehydroxylated. Those that lack the 7α-hydroxyl group are called **secondary bile salts.**

d. The **liver recycles** about 95% of the bile salts each day; 5% are lost in the feces.

---

cc 14.4 **Bile acid sequestrants,** such as cholestyramine, **bind with bile acids that are bound to low-density lipoprotein (LDL).** The insoluble complex of bile acid sequestrant, bile acid, and LDL is eliminated in the stool. This **causes fecal loss of LDL.**

C. **Steroid hormones** are synthesized from cholesterol, and 1,25-dihydroxychole-calciferol (active **vitamin D₃**) is synthesized from a precursor of cholesterol.

II. Blood Lipoproteins

A. Composition of the blood lipoproteins (Table 14-1)

1. The major components of lipoproteins are triacylglycerols, cholesterol, cholesterol esters, phospholipids, and proteins. The protein components (called apoproteins) are designated A, B, C, and E.
2. **Chylomicrons** are the least dense of the blood lipoproteins because they have the most triacylglycerol and the least protein.
3. **Very low–density lipoprotein (VLDL)** is more dense than chylomicrons but still has a high content of triacylglycerol.
4. **Intermediate-density lipoprotein (IDL),** which is derived from VLDL, is denser than VLDL and has less than one half the amount of triacylglycerol.
5. **LDL** has less triacylglycerol and more protein and, therefore, is denser than the IDL from which it is derived. LDL has the highest content of cholesterol and its esters.
6. **High-density lipoprotein (HDL)** is the densest lipoprotein. It has the lowest triacylglycerol content and the highest protein content.

B. Metabolism of chylomicrons (Figure 14-4)

1. Chylomicrons are **synthesized in intestinal epithelial cells.** Their triacylglycerols are derived from dietary lipid, and their major apoprotein (apo) is apo B-48.
2. Chylomicrons travel through the lymph into the blood. (Step 1) **Apo C$_{II}$,** the activator of lipoprotein lipase, and **apo E** are transferred to nascent chylomicrons from HDL, and mature chylomicrons are formed. (Step 2)

TABLE 14-1 *Composition of the Blood Lipoproteins*

Component	Chylomicrons	VLDL	IDL	LDL	HDL
Triacylglycerol	85%	55%	26%	10%	8%
Protein	2%	9%	11%	20%	45%
Type	B, C, E	B, C, E	B, E	B	A, C, E
Cholesterol	1%	7%	8%	10%	5%
Cholesterol ester	2%	10%	30%	35%	15%
Phospholipid	8%	20%	23%	20%	25%

HDL = high-density lipoprotein; IDL = intermediate-density lipoprotein; LDL = low-density lipoprotein; VLDL = very low–density lipoprotein.

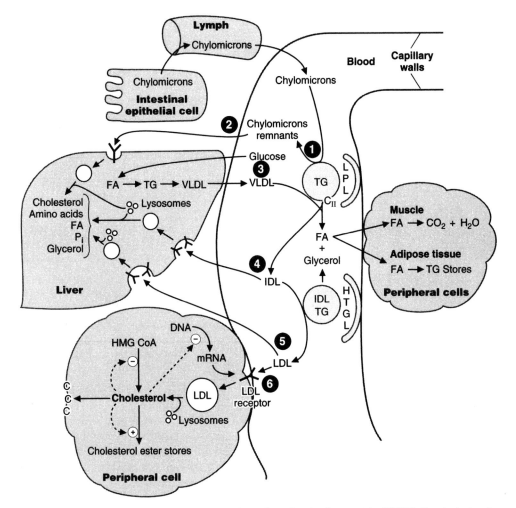

Figure 14-4 Metabolism of chylomicrons and very low–density lipoprotein (VLDL). C = cholesterol; FA = fatty acid; LPL = lipoprotein lipase; HTGL = hepatic triglyceride lipase; TG = triacylglycerol; circled TG = triacylglycerol of chylomicrons and VLDL; ⊖ = inhibits; ⊕ = stimulates. ❶ to ❷ = fate of chylomicrons; ❸ to ❻ = fate of VLDL.

3. In peripheral tissues, particularly adipose and muscle, the triacylglycerols are **digested by lipoprotein lipase.**

4. The chylomicron remnants interact with receptors on liver cells and are taken up by **endocytosis.** The contents are degraded by **lysosomal enzymes,** and the products (amino acids, fatty acids, glycerol, cholesterol, and phosphate) are released into the cytosol and reused.

C. Metabolism of VLDL (see Figure 14-4)

1. **VLDL** is synthesized in the **liver,** particularly after a high-carbohydrate meal. It is formed from triacylglycerols that are packaged with cholesterol, apoproteins (particularly apo B-100), and phospholipids, and it is released into the blood. (Step 3)

2. In **peripheral tissues,** particularly adipose and muscle, VLDL triacylglycerols are **digested by lipoprotein lipase,** and VLDL is converted to IDL.

> cc *14.5* The agent **gemfibrozil,** a member of the **fibrate** class of lipid-lowering agents, **activates lipoprotein lipase.** Therefore, it **decreases VLDLs** and other triglyceride-rich lipoproteins.

3. **IDL** returns to the liver, is taken up by endocytosis, and is degraded by **lysosomal enzymes.** (Step 4) IDL can also be further degraded, forming LDL. (Step 5)

4. **LDL** reacts with receptors on various cells, is taken up by endocytosis, and is digested by **lysosomal enzymes.** (Step 6)

   a. **Cholesterol,** released from cholesterol esters by a lysosomal esterase, can be used for the synthesis of cell **membranes** or for the synthesis of bile salts in the liver or **steroid hormones** in endocrine tissue.

   b. Cholesterol **inhibits HMG-CoA reductase** (a key enzyme in cholesterol biosynthesis) and, thus, decreases the rate of cholesterol synthesis by the cell.

   c. Cholesterol **inhibits synthesis of LDL receptors** (downregulation), and, thus, reduces the amount of cholesterol taken up by cells.

   d. Cholesterol **activates acyl:cholesterol acyltransferase (ACAT),** which converts cholesterol to cholesterol esters for storage in cells.

D. Familial hypercholesterolemia (types I, IIa, IIb, III, IV, V) (Table 14-2)

E. Metabolism of HDL (Figure 14-5)

   1. **HDL** is synthesized by the **liver** and released into the blood as small, disk-shaped particles. The major **protein** of HDL is **apo A.**

TABLE 14-2	*Hyperlipidemias*			
	Disease	Description	Etiology of Lipid Disorder	Biochemical Finding
cc *14.6*	Type I	Rare genetic disorders of lipoprotein lipase deficiency or apo C_{II} deficiency	Deficiency of LDL receptors	Cholesterol high Chylomicrons high Triglycerides extremely elevated at 1000–10,000 mg/dL
cc *14.7*	Type IIa	Common familial	Complete block in LDL receptor transport between the endoplasmic reticulum and the Golgi apparatus	Cholesterol high LDL high Triglycerides normal Autosomal dominant inheritance
cc *14.8*	Type IIb	Classic mixed hyperlipidemia	Partial block in LDL receptor transport between the endoplasmic reticulum and the Golgi apparatus	Cholesterol high LDL and VLDL high Triglycerides < 1000 mg/dL Autosomal dominant inheritance

(continued)

TABLE 14-2	Hyperlipidemias *(Continued)*			
	Disease	Description	Etiology of Lipid Disorder	Biochemical Finding
cc 14.9	Type III	Dysbetalipo-proteinemia	Mutated LDL receptor that cannot bind to LDL normally	Cholesterol high IDL (a VLDL remnant) high Triglycerides < 1000 mg/dL Less common familial
cc 14.10	Type IV	Endogenous hyper-triglyceridemia, hyperprebeta-lipoproteinemia	Block in internalization of the complex (LDL bound to the LDL receptor)	Cholesterol normal LDL high Triglycerides < 1000 mg/dL Common familial
cc 14.11	Type V	Hyperprebetalipo-proteinemia with chylo-micronemia	Block in release of LDL intracellularly after internalization, preventing recycling of the LDL receptor back to the cell surface	Cholesterol high Chylomicrons and VLDL high Triglycerides extremely elevated at 1,000–10,000 mg/dL Uncommon familial

HDL = high-density lipoprotein; LDL = low-density lipoprotein; VLDL = very low–density lipoprotein; IDL = intermediate-density lipoprotein.

cc 14.12 **Tangier disease** is a disease of **cholesterol transport.** The first case was identified in a patient who lived on the island of Tangier and who had characteristic **orange-colored tonsils,** a **very low HDL** level, and an **enlarged liver and spleen.** Due to a mutation in a transport protein, **cholesterol cannot properly exit the cell to bind to apo A** (forming HDL). This results in a very low HDL level.

2. Apo C_{II}, which is transferred by HDL to chylomicrons and VLDL, serves as an **activator of lipoprotein lipase.**
   a. Apo E is also transferred and serves as a **recognition factor** for **cell surface receptors.**
   b. Apo C_{II} and apo E are transferred back to HDL following digestion of triacylglycerols of chylomicrons and VLDL.
3. **Cholesterol**, obtained by HDL from cell membranes or from other lipoproteins, is converted to **cholesterol esters** by the **lecithin:cholesterol acyltransferase (LCAT) reaction,** which is activated by apo A_I.
   a. A fatty acid from position 2 of lecithin (phosphatidylcholine), a component of HDL, forms an ester with the 3-hydroxyl group of cholesterol, producing lysolecithin and a cholesterol ester.
   b. As cholesterol esters accumulate in the core of the lipoprotein, HDL particles become spheroids.

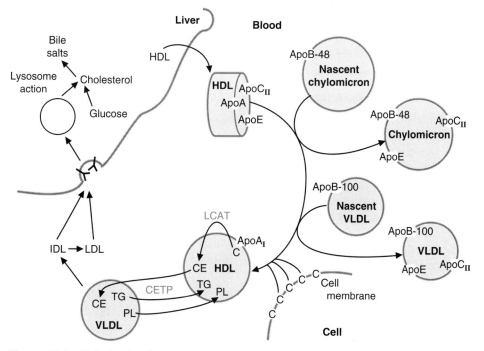

Figure 14-5 High-density lipoprotein (HDL) function and metabolism. apo = apoprotein; C = cholesterol; CE = cholesterol ester; CETP = cholesterol ester transfer protein; IDL = intermediate-density lipoprotein; LCAT = lecithin:cholesterol acyltransferase; LDL = low-density lipoprotein; PL = phospholipid; TG = triacylglycerol; VLDL = very low–density lipoprotein.

> *cc 14.13* **LCAT deficiency** results in an **inability to convert cholesterol on HDL to cholesterol esters.** Ordinarily, these **cholesterol esters would be transferred to other lipoproteins,** which would then be **taken up by receptors in the liver.** Therefore, by inducing esterification of cholesterol, LCAT is important for the **continued removal of cholesterol from the periphery.** Clinical manifestations include defects in the kidneys, red blood cells, and the cornea of the eyes.

4. **HDL transfers cholesterol esters** to other lipoproteins in exchange for various lipids. Cholesterol ester transfer protein (CETP) mediates this exchange. HDL and other lipoproteins carry the cholesterol esters back to the liver.
5. **HDL particles** and other lipoproteins are taken up by the liver by endocytosis and **hydrolyzed by lysosomal enzymes.**
6. Cholesterol, released from cholesterol esters, can be packaged by the liver in VLDL and released into the blood or converted to bile salts and secreted into the bile.

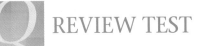

Directions: Each of the numbered questions or incomplete statements in this section is followed by answers or by completions of the statement. Select the **one** lettered answer or completion that is **best** in each case.

1. A gallstone that blocked the upper part of the bile duct would cause an increase in which of the following?

(A) The formation of chylomicrons
(B) The recycling of bile salts
(C) The excretion of bile salts
(D) Increased conjugation of bile salts
(E) The excretion of fat in the feces

2. Which of the following statements concerning the liver and adipose cells is correct?

(A) Adipose cells contain glycerol kinase.
(B) Liver cells contain a hormone-sensitive lipase.
(C) Adipose cells have a transport system for glucose that is not regulated by insulin.
(D) Liver cells secrete lipoproteins when blood insulin levels are low.
(E) Adipose cells secrete lipoprotein lipase when blood insulin levels are high.

3. In the conversion of cholesterol to bile salts, which of the following statements best describes the process?

(A) Carbon 8 is hydroxylated.
(B) The side chain can be conjugated with glycine or taurine.
(C) The double bond is oxidized.
(D) The hydroxyl group on carbon 3 remains in the β-position.
(E) It occurs in the bile duct.

4. Which of the following statements best describes low-density lipoprotein (LDL)?

(A) It has the most triacylglycerol and the least protein.
(B) It has more triacylglycerol than very low–density lipoprotein (VLDL).
(C) It has the highest content of cholesterol and its esters.
(D) It has the lowest triacylglycerol content.
(E) It has the highest protein content.

5. Which lipoprotein has the lowest triacylglycerol content?

(A) Chylomicrons
(B) VLDL
(C) Intermediate-density lipoprotein (IDL)
(D) LDL
(E) High-density lipoprotein (HDL)

6. In contrast to secondary bile salts, which of the following is characteristic of primary bile salts?

(A) Are hydroxylated at carbon 7
(B) Have an oxidized side chain
(C) Form coenzyme A (CoA) derivatives
(D) Can be conjugated to glycine or taurine
(E) Are resorbed in the intestine

7. Concerning metabolism of VLDL, which of the following converts VLDL to IDL?

(A) Lipoprotein lipase
(B) Hydroxymethylglutaryl CoA (HMG-CoA) reductase
(C) Acyl:cholesterol acyltransferase (ACAT)
(D) Lecithin:cholesterol acyltransferase (LCAT)
(E) Cholesterol ester transfer protein (CETP)

8. Which of the following apoproteins is an activator of lipoprotein lipase?

(A) Apo A
(B) Apo B
(C) Apo C_{II}
(D) Apo D
(E) Apo E

9. Which of the following statements best describes CETP?

(A) It converts cholesterol from LDL to cholesterol esters.
(B) It is the major protein of HDL.
(C) It exchanges cholesterol esters from HDL for other lipids.

(D) It converts mevalonic acid to isopentenyl pyrophosphate.

(E) It converts squalene to lanosterol.

10. The major carriers of triacylglycerols are which of the following?

(A) Chylomicrons and VLDL
(B) IDL and LDL
(C) VLDL and LDL
(D) HDL and LDL
(E) Chylomicrons and LDL

11. A 40-year-old, obese woman presents with acute pain in the right upper quadrant of her abdomen as well as vomiting. She is diagnosed with having gallstones and is placed on ursodeoxycholate, a bile salt used to inhibit the formation of cholesterol gallstones by facilitating dissolution of cholesterol. Which of the following is a bile salt?

(A) HMG-CoA
(B) Mevalonate
(C) Squalene
(D) Lanosterol
(E) Chenocholic acid

12. An 8-year-old boy presents with orange-colored tonsils, a very low HDL level, and an enlarged liver and spleen. He is diagnosed with Tangier disease. Tangier disease is a disease of cholesterol transport, such that cholesterol cannot properly exit the cell and form HDL. Which the following statements describes HDL?

(A) It is produced in skeletal muscle.
(B) It scavenges cholesterol from cell membranes.
(C) Its major protein is apo E.
(D) It is formed when VLDL is digested by lipoprotein lipase.
(E) It activates ACAT.

13. A 40-year-old man presents with chest pain that radiates to his left jaw and shoulder. He is diagnosed with a myocardial infarct (heart attack) and is prescribed a statin medication. Statins are competitive inhibitors of HMG-CoA reductase, which converts HMG-CoA to which of the following?

(A) Mevalonate
(B) Isopentenyl pyrophosphate

(C) Geranyl pyrophosphate
(D) Farnesyl pyrophosphate
(E) Cholesterol

14. A 45-year-old woman presents with oily, foul-smelling stool. Gallstones can obstruct the bile duct, leading to an inadequate concentration of bile salts in the intestines. Which of the following statements describes bile salts?

(A) They can act as detergents, aiding in lipid digestion.
(B) They are stored in the intestines.
(C) Ninety-five percent of bile salts are excreted in the feces, and 5% are recycled back to the liver.
(D) Bile salts are synthesized in the intestines.
(E) Squalene and lanosterol are examples of bile salts.

15. A 60-year-old woman presents with chest pain radiating to her left arm. She is diagnosed with a having had a myocardial infarct (heart attack) and is prescribed a statin medication. Statins inhibit HMG-CoA reductase. How does inhibition of HMG-CoA reductase lower cholesterol and LDL levels?

(A) It inhibits the rate-limiting step in cholesterol biosynthesis.
(B) It increases synthesis of bile salts to digest cholesterol.
(C) It increases the serum level of HDL.
(D) It inhibits formation of LDL from IDL.
(E) It inhibits synthesis of LDL receptors.

16. A 55-year-old woman presents with crushing substernal chest pain and shortness of breath. A coronary artery is occluded due to an atherosclerotic plaque, and she is diagnosed with a having had a myocardial infarct. High serum HDL levels are protective against the development of atherosclerosis because HDL does which of the following?

(A) Inhibits cholesterol production by the liver
(B) Inhibits HMG-CoA reductase
(C) Increases VLDL production
(D) Increases LDL production
(E) Brings cholesterol esters back to the liver

17. A 30-year-old man presents with weakness in his right leg. He is diagnosed with a stroke, an occlusion of a cerebral artery due to atherosclerosis. Genetic studies show that he has familial hypercholesterolemia, type I, a disorder caused by a deficiency of LDL receptors. Which of the following statements describes patients with familial hypercholesterolemia, type I?

(A) After LDL binds to the LDL receptor, the LDL is degraded extracellularly.

(B) The number of LDL receptors on the surface of hepatocytes increases.

(C) Cholesterol synthesis by hepatocytes increases.

(D) Excessive cholesterol is released by LDL.

(E) The cholesterol level in the serum decreases.

18. A 40-year-old woman presents with an LDL serum level of 400 (recommended level is <160), and a triglyceride (triacylglycerol) level of 170 (recommended level is <140). She is diagnosed with type III familial hypercholesterolemia. In this disorder, a mutated LDL receptor is formed, such that it cannot bind to LDL. Which of the following would result?

(A) HMG-CoA reductase activity is not inhibited.

(B) Chylomicrons cannot be degraded to triacylglycerols.

(C) VLDL level in the serum increases.

(D) HDL level in the serum increases.

(E) VLDL cannot be converted to IDL.

19. A 25-year-old woman presents with a low red blood cell count, corneal opacities, and kidney insufficiency. She is diagnosed with lecithin:cholesterol acyltransferase (LCAT) deficiency. Which of the following is LCAT involved in?

(A) Converting cholesterol to cholesterol esters

(B) The transfer of cholesterol esters from HDL to other lipoproteins

(C) Endocytosis of HDL particles into hepatocytes

(D) Hydrolysis of HDL

(E) Decreased uptake of cholesterol by hepatocytes

20. A 40-year-old man presents with severe pain in his legs upon walking. He is diagnosed with atherosclerotic plaques in the arteries of his legs. High levels of cholesterol and LDL contribute to the formation of atherosclerosis. Which of the following is digested to form LDL?

(A) IDL

(B) Cholesterol

(C) Cholesterol esters

(D) HDL

(E) Chylomicrons

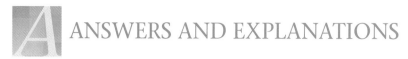

ANSWERS AND EXPLANATIONS

1–E. In this situation, bile salts could not enter the digestive tract. Therefore, recycling and excretion of bile salts, digestion of fats, and formation of chylomicrons would all decrease. As a consequence, fat in the feces would increase (steatorrhea).

2–E. Adipose cells lack glycerol kinase but have a hormone-sensitive lipase. The glucose transport system of adipose cells (and muscle) is stimulated by insulin. When insulin levels are elevated, liver cells secrete very low–density lipoprotein (VLDL), and adipose cells secrete lipoprotein lipase, which cleaves the triacylglycerols of chylomicrons and VLDL.

3–B. During the conversion of cholesterol to bile salts, carbon 7 is hydroxylated. All hydroxyl groups, including the one on carbon 3, assume an α-configuration. The double bond is reduced, and the side chain can be oxidized and conjugated with glycine to form glycocholic acid or glycochenocholic acid, or with taurine to form taurocholic acid or taurochenocholic acid.

4–C. Low-density lipoprotein (LDL) has the highest content of cholesterol and its esters. Chylomicrons have the most triacylglycerol and the least protein content. VLDL has a high content of triacylglycerol but less than chylomicrons. Intermediate-density lipoprotein (IDL) carries less than half the amount of triacylglycerols as VLDL. LDL carries less triacylglycerols and more protein than IDL. High-density lipoprotein (HDL) has the lowest triacylglycerol content and the highest protein content.

5–E. HDL has the lowest triacylglycerol content and is the densest lipoprotein. The order of the least to most dense lipoprotein is: chylomicrons, VLDL, IDL, LDL, and HDL.

6–A. Primary bile salts include cholic acid, chenocholic acid, and their conjugates. They are synthesized from cholesterol by hydroxylation at carbon 7. The side chain is oxidized. They are activated to form coenzyme A (CoA) derivatives and can form conjugates with glycine or taurine. Primary bile salts are secreted via the bile to the intestine, where they are deconjugated and dehydroxylated. These bile salts are then resorbed and reconjugated, but they cannot be rehydroxylated. Bile salts that lack the hydroxyl group at carbon 7 are called secondary bile salts.

7–A. When VLDL triacylglycerols are digested by lipoprotein lipase, VLDL is converted to IDL. Hydroxymethylglutaryl CoA (HMG-CoA) reductase is the rate-limiting enzyme in cholesterol biosynthesis. Acyl:cholesterol acyltransferase (ACAT) converts cholesterol (derived from LDL) to cholesterol esters for storage in cells. Lecithin:cholesterol acyltransferase (LCAT) converts cholesterol (derived from HDL) to cholesterol esters. Cholesterol ester transfer protein (CETP) mediates the exchange of cholesterol esters from HDL to other lipoproteins.

8–C. Apoprotein (apo) C_{II} is an activator of lipoprotein lipase. Apo A is the major apolipoprotein of HDL. Apo B is the major apolipoprotein of LDL and VLDL. There is no Apo D. Apo E is transferred by HDL to nascent chylomicrons, to form mature chylomicrons.

9–C. CETP mediates the exchange of cholesterol esters from HDL to other lipoproteins in exchange for various lipids. ACAT converts cholesterol from LDL to cholesterol esters. Apo A is the major protein of HDL. Mevalonic acid, isopentenyl pyrophosphate, squalene, and lanosterol are intermediates in cholesterol synthesis.

10–A. The major carriers of triacylglycerols are chylomicrons and VLDL. The triacyl-glycerols are digested in capillaries by lipoprotein lipase. The fatty acids that are produced are used for energy by cells or are converted to triacylglycerols and stored.

11–E. Chenocholic acid is an example of a bile salt. HMG-CoA, mevalonate, squalene, and lanosterol are intermediates in cholesterol synthesis. Bile salts are synthesized from cholesterol in the liver and facilitate lipid digestion in the intestines.

12–B. HDL scavenges cholesterol from cell membranes and lipoproteins. HDL is produced in the liver, and its major protein is apo A. IDL is formed when VLDL is digested by lipoprotein lipase. Cholesterol activates ACAT, which converts cholesterol to cholesterol esters for storage in cells.

13–A. HMG-CoA reductase converts HMG-CoA to mevalonate, using 2 NADPH as cofactor. Isopentenyl pyrophosphate, geranyl pyrophosphate, and farnesyl pyrophosphate are intermediates in cholesterol synthesis.

14–A. Bile salts can act as detergents, aiding in lipid digestion. They are synthesized in the liver (not in the intestines). Bile salts are stored in the gallbladder and are secreted into the intestines. An inadequate concentration of bile salts in the intestines can lead to oily, foul-smelling stool with a high fat content. Ninety-five percent of bile salts are recycled back to the liver, and 5% are excreted in the feces. Squalene and lanosterol are intermediary compounds in cholesterol synthesis.

15–A. HMG-CoA reductase is the rate-limiting enzyme in cholesterol biosynthesis. Inhibition of HMG-CoA reductase results in decreased intracellular cholesterol levels. Decreased intracellular cholesterol levels result in an increased expression of LDL receptors on the surface of hepatocytes. This results in increased intracellular uptake of serum LDL, leading to decreased serum LDL levels. Inhibition of HMG-CoA reductase does not directly affect synthesis of bile salts, HDL, or IDL.

16–E. HDL is known as the "good" lipoprotein because HDL scavenges cholesterol from the periphery (from cell membranes and from other lipoproteins) and brings cholesterol esters back to the liver, where they can be excreted as bile salts. HDL does not inhibit cholesterol production by the liver. Statin medications inhibit HMG-CoA reductase. Increasing VLDL or LDL will facilitate the development of atherosclerosis.

17–C. Cholesterol synthesis by hepatocytes increases in patients with familial hyper-cholesterolemia type I because HMG-CoA reductase is not properly inhibited. Normally, after LDL binds to the LDL receptor, LDL is degraded intracellularly, and cholesterol is released by LDL in the cytosol. Intracellular cholesterol inhibits HMG-CoA reductase, resulting in decreased cholesterol synthesis by hepatocytes. Because the LDL receptor is deficient in patients with this disease, LDL cannot be taken up by hepatocytes (to release cholesterol), and an extremely high serum cholesterol level results.

18–A. Normally, LDL is digested by lysosomal enzymes to release cholesterol. High levels of intracellular cholesterol inhibit HMG-CoA reductase, and cholesterol synthesis decreases in hepatocytes. In familial hypercholesterolemia type III, LDL cannot be taken up into hepatocytes. Since HMG-CoA reductase is not properly inhibited, excessive cholesterol levels result. Chylomicron degradation, the level of VLDL, the level of HDL, and conversion of VLDL to IDL are not affected.

19–A. LCAT converts cholesterol to cholesterol esters, which accumulate in the core of HDL. These cholesterol esters are transferred from HDL to VLDL and LDL, which are then taken up by receptors in the liver. Therefore, LCAT is important for removing cholesterol from peripheral cells by inducing esterification of cholesterol, thus allowing eventual cholesterol uptake by the liver. LCAT is not involved in endocytosis of HDL into hepatocytes or hydrolysis of HDL.

20–A. IDL is degraded to form LDL. Cholesterol is converted to cholesterol esters for storage in cells. HDL is synthesized by the liver. Chylomicrons are synthesized by intestinal epithelial cells.

Ketones and Other Lipid Derivatives

I. Ketone Body Synthesis and Utilization (Figure 15-1)

A. **Synthesis of ketone bodies** (Figure 15-1, *top*) occurs in **liver mitochondria** when fatty acids are in high concentration in the blood (during fasting, starvation, or as a result of a high-fat diet).

1. **β-Oxidation** produces NADH and adenosine triphosphate (ATP) and results in the accumulation of acetyl coenzyme A (CoA). The liver is producing glucose using oxaloacetate (OAA), so there is decreased condensation of acetyl CoA with OAA to form citrate.
2. **Two molecules of acetyl CoA** condense to produce acetoacetyl CoA. This reaction is catalyzed by thiolase or an isoenzyme of **thiolase.**
3. Acetoacetyl CoA and acetyl CoA form HMG CoA in a reaction catalyzed by hydroxymethylglutaryl CoA (HMG-CoA) synthetase.
4. **HMG-CoA** is cleaved by HMG-CoA lyase to form acetyl CoA and acetoacetate.
5. **Acetoacetate** can be reduced by an NAD-requiring dehydrogenase (3-hydroxybutyrate dehydrogenase) to **3-hydroxybutyrate.** This is a reversible reaction.
6. Acetoacetate is also spontaneously **decarboxylated** in a nonenzymatic reaction, forming **acetone** (the source of the odor on the breath of ketotic diabetics).

> *cc 15.1* **Type 1 diabetes mellitus** is due to a **deficiency of insulin,** which is caused by autoimmune destruction of insulin-producing cells in the pancreas. Insulin is required for glucose to be used by cells. Deficiency of insulin leads to a state known as **diabetic ketoacidosis,** which manifests as a **severely elevated serum glucose level, increased ketone body synthesis,** and formation of **acetone** due to decarboxylation of acetoacetate.

7. The **liver** lacks succinyl CoA-acetoacetate-CoA transferase (a thiotransferase) so it **cannot use ketone bodies.** Therefore, acetoacetate and 3-hydroxybutyrate are released into the blood by the liver.

B. **Utilization of ketone bodies** (Figure 15-1, *bottom*)

1. When ketone bodies are released from the liver into the blood, they are taken up by peripheral tissues such as **muscle and kidney,** where they are oxidized for

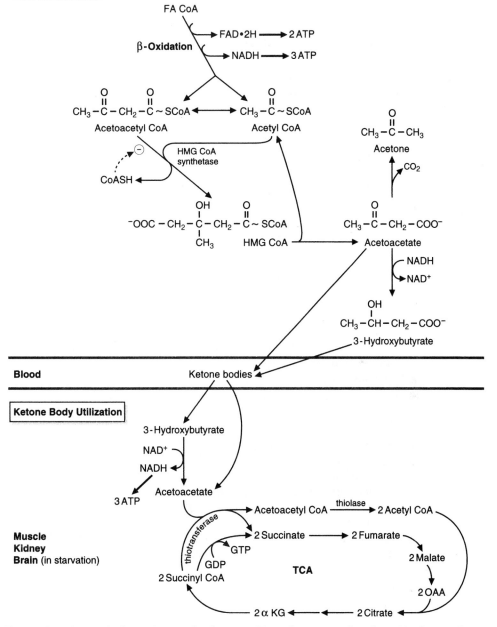

Figure 15-1 Ketone body synthesis and utilization. ATP = adenosine triphosphate; FA = fatty acid; FAD = flavin adenine dinucleotide; αKetone = α-ketoglutarate; HMG-CoA = hydroxymethylglutaryl coenzyme A; OAA = oxaloacetate; TCA = tricarboxylic acid. The thiotransferase is succinyl CoA–acetone-CoA transferase.

energy. During **starvation**, ketone bodies in the blood increase to a level that permits entry into **brain** cells, where they are oxidized.

2. **Acetoacetate** can enter cells directly, or it can be produced from the oxidation of 3-hydroxybutyrate by 3-hydroxybutyrate dehydrogenase. NADH is produced by this reaction and can generate ATP.

3. Acetoacetate is activated by reacting with succinyl CoA to form **acetoacetyl CoA** and succinate. The enzyme is succinyl CoA-acetoacetate-CoA transferase (a thiotransferase).

4. Acetoacetyl CoA is cleaved by **thiolase** to form two acetyl CoAs, which enter the tricarboxylic acid (TCA) cycle and are oxidized to CO_2 and H_2O.

5. **Energy is produced** from the oxidation of ketone bodies.
   a. One acetoacetate produces 2 acetyl CoAs, each of which can generate about 12 ATP, or a total of about 24 ATP via the TCA cycle.
   b. However, activation of acetoacetate results in the generation of one less ATP because guanosine triphosphate (GTP), the equivalent of ATP, is not produced when succinyl CoA is used to activate acetoacetate. (In the TCA cycle, when succinyl CoA forms succinate, GTP is generated.) Therefore, the oxidation of acetoacetate produces a net yield of only 23 ATP.
   c. When **3-hydroxybutyrate** is oxidized, three additional ATP are formed because the oxidation of 3-hydroxybutyrate to acetoacetate produces NADH.

II.   Phospholipid and Sphingolipid Metabolism

A. Synthesis and degradation of phosphoglycerides

1. The phosphoglycerides are synthesized by a process similar in its initial steps to triacylglycerol synthesis (glycerol 3-phosphate combines with two fatty acyl CoAs to form **phosphatidic acid**).

2. *Synthesis of phosphatidylinositol*
   a. **Phosphatidic acid** reacts with cytosine triphosphate (CTP) to form cytosine diphosphate (CDP)-diacylglycerol, which reacts with inositol to form phosphatidylinositol.
   b. **Phosphatidylinositol** can be further phosphorylated to form phosphatidylinositol 4,5-bisphosphate, which is cleaved in response to various stimuli to form the compounds inositol 1,4,5-trisphosphate (IP_3) and diacylglycerol (DAG), which serve as second messengers.

3. *Synthesis of phosphatidylethanolamine, phosphatidylcholine, and phosphatidylserine* (Figure 15-2)
   a. **Phosphatidic acid** releases inorganic phosphate, and diacylglycerol is produced. **DAG** reacts with compounds containing cytosine nucleotides to form **phosphatidylethanolamine** and **phosphatidylcholine.**
   b. **Phosphatidylethanolamine**
      (1) DAG reacts with CDP-ethanolamine to form phosphatidylethanolamine.
      (2) Phosphatidylethanolamine can also be formed by decarboxylation of phosphatidylserine.
   c. **Phosphatidylcholine**
      (1) DAG reacts with CDP-choline to form **phosphatidylcholine (lecithin).**
      (2) Phosphatidylcholine can also be formed by methylation of phosphatidylethanolamine. *S*-Adenosylmethionine (SAM) provides the methyl groups.
      (3) In addition to being an important component of cell membranes and the blood lipoproteins, phosphatidylcholine provides the fatty acid for the syn-

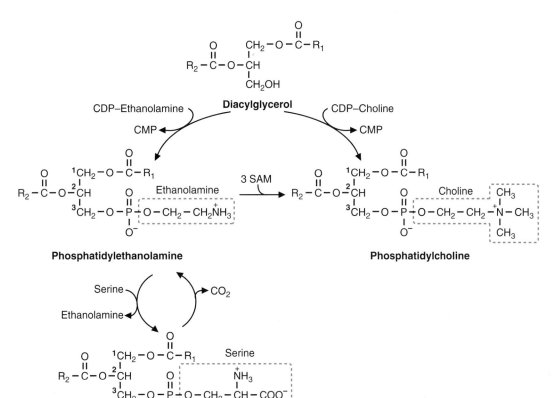

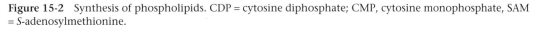

Figure 15-2   Synthesis of phospholipids. CDP = cytosine diphosphate; CMP, cytosine monophosphate, SAM = *S*-adenosylmethionine.

thesis of cholesterol esters in high-density lipoprotein (HDL) by the **lecithin:cholesterol acyltransferase (LCAT) reaction** and, as the dipalmitoyl derivative, serves as **lung surfactant.** If choline is deficient in the diet, phosphatidylcholine can be synthesized de novo from glucose (see Figure 15-2).

> *cc* **15.2**   **Respiratory distress syndrome** (RDS) of the newborn occurs in **premature infants** due to a **deficiency of surfactant in the lungs,** which leads to a decrease in lung compliance. **Dipalmitoyl phosphatidylcholine** (DPPC, also called lecithin), is the **primary phospholipid in surfactant,** which lowers surface tension at the alveolar air-fluid interface. Surfactant is normally produced at gestation week 30.

d. **Phosphatidylserine**
   (1) Phosphatidylserine is formed when phosphatidylethanolamine reacts with serine.
   (2) Serine replaces the ethanolamine moiety (see Figure 15-2).
4. *Degradation of phosphoglycerides*
   a. Phosphoglycerides are hydrolyzed by phospholipases.
   b. Phospholipase A_1 releases the fatty acid at position 1 of the glycerol moiety; phospholipase A_2 releases the fatty acid at position 2; phospholipase C releases the phosphorylated base (e.g., choline) at position 3; and phospholipase D releases the free base.

B. **Synthesis and degradation of sphingolipids** (Figure 15-3)

1. Sphingolipids are derived from **serine** rather than glycerol.
2. **Serine** condenses with **palmitoyl CoA** in a reaction in which the serine is decarboxylated by a pyridoxal phosphate–requiring enzyme.
3. The product is converted to a derivative of **sphingosine**.
4. A fatty acyl CoA forms an amide with the nitrogen, and the resulting compound is **ceramide**.
5. The hydroxymethyl moiety of ceramide combines with various compounds to form **sphingolipids**.
   a. **Phosphatidylcholine** reacts with ceramide to form **sphingomyelin**.
   b. Uridine diphosphate (UDP)-galactose, or UDP-glucose, reacts with ceramide to form galactocerebrosides or glucocerebrosides.
   c. A series of sugars can add to ceramide, with UDP-sugars serving as precursors. **CMP-NANA** (*N*-acetylneuraminic acid, a sialic acid) can form branches

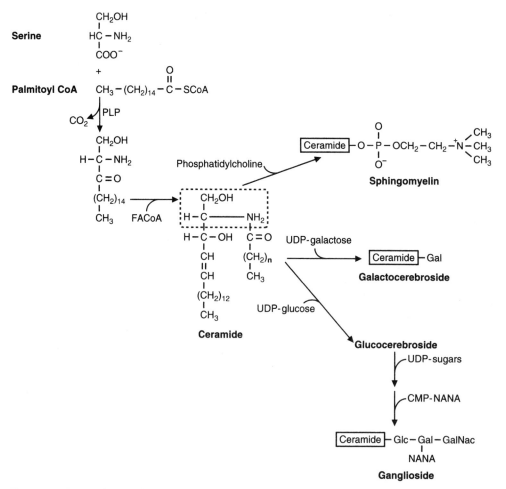

Figure 15-3 Synthesis of sphingolipids. FA = fatty acyl groups; Gal = galactose; GalNAc = *N*-acetylgalactosamine; Glc = glucose; NANA = *N*-acetylneuraminic acid; PLP = pyridoxal phosphate. The *dashed box* contains the protein of ceramide derived from serine.

from the carbohydrate chain. These ceramide-oligosaccharide compounds are **gangliosides.**

6. Sphingolipids are degraded by **lysosomal enzymes.** Genetic deficiencies of enzymes involved in the degradation of sphingolipids are well characterized (Table 15-1).

TABLE 15-1	*Sphingolipidoses*			
	Disease	Enzyme Deficiency	Accumulated Products	Clinical Consequence
cc **15.3**	Niemann-Pick disease	Sphingomyelinase	Sphingomyelin in the brain and blood cells	**Mental retardation, spasticity, seizures,** and **ataxia.** Death usually results by age 2–3 years. Inheritance is **autosomal recessive.**
cc **15.4**	Fabry disease	α-galactosidase A	Glycolipids in brain, heart, and kidney, resulting in ischemia of affected organs	Severe pain in the extremities (**acroparesthesia**), skin lesions (**angiokeratomas**), **hypohidrosis,** and ischemic infarction of the kidney, heart, and brain.
cc **15.5**	Krabbe disease	β-Galactosidase	Glycolipids causing destruction of myelin-producing oligodendrocytes	Clinical consequences of demyelination include **spasticity** and rapid neurodegeneration leading to death. Clinical signs include **hypertonia, hyperreflexia,** leading to **decerebrate posturing,** blindness, and deafness. Inheritance is autosomal recessive.
cc **15.6**	Gaucher disease	Glucocerebrosidase	Glucocerebrosides in blood cells, liver, and spleen	Enlarged liver and spleen (**hepatosplenomegaly**), anemia, low platelet count (**thrombocytopenia**), bone pain, and Erlenmeyer flask deformity of the distal femur. This **autosomal recessive** deficiency is prevalent in Ashkenazi Jews.

(continued)

TABLE 15-1	Sphingolipidoses (Continued)			
	Disease	Enzyme Deficiency	Accumulated Products	Clinical Consequence
cc 15.7	Tay-Sachs disease	Hexosaminidase A	GM2 gangliosides in neurons	Progressive **neurodegeneration, developmental delay,** and early death. This **autosomal recessive** deficiency is prevalent in Ashkenazi Jews.
cc 15.8	Metachromatic leukodystrophy	Arylsulfatase A	Sulfated glycolipid (sulfatide) compounds accumulate in neural tissue, causing demyelination of CNS and peripheral nerves.	Clinical consequences of demyelination include loss of cognitive and motor functions, intellectual decline in school performance, **ataxia, hyporeflexia,** and seizures.

CNS = central nervous system.

III.   Metabolism of the Eicosanoids

A. Prostaglandins, prostacyclins, and thromboxanes (Figure 15-4)

1. **Polyunsaturated fatty acids** containing 20 carbons and three to five double bonds (e.g., arachidonic acid) are usually esterified to position 2 of the glycerol moiety of phospholipids in cell membranes. These fatty acids require **essential fatty acids,** such as dietary linoleic acid ($18:2,\Delta^{9,12}$), for their synthesis.
2. The polyunsaturated fatty acid is cleaved from the membrane phospholipid by **phospholipase A_2,** which is inhibited by the steroidal anti-inflammatory agents (steroids).

 Steroids, such as cortisone and prednisone, are often prescribed for **inflammatory or autoimmune diseases,** such as rheumatoid arthritis, a debilitating inflammatory joint disease.

3. Oxygen is added and a 5-carbon ring is formed by a **cyclo-oxygenase** that produces the initial prostaglandin, which is converted to other classes of **prostaglandins** and to the **thromboxanes.**
   a. **Aspirin, acetaminophen,** and other nonsteroidal anti-inflammatory agents **inhibit** this cyclo-oxygenase.
   b. The **prostaglandins** have a multitude of effects that differ from one tissue to another and include inflammation, pain, fever, and aspects of reproduction. These compounds are known as **autocoids** because they exert their effects primarily in the tissue in which they are produced.
   c. Certain **prostacyclins** (PGI_2), produced by vascular endothelial cells, **inhibit platelet aggregation,** while certain **thromboxanes** (TXA_2) **promote platelet aggregation.**

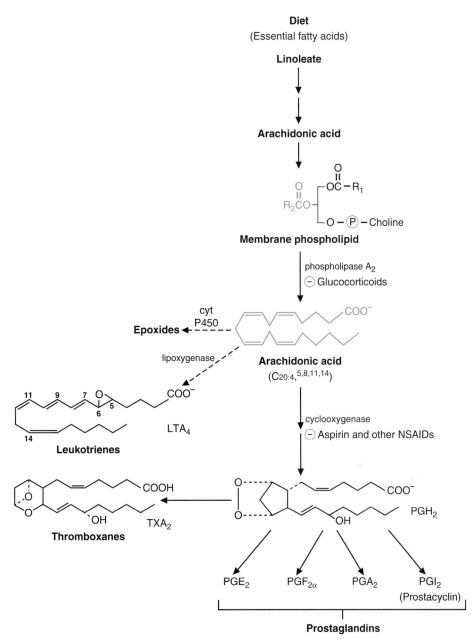

Figure 15-4 Overview of eicosanoid metabolism. Arachidonic acid is the major precursor of the eicosanoid including leukotriene (LT), prostaglandin (PG), and thromboxane (TX). NSAIDs = nonsteroidal anti-inflammatory drugs; ⊖ = inhibits.

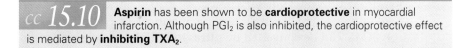

cc 15.10 **Aspirin** has been shown to be **cardioprotective** in myocardial infarction. Although PGI_2 is also inhibited, the cardioprotective effect is mediated by **inhibiting TXA_2**.

4. Inactivation of the prostaglandins occurs when the molecule is oxidized from the carboxyl and ω-methyl ends to form **dicarboxylic acids** that are excreted in the urine.

B. Leukotrienes

1. **Arachidonic acid**, derived from membrane phospholipids, is the major precursor for synthesis of the leukotrienes.
2. In the first step, oxygen is added by lipoxygenases, and a family of linear molecules, hydroperoxyeicosatetraenoic acids (**HPETEs**), is formed.
3. A series of compounds, comprising the family of leukotrienes, is produced from these HPETEs. The leukotrienes are involved in **allergic reactions.**

> *cc* **15.11** **Asthma** causes severe difficulty breathing due to **hyperreactivity and narrowing of the airways.** Since leukotrienes cause bronchoconstriction, **leukotriene receptor antagonists** can be prescribed as treatment.

IV. Synthesis of the Steroid Hormones

A. Steroid hormones are derived from **cholesterol** (Figure 15-5), which forms **pregnenolone** by cleavage of its side chain.

B. Progesterone is produced by oxidation of the A ring of **pregnenolone.**

C. Testosterone is produced from **progesterone** by removal of the side chain of the D ring. Testosterone is also produced from **pregnenolone** via dehydroepiandrosterone (DHEA).

D. 17β-Estradiol (E₂) is produced from **testosterone** by aromatization of the A ring.

E. **Cortisol** and **aldosterone**, the adrenal steroids, are produced from **progesterone.**

> *cc* **15.12** **3-β Hydroxylase deficiency** is a disease resulting in decreased production of aldosterone, cortisol, and androgens. (3-β Hydroxylase is required for production of all three types of steroids.) **Male infants** manifest with **ambiguous genitalia** (due to lack of androgens), and both males and females show salt wasting (due to lack of aldosterone).

> *cc* **15.13** *cc 15.13* **17-α Hydroxylase deficiency** is a disease resulting in decreased production of cortisol and androgens but increased production of aldosterone. Male and female teenagers are usually diagnosed during **puberty** with **lack of secondary sexual characteristics.** Increased aldosterone can cause excessive salt absorption.

F. **1,25-Dihydroxycholecalciferol** (1,25-DHC or calcitriol) (Figure 15-6), the active form of vitamin D_3, can be produced by two hydroxylations of **dietary vitamin D_3** (cholecalciferol).

1. The first hydroxylation occurs at position 25 (in the liver), and the second occurs at position 1 (in the kidney).
2. In addition, 7-dehydrocholesterol, a precursor of cholesterol produced from acetyl CoA, can be converted by **ultraviolet light** in the **skin** to cholecalciferol and then hydroxylated to form 1,25-DHC.

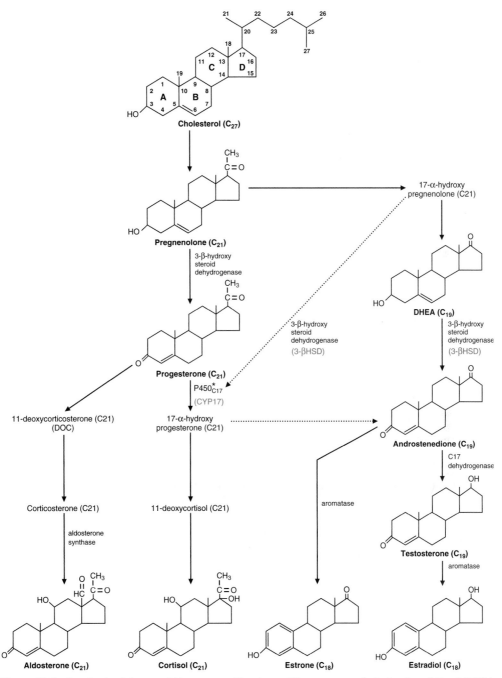

Figure 15-5   Synthesis of the steroid hormones. The rings of the precursor cholesterol are *lettered*. DHEA = dehydroepiandrosterone.

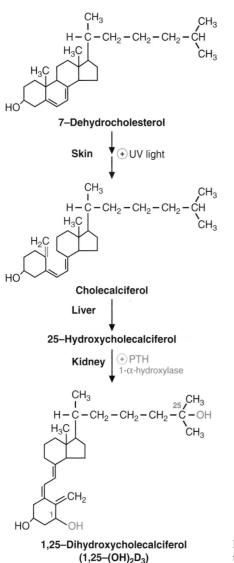

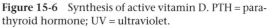

1,25–Dihydroxycholecalciferol
(1,25–(OH)₂D₃)

Figure 15-6 Synthesis of active vitamin D. PTH = parathyroid hormone; UV = ultraviolet.

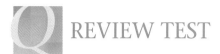

*Directions: Each of the numbered questions or incomplete statements in this section is followed by answers or by completions of the statement. Select the **one** lettered answer or completion that is **best** in each case.*

1. Which of the following are ketone bodies?

(A) Acetoacetate and β-hydroxybutyrate
(B) Ethanol and acetaldehyde
(C) β-Hydroxyacyl coenzyme A (CoA) and β-ketoacyl CoA
(D) Acetyl CoA and propionyl CoA
(E) Lecithin and lysolecithin

2. Which of following tissues lacks a thio-transferase enzyme that allows it to activate acetoacetate?

(A) Skeletal muscle
(B) Heart muscle
(C) Brain
(D) Kidney
(E) Liver

3. Which of the following statements best describes the conversion of fatty acids to ketone bodies?

(A) Carnitine transports the fatty acid across the plasma membrane.
(B) Three acetyl CoA molecules condense to form acetoacetyl CoA.
(C) Thiolase cleaves hydroxymethylglu-taryl CoA (HMG-CoA).
(D) HMG-CoA is cleaved to form acetyl CoA and acetoacetate.
(E) The reduction of acetoacetate to 3-hydroxybutyrate is an irreversible reaction.

4. When ketone bodies are used, thiolase cleaves acetoacetyl CoA into which of the following?

(A) 2 Acetyl CoA
(B) 2 Succinates
(C) 2 Fumarates
(D) 2 Malates
(E) 2 Oxaloacetates

5. When acetoacetate is oxidized, how many adenosine triphosphates (ATP) (or equivalents) are produced?

(A) 2
(B) 12
(C) 23
(D) 46
(E) 52

6. Which of the following statements best describes sphingolipids?

(A) Sphingolipids are derived from glycerol rather than serine.
(B) Sphingolipids are degraded by lyso-somal enzymes.
(C) Sphingomyelin contains a sugar residue.
(D) Galactocerebrosides and glucocerebro-sides contain phosphatidylcholine.
(E) Sphingolipids are synthesized but cannot be degraded and thus accu-mulate in cells.

7. Sphingolipids accumulate in what part of the cell?

(A) Lysosome
(B) Peroxisome
(C) Plasma membrane
(D) Outer mitochondrial membrane
(E) Inner mitochondrial membrane

8. Phospholipids have which of the following characteristics?

(A) They always contain choline and glycerol.
(B) They are an important source of energy during fasting.
(C) They are a major component of membranes.
(D) They are not charged in the body.
(E) They are not soluble in water.

9. Which of the following statements describes phosphatidylcholine?

(A) It can transfer a fatty acyl group to cholesterol.
(B) It can be synthesized by methylation of phosphatidylserine.

(C) It is not produced in the lung.

(D) It requires dietary choline for its synthesis.

(E) It can be directly converted to phosphatidylserine.

10. A 16-year-old girl presents with severe menstrual cramping, caused by increased prostaglandin production. Prostaglandin are synthesized from which of the following?

(A) Arachidonic acid

(B) Glucose

(C) Acetyl CoA

(D) Oleic acid

(E) Leukotrienes

11. A 12-year-old boy presents with fatigue, polydipsia (excessive drinking), polyuria (excessive urination), and polyphagia (excessive eating). A fingerstick glucose measurement shows a glucose level of 350 mg/dL in his serum. He is diagnosed with type 1 diabetes mellitus, a disease characterized by a deficiency of insulin. Which of the following would occur in this patient?

(A) Increased fatty acid synthesis from glucose in liver

(B) Decreased conversion of fatty acids to ketone bodies

(C) Increased stores of triacylglycerol in adipose tissue

(D) Increased production of acetone

(E) Chronic pancreatitis

12. A 20-year-old woman has a myocardial infarct (heart attack) and is given an aspirin to chew. Taking an aspirin has been shown to be cardioprotective in myocardial infarction. Aspirin is a nonsteroidal anti-inflammatory drug (NSAID) that inhibits cyclo-oxygenase (COX). COX is required for the production of which of these?

(A) Thromboxanes from arachidonic acid

(B) Leukotrienes from arachidonic acid

(C) Phospholipids from arachidonic acid

(D) Arachidonic acid from linoleic acid

(E) Hydroperoxyeicosatetraenoic acids (HPETEs) and subsequently hydroxyeicosatetraenoic acids (HETEs)

13. A 40-year-old woman has rheumatoid arthritis, a crippling disease causing severe pain and deformation in the joints of the fingers. She is prescribed prednisone, a steroidal anti-inflammatory drug. What is the mechanism of steroidal anti-inflammatory agents?

(A) Prevent conversion of arachidonic acid to epoxides

(B) Inhibit phospholipase A_2

(C) Promote activation of prostacyclins

(D) Degrade thromboxanes

(E) Promote leukotriene formation from HPETEs

14. An infant is born prematurely at 28 weeks and increasingly has great difficulty breathing, taking rapid breaths with intercostal retractions. His skin starts to turn blue from lack of oxygen (cyanosis). He is diagnosed with respiratory distress syndrome due to a deficiency of surfactant. Which of the following is the phospholipid of primary importance in surfactant?

(A) Dipalmitoyl phosphatidylcholine

(B) Dipalmitoyl phosphatidylethanolamine

(C) Dipalmitoyl phosphoglyceride

(D) Dipalmitoyl phosphatidylinositol

(E) Dipalmitoyl phosphatidylserine

15. A 16-year-old girl has never had menses. She also shows a lack of secondary sexual characteristics, such as age-appropriate pubic hair growth and breast development. She is diagnosed with 17-α hydroxylase deficiency. The levels of various steroid hormones in her serum are found to be abnormal. Steroid hormones are derived from which of the following?

(A) Acetyl CoA

(B) Cholesterol

(C) Fatty acids

(D) Glucose

(E) Oleic acid

16. An 11-year-old Ashkenazi Jewish girl presents with an enlarged liver and spleen, low white and red blood cell counts, bone pain, and bruising. She is diagnosed with Gaucher disease, a disease resulting in accumulation of glucocerebrosides in cells. Which of the following combine to directly form glucocerebrosides?

(A) Uridine diphosphate (UDP)-glucose and serine
(B) UDP-glucose and palmitoyl CoA
(C) UDP-glucose and ceramide
(D) UDP-galactose and serine
(E) UDP-galactose and ceramide

17. A 1-year-old infant's arms and legs have become spastic and rigid. Analysis shows an abnormally low level of the sphingomyelinase enzyme, causing accumulation of sphingomyelins. Which of the following combine to directly form sphingomyelin?

(A) Serine and palmitoyl CoA
(B) Fatty acyl CoA and sphingosine
(C) Palmitoyl CoA and ceramide
(D) Phosphatidylcholine and ceramide
(E) UDP-galactose and ceramide

18. A 4-month-old infant presents with muscular weakness that is progressing to paralysis. Examination of the back of the eye shows a cherry-red spot on the macula. An abnormally low level of hexosaminidase A is present, causing deposition of gangliosides in neurons. Gangliosides are formed when ceramide reacts with a compound derived from which of the following?

(A) Serine
(B) Palmitoyl CoA
(C) Sphingomyelin
(D) Galactocerebroside
(E) Glucocerebroside

19. A male infant is born with ambiguous genitalia (from lack of androgens such as testosterone) and severe salt wasting (due to lack of aldosterone). He is diagnosed with 3-β hydroxylase deficiency. Testosterone is produced by which of the following?

(A) Oxidation of the A ring of pregnenolone
(B) Removal of the side chain of the D ring of progesterone
(C) Aromatization of the A ring of estradiol
(D) Cleavage of the side chain of cortisol
(E) Oxidation of aldosterone

20. A 2-year-old girl presents with progressive difficulty walking, and she no longer is meeting motor and cognitive milestones appropriate for her age. An abnormally low level of arylsulfatase A is present, causing accumulation of sulfated glycolipids in neurons. She dies 5 years later. Which is the following is the most likely diagnosis?

(A) Fabry disease
(B) Gaucher disease
(C) Niemann-Pick disease
(D) Tay-Sachs disease
(E) Metachromatic leukodystrophy

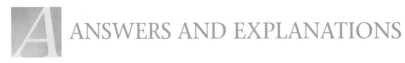

1–A. Acetoacetate and β-hydroxybutyrate are ketone bodies, which serve as a source of fuel during fasting, starvation, or a high-fat diet. They are synthesized mainly in liver mitochondria whenever fatty acids are high in the blood. Acetaldehyde is produced in the metabolism of ethanol. β-Hydroxyacyl coenzyme A (CoA) and β-ketoacyl CoA are intermediates in fatty acid oxidation. Acetyl CoA and propionyl CoA are produced in odd-chain fatty acid oxidation. Lecithin and lysolecithin are phosphatidylcholine and a derivative.

2–E. The liver lacks succinyl CoA-acetoacetate-CoA transferase (a thiotransferase), so the liver cannot use the ketone bodies that it produces. Instead, ketone bodies are released into the blood by the liver for use as fuel by the heart, brain, kidney, and skeletal muscle.

3–D. Two acetyl CoA molecules condense to form acetoacetyl CoA. Hydroxymethyl-glutaryl CoA (HMG-CoA) lyase cleaves HMG-CoA to form acetyl CoA and acetoacetate. The reduction of acetoacetate to 3-hydroxybutyrate is a reversible reaction.

4–A. Thiolase cleaves acetoacetyl CoA into 2 acetyl CoA molecules, which then enter the (tricarboxylic acid) TCA cycle and are oxidized to CO_2 and H_2O, generating adenosine triphosphate (ATP). Succinate, fumarate, malate, and oxaloacetate are intermediates in the TCA cycle.

5–C. One acetoacetate produces 2 acetyl CoA molecules, each of which generates about 12 ATP via the TCA cycle, for a total of about 24 ATP. However, the activation of acetoacetate results in the generation of 1 less ATP equivalent because guanosine triphosphate (GTP) is not produced when succinyl CoA is used to activate acetoacetate. Thus, a total of about 23 ATP are produced from 1 acetoacetate molecule.

6–B. Sphingolipids are degraded by lysosomal enzymes, and genetic deficiency of a given lysosomal enzyme can cause a sphingolipidosis disease. Sphingolipids are derived from serine, rather than from glycerol. Sphingomyelin contains phosphatidylcholine. Galactocerebrosides and glucocerebrosides contain a sugar residue of uridine diphosphate (UDP)-galactose or UDP-glucose, respectively.

7–A. In a group of diseases called sphingolipidoses, sphingolipids accumulate in the lysosomes of cells. The sphingolipidoses include a group of diseases in which various lysosomal enzymes are deficient. Very long–chain fatty acids are oxidized in peroxisomes. Long-chain fatty acids must pass from the cytosol through the outer and inner mitochondrial membranes for oxidation.

8–C. Phospholipids are important components of membranes but are also found in blood lipoproteins and in lung surfactant. They are amphipathic molecules that are not involved in storing energy but in interfacing between body lipids and their aqueous environment. They are soluble in water because they contain a phosphate residue that is negatively charged, and they often contain choline, ethanolamine, or serine residues that have a positive charge at physiologic pH. (A serine residue will contain both a negative charge and a positive charge.)

9–A. In the absence of dietary choline, phosphatidylcholine can be synthesized de novo from glucose. The last step in this pathway involves methylation of phosphatidylethanolamine by *S*-adenosylmethionine (SAM). As dipalmitoylphosphatidylcholine, phosphatidylcholine serves as a major component of lung surfactant. Phosphatidylcholine, also called lecithin, transfers a fatty acyl group in the lecithin:cholesterol acyltransferase (LCAT) reaction that occurs in high-density lipoprotein (HDL) and produces cholesterol esters. Phosphatidylcholine cannot be directly converted to phosphatidylserine but phosphatidylethanolamine can.

10–C. Prostaglandins can be synthesized from arachidonic acid (which requires the essential fatty acid, linoleate, for its synthesis). They cannot be synthesized from glucose, and they cannot be made from acetyl CoA or oleic acid. Leukotrienes are also derived from arachidonic acid.

11–D. Decreased insulin levels cause fatty acid synthesis to decrease and glucagon levels to increase. Adipose triacylglycerols are degraded, and fatty acids are released. In liver mitochondria, fatty acids undergo β-oxidization into the ketone bodies of acetoacetate and β-hydroxybutyrate. These ketone bodies are used as fuel by extrahepatic cells, such as heart, muscle, and brain. Nonenzymatic decarboxylation of acetoacetate forms acetone, which can be smelled on the breath of patients in diabetic ketoacidosis (a state of very elevated serum glucose).

12–A. Prostaglandins, prostacyclins, and thromboxanes are synthesized from arachidonic acid by the action of cyclo-oxygenases (COX). Inhibiting COX decreases the synthesis of prostaglandins.

13–B. Steroidal anti-inflammatory agents, such as cortisone and prednisone, inhibit phospholipase A_2, which cleaves arachidonic acid from a membrane phospholipid. Prostaglandins are formed from arachidonic acid. Leukotrienes are formed from arachidonic acid plus oxygen plus HPETEs.

14–A. Dipalmitoyl phosphatidylcholine (DPPC), also called lecithin, is the phospholipid in surfactant that lowers surface tension at the alveolar air-fluid interface. Phosphoglycerides are the group of the major phospholipids (which contain glycerol, fatty acids, and phosphate). To create each of the phospholipids, the phosphate can be esterified to choline, serine, ethanolamine, or inositol. Respectively, this creates phosphatidylcholine, phosphatidylserine, phosphatidylethanolamine, and phosphatidylinositol.

15–B. Steroid hormones, such as progesterone, testosterone, 17β-estradiol, cortisol, and aldosterone, are formed from cholesterol. Cholesterol forms pregnenolone by cleavage of its side chain.

16–C. Patients with Gaucher disease have a deficiency of β-glucocerebrosidase, resulting in glucocerebroside accumulation in cells of the liver, spleen, and bone marrow cells. Glucocerebrosides are formed when UDP-glucose reacts with ceramide. Sphingolipids, in general, are formed from serine. When serine condenses with palmitoyl CoA, the product is converted into a derivative of sphingosine.

17–D. Patients with Niemann-Pick disease have a deficiency of sphingomyelinase. The mechanism of disease is due to accumulation of sphingomyelin in the brain and blood cells. Sphingomyelin is formed when phosphatidylcholine reacts with ceramide. Serine and palmitoyl CoA condense to form a derivative of sphingosine. A fatty acyl CoA combines with this sphingosine product and forms ceramide. UDP-galactose and ceramide combine to form galactocerebroside.

18–E. This patient has Tay-Sachs disease. Patients with this disease have a deficiency of hexosaminidase A, resulting in buildup of gangliosides in neurons, which can result in neurodegeneration and early death. Gangliosides are formed when a glucocerebroside reacts with a series of sugars and combines with ceramide. The initial precursors of gangliosides are serine and palmitoyl CoA. Sphingomyelin, galactocerebroside, and glucocerebroside are other types of sphingolipids.

19–B. 3-β Hydroxylase deficiency is a disease resulting in decreased production of aldosterone, cortisol, and androgens (3-β hydroxylase is required for production of all three types of steroids). Male infants manifest with ambiguous genitalia (due to lack of androgens and testosterone), and both males and females show salt wasting (due to lack of aldosterone). Testosterone is produced by the removal of the side chain of the D ring of progesterone.

20–E. Metachromatic leukodystrophy is due to a deficiency in arylsulfatase A, a lysosomal enzyme that degrades sulfated glycolipids. These sulfatide compounds accumulate in neural tissue, causing demyelination of central nervous system and peripheral nerves, with resultant loss of cognitive and motor functions. Fabry disease is a result of a deficiency in α-galactosidase A; Niemann-Pick is a result of a deficiency in sphingomyelinase; Gaucher disease is a result of a deficiency in glucocerebroside; and Tay-Sachs is a result of a deficiency in hexosaminidase A.

Amino Acid Metabolism

I. Addition and Removal of Amino Acid Nitrogen

A. Transamination reactions (Figure 16-1)

1. Transamination involves the **transfer of an amino group** from one amino acid (which is converted to its corresponding α-ketoacid) to an α-ketoacid (which is converted to its corresponding α-amino acid). Thus, the nitrogen from one amino acid appears in another amino acid.

2. The enzymes that catalyze transamination reactions are known as **transaminases** or **aminotransferases.**

> **cc 16.1** Transaminases are important and common serum diagnostic markers of liver damage. The cytosolic **alanine aminotransferase (ALT),** also known as **serum glutamate pyruvate transaminase (SGPT)** and **aspartate aminotransferase (AST),** are released from cells upon insult.

3. **Glutamate** and **α-ketoglutarate** are often involved in transamination reactions, serving as one of the amino acid/α-ketoacid pairs (see Figure 16-1B).

4. Transamination reactions are readily reversible and can be used in the **synthesis** or the **degradation** of amino acids.

5. Most amino acids participate in transamination reactions. **Lysine** is an exception; it **is not transaminated.**

6. **Pyridoxal phosphate (PLP)** serves as the cofactor for transamination reactions. PLP is derived from vitamin B_6.

B. Removal of amino acid nitrogen as ammonia

1. A number of amino acids undergo reactions in which their nitrogen is released as ammonia (NH_3) or ammonium ion (NH_4^+).

2. **Glutamate dehydrogenase** catalyzes the oxidative deamination of glutamate (Figure 16-2). Ammonium ion is released, and α-ketoglutarate is formed. The glutamate dehydrogenase reaction, which is readily reversible, requires NAD or NADP.

3. **Histidine** is deaminated by histidase to form NH_4^+ and urocanate.

4. **Serine** and **threonine** are deaminated by serine dehydratase, which requires PLP. Serine is converted to pyruvate, and threonine is converted to α-ketobutyrate; NH_4^+ is released.

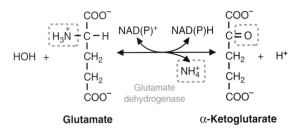

Figure 16-1 The glutamate dehydrogenase reaction. The reaction is readily reversible and uses NAD or NADP as a cofactor. The origin of the oxygen in α-ketoglutarate is from H_2O.

5. The amide groups of **glutamine** and **asparagine** are released as ammonium ions by hydrolysis. Glutaminase converts glutamine to glutamate and NH_4^+. Asparaginase converts asparagine to aspartate and NH_4^+.

6. The **purine nucleotide cycle** serves to release NH_4^+ from amino acids, particularly in muscle.

   a. Glutamate collects nitrogen from other amino acids and transfers it to aspartate by a transamination reaction.

   b. Aspartate reacts with inosine monophosphate (IMP) to form adenosine monophosphate (AMP) and generate fumarate.

   c. NH_4^+ is released from AMP, and IMP is re-formed.

C. **The role of glutamate** (Figure 16-3)

   1. **Glutamate provides nitrogen for synthesis** of many amino acids.

      a. NH_4^+ provides the nitrogen for amino acid synthesis by reacting with α-ketoglutarate to form glutamate in the glutamate dehydrogenase reaction.

      b. Glutamate transfers nitrogen by transamination reactions to α-ketoacids to form their corresponding α-amino acids.

   2. **Glutamate plays a key role in removing nitrogen** from amino acids.

      a. Glutamate collects nitrogen from other amino acids by means of transamination reactions.

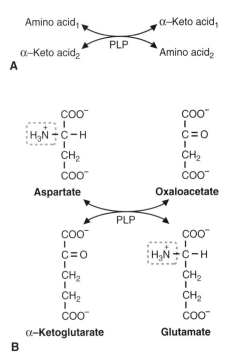

Figure 16-2 Transamination. The amino group from one amino acid is transferred to another. The enzymes mediating this reaction are termed transaminases or aminotransferases. **(A)** The generalized reaction uses pyridoxal phosphate (PLP) as a coenzyme. **(B)** The aspartyl transaminase reaction.

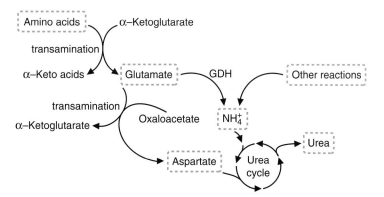

Figure 16-3   The role of glutamate in urea production. By transamination reactions, glutamate collects nitrogen from other amino acids. Nitrogen is released as NH_4^+ (ammonium ion) by glutamate dehydrogenase (GDH). NH_4^+ provides 1 nitrogen for urea synthesis (the other is from glutamate from transamination of oxaloacetate).

   b. The nitrogen of glutamate is released as NH_4^+ via the glutamate dehydrogenase reaction.
   c. NH_4^+ and aspartate provide nitrogen for urea synthesis via the urea cycle. Aspartate obtains its nitrogen from glutamate by transamination of oxalo-acetate.

II.   Urea Cycle

A.   Transport of nitrogen to the liver

   1. Ammonia is **very toxic**, particularly to the central nervous system (CNS).
   2. The concentration of ammonia and ammonium ions in the blood is normally very low. ($NH_3 + H^+ \leftrightarrow NH_4^+$) NH_3 is freely diffusible across membranes, but because the pK_a of the reaction is 9.3, at physiological pH, it is 1/100 the concentration of the NH_4^+ ion. Remember the Henderson-Hesselbach equation.
   3. Ammonia travels to the **liver** from other tissues, mainly in the form of **alanine and glutamine.** It is released from amino acids in the liver by a series of transamination and deamination reactions.
   4. Ammonia is also produced **by bacteria in the gut** and travels to the liver via the hepatic portal vein. The agent lactulose is used to treat this condition and is thought to work reducing ammonia by either increasing bacterial assimilation of ammonia or reducing deamination of nitrogenous compounds.

> *cc 16.2*   Patients with severe liver disease can not detoxify ammonia and thus develop **hepatic encephalopathy** from the accumulation of **ammonia in the CNS. Lactulose** is used to treat this condition and **reduces ammonia** by either increasing bacterial assimilation of ammonia or reducing deamination of nitrogenous compounds.

B.   Reactions of the urea cycle (Figure 16-4)

   1. NH_4^+ and **aspartate** provide the nitrogen that is used to produce **urea,** and CO_2 provides the carbon. Ornithine serves as a carrier that is regenerated by the cycle.

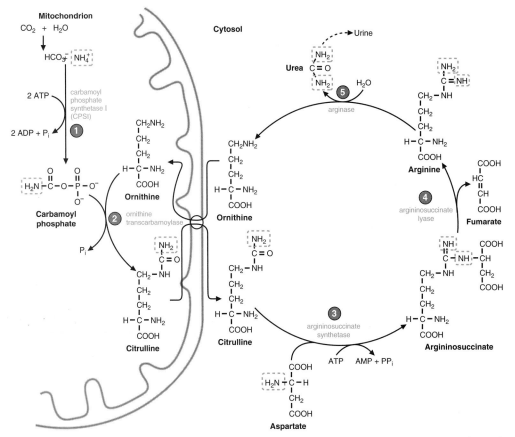

Figure 16-4 Urea cycle. Dashed boxes depict nitrogen-containing groups from which urea is formed. Numbers refer to reaction steps described in the text in section II B. ADP = adenosine diphosphate; AMP = adenosine monophosphate; ATP = adenosine triphosphate; P_i = inorganic phosphate.

2. **Carbamoyl phosphate** is synthesized in the first reaction from NH_4^+, CO_2, and 2 adenosine triphosphates (ATP).
   a. Inorganic phosphate and 2 adenosine triphosphates (ADP) are also produced.
   b. Enzyme: **carbamoyl phosphate synthetase I**, which is located in mitochondria and is activated by *N*-acetylglutamate. (Reaction 1)

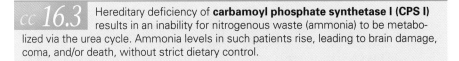

cc *16.3* Hereditary deficiency of **carbamoyl phosphate synthetase I (CPS I)** results in an inability for nitrogenous waste (ammonia) to be metabolized via the urea cycle. Ammonia levels in such patients rise, leading to brain damage, coma, and/or death, without strict dietary control.

3. **Ornithine** reacts with carbamoyl phosphate to form citrulline. Inorganic phosphate is released.
   a. Enzyme: **ornithine transcarbamoylase**, which is found in mitochondria. (Reaction 2)
   b. The product, citrulline, is transported to the cytosol.

Deficiency of **ornithine transcarbamoylase** results in similar neurologic sequelae as CPS I deficiency, although it is inherited as an X-linked trait.

4. **Citrulline** combines with aspartate—using the enzyme **argininosuccinate synthetase** (Reaction 3)—to form argininosuccinate in a reaction that is driven by the hydrolysis of ATP to AMP and inorganic pyrophosphate.

cc 16.5 Citrullinemia results from a deficiency of the enzyme **argininosuccinate synthetase,** causing an elevation in serum levels of citrulline. Again, without dietary management, the manifestations of this disease include lethargy, hypotonia, seizures, ataxia, and behavioral changes.

5. **Argininosuccinate** is cleaved to form arginine and fumarate.
   a. Enzyme: **argininosuccinate lyase.** (Reaction 4) This reaction occurs in the cytosol.

cc 16.6 Argininosuccinate aciduria results from a deficiency of the enzyme **argininosuccinate lyase** in the urea cycle, resulting in hyperammonemia with grave effects on the CNS.

   b. The carbons of fumarate, which are derived from the aspartate added in reaction 3, can be converted to malate.
   c. In the fasting state in the liver, malate can be converted to glucose or to oxaloacetate, which is transaminated to regenerate the aspartate required for reaction 3.
6. **Arginine** is cleaved, with the help of the enzyme, **arginase**, to form urea and regenerate ornithine. (Reaction 5) **Arginase** is located primarily in the liver and is inhibited by ornithine.

cc 16.7 Unlike deficiencies of other enzymes in the urea cycle, **arginase deficiency** does not result in severe hyperammonemia. The reason is twofold. First, the formed arginine, containing 2 "waste" nitrogens, can be excreted in the urine. Second, there are two isozymes, and in the event that the predominant liver enzyme is dysfunctional, the peripheral isozyme is inducible, leading to adequate restoration of the pathway.

7. **Urea** passes into the blood and is excreted by the kidneys. The urea excreted each day by a healthy adult (about 30 g) accounts for about 90% of the nitrogenous excretory products.

 The **blood urea nitrogen (BUN)** is a widely used measure of the kidney's functional ability to excrete the nitrogenous waste produced by the body.

8. **Ornithine** is transported back into the mitochondrion where it can be used for another round of the cycle.
   a. When the cell requires additional **ornithine**, it is synthesized from glucose via glutamate (Figure 16-5).
   b. **Arginine** is a nonessential amino acid. It is synthesized from glucose via ornithine and the first four reactions of the urea cycle.

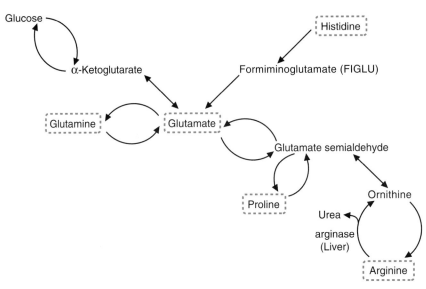

Figure 16-5 Amino acids related through glutamate. These amino acids contain carbons convertible to glutamate that can then be converted to glucose in the liver. Except for histidine, all of these amino acids can be synthesized from glucose.

C. Regulation of the urea cycle

1. **N-Acetylglutamate** is an activator of CPS I, the first enzyme of the urea cycle.
2. **Arginine** stimulates the synthesis of N-acetylglutamate from acetyl coenzyme A (CoA) and glutamate.
3. Although the liver normally has a great capacity for urea synthesis, the enzymes of the urea cycle are induced if a high-protein diet is consumed for 4 days or more.
4. The key relationship between the urea cycle and the tricarboxylic acid (TCA) cycle is that one of the urea nitrogens is supplied to the urea cycle as aspartic acid formed from the TCA cycle intermediate, oxaloacetic acid.

III. Synthesis and Degradation of Amino Acids

A. Synthesis of amino acids

1. Messenger RNA contains codons for 20 amino acids. Eleven of these amino acids can be synthesized in the body. The carbon skeletons of 10 of these amino acids can be derived from **glucose [S, G, C, A, E, Q, D, N, P, and R]. The essential amino acids derived from diet are: K, I, L, T, V, M, H, W, and F; Y is derived from F** (Table 16-1).
2. *Amino acids derived from intermediates of glycolysis* (Figure 16-6)
   a. Intermediates of glycolysis serve as precursors for serine, glycine, cysteine, and alanine.
   b. **Serine** can be synthesized from the glycolytic intermediate 3-phosphoglycerate, which is oxidized, transaminated by glutamate, and dephosphorylated.
   c. **Glycine** and **cysteine** can be derived from serine.
      (1) **Glycine** can be produced from serine by a reaction in which a methylene group is transferred to tetrahydrofolate (FH_4).

TABLE 16-1	*Amino Acid Abbreviations*	
Amino Acid	**Single-Letter Code**	**Three-Letter Code**
Derived from Glucose		
Serine	S	Ser
Glycine	G	Gly
Cysteine	C	Cys
Alanine	A	Ala
Glutamic acid	E	Glu
Glutamine	Q	Gln
Aspartic acid	D	Asp
Asparagine	N	Asn
Proline	P	Pro
Arginine	R	Arg
Derived from Diet		
Lysine	K	Lys
Isoleucine	I	Ile
Leucine	L	Leu
Threonine	T	Thr
Valine	V	Val
Methionine	M	Met
Histidine	H	HisI
Tryptophan	W	Trp
Other	Y	
Tyrosine	Y*	Tyr
Phenylalanine	F	Phe

*Y is derived from F.

    (2) **Cysteine** derives its carbon and nitrogen from serine. The essential amino acid **methionine** supplies the sulfur.

    d. **Alanine** can be derived by transamination of pyruvate.

3. *Amino acids derived from TCA cycle intermediates* (Figure 16-7)

    a. **Aspartate** can be derived from oxaloacetate by transamination.

    b. **Asparagine** is produced from aspartate by amidation.

    c. **Glutamate** is derived from α-ketoglutarate by the addition of NH_4^+ via the glutamate dehydrogenase reaction or by transamination. **Glutamine, proline, and arginine** can be derived from glutamate (see Figure 16-5).

    (1) **Glutamine** is produced by amidation of glutamate.

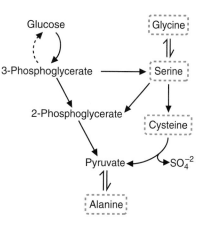

Figure 16-6 Amino acids derived from intermediates in glycolysis (synthesized from glucose). Their carbons can be reconverted to glucose in the liver. FH_4 = tetrahydrofolate; SO_4^{-2} = sulfate anion; PLP = pyridoxal phosphate.

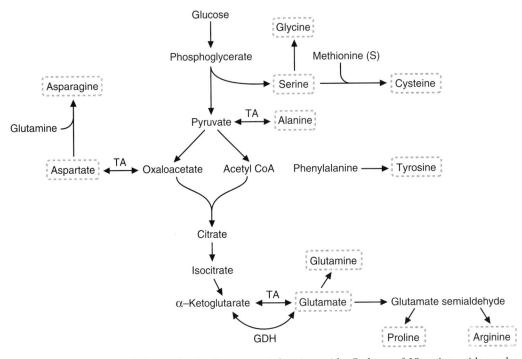

Figure 16-7 Overview of the synthesis of nonessential amino acids. Carbons of 10 amino acids can be produced from glucose via intermediates of glycolysis or the tricarboxylic acid (TCA) cycle. The 11th nonessential amino acid, tyrosine, is synthesized by hydroxylation of the essential amino acid, phenylalanine. The source of sulfur for cysteine is the essential amino acid methionine (its carbons and nitrogens from serine). CoA = coenzyme A; GDH = glutamate dehydrogenase; TA = transamination.

        (2) Proline and arginine can be derived from **glutamate semialdehyde**, which is formed by reduction of glutamate.

        (3) **Proline** can be produced by cyclization of glutamate semialdehyde.

        (4) **Arginine,** via three reactions of the urea cycle, can be derived from ornithine, which is produced by transamination of glutamate semialdehyde.

    4. Tyrosine, the eleventh nonessential amino acid, is synthesized by hydroxylation of the essential amino acid phenylalanine in a reaction that requires tetrahydrobiopterin.

B. Degradation of amino acids

    1. When the carbon skeletons of amino acids are degraded, the major products are **pyruvate**, intermediates of the TCA cycle, **acetyl CoA**, and **acetoacetate** (Figure 16-8).

        a. Amino acids that form pyruvate or intermediates of the TCA cycle in the liver are **glucogenic** (or gluconeogenic); that is, they provide carbon for the synthesis of glucose (see Figure 16-8A).

        b. Amino acids that form acetyl CoA or acetoacetate are **ketogenic;** that is, they form ketone bodies (see Figure 16-8B).

        c. Some amino acids (isoleucine, tryptophan, phenylalanine, and tyrosine) are both glucogenic and ketogenic.

    2. *Amino acids that are converted to pyruvate* (see Figure 16-6)

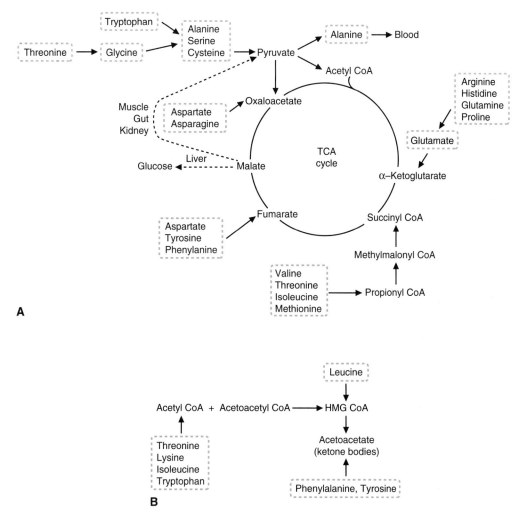

Figure 16-8 Degradation of amino acids. **(A)** Amino acids producing pyruvate or intermediates of the tricarboxylic acid (TCA) cycle. These amino acids are glucogenic, producing glucose in the liver. **(B)** Amino acids producing acetyl coenzyme A (CoA) or ketone bodies. These amino acids are ketogenic. HMG CoA = hydroxymethylglutaryl CoA.

a. The amino acids that are synthesized from intermediates of glycolysis (serine, glycine, cysteine, and alanine) are degraded to form pyruvate.

b. **Serine** is converted to 2-phosphoglycerate, an intermediate of glycolysis, or directly to pyruvate and NH_4^+ by serine dehydratase, which is an enzyme that requires PLP.

c. **Glycine**, in a reversal of the reaction used for its synthesis, reacts with methylene FH_4 to form serine.

   (1) Glycine also reacts with FH_4 and NAD^+ to produce CO_2 and NH_4^+.

   (2) Glycine can be converted to glyoxylate, which can be oxidized to CO_2 and H_2O, or converted to oxalate.

> *cc 16.9* **Renal calculi** (kidney stones) often occur from accumulated oxalate that precipitates with calcium.

> *cc 16.10*   **Type I primary oxaluria** results from the absence of the transaminase, which converts glyoxylate to glycine, resulting in renal failure due to excess oxalate in the kidney.

   d. Cysteine forms pyruvate. Its sulfur, which was derived from methionine, is converted to sulfuric acid (H_2SO_4), which is excreted by the kidneys.

   e. Alanine can be transaminated to pyruvate.

3. *Amino acids that are converted to intermediates of the TCA cycle* (see Figure 16-8).

   a. Carbons from four groups of amino acids form the TCA cycle intermediates **α-ketoglutarate, succinyl CoA, fumarate**, and **oxaloacetate**.

   b. Amino acids that form α-ketoglutarate (see Figure 16-5).

   (1) Glutamate can be deaminated by glutamate dehydrogenase or transaminated to form α-ketoglutarate.

   (2) Glutamine is converted by glutaminase to glutamate with the release of its amide nitrogen as NH_4^+.

   (3) Proline is oxidized so that its ring opens, forming glutamate semialdehyde, which is reduced to glutamate.

   (4) Arginine is cleaved by arginase in the liver to form urea and ornithine. Ornithine is transaminated to glutamate semialdehyde, which is oxidized to glutamate.

   (5) Histidine is converted to formiminoglutamate (FIGLU). The formimino group is transferred to FH_4, and the remaining 5 carbons form glutamate.

> *cc 16.11*   In the rare hereditary metabolic disorder of **histidinemia,** histidase, which converts histidine to urocanate, is defective. Early cases were reported to be associated with mental retardation, but more recently, deleterious consequences have not been observed.

   c. Amino acids that form succinyl CoA (Figure 16-9)

   (1) Four amino acids (**threonine, methionine, valine**, and **isoleucine**) are converted to **propionyl CoA.**

   • Propionyl CoA is carboxylated in a biotin-requiring reaction to form methylmalonyl CoA.

   • Methylmalonyl CoA is rearranged to form succinyl CoA in a reaction that requires vitamin B_{12}.

> *cc 16.12*   The hereditary deficiency of **methylmalonyl CoA mutase** results in failure to thrive, vomiting, dehydration, developmental delay, and seizures. Consequences of this deficiency are compounded by accumulation of propionyl CoA, a substrate for the TCA cycle enzyme, and of citrate synthase, leading to accumulation of the TCA toxin, methyl citrate.

   (2) Threonine is converted by a dehydratase to NH_4^+ and α-ketobutyrate, which is oxidatively decarboxylated to propionyl CoA. In a different set of reactions, threonine is converted to glycine and acetyl CoA.

   (3) Methionine provides **methyl groups** for the synthesis of various compounds; its sulfur is incorporated into **cysteine;** and the remaining carbons form **succinyl CoA.**

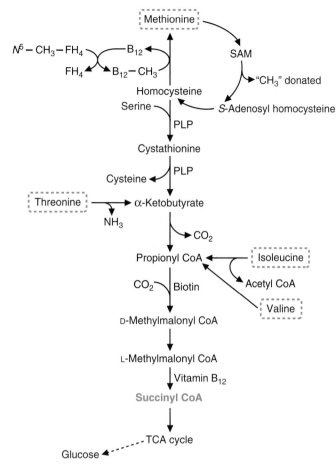

Figure 16-9 Amino acid conversion to succinyl coenzyme A (CoA). Methionine, threonine, isoleucine, and valine all form succinyl CoA via methylmalonyl CoA and are essential in the diet. Carbons of serine are converted to cysteine and thus do not form succinyl CoA by this pathway. PLP = pyridoxal phosphate; SAM = S-adenosylmethionine; TCA = tricarboxylic acid.

- Methionine and ATP form **S-adenosylmethionine (SAM)**, which donates a methyl group and forms homocysteine.
- **Homocysteine** is reconverted to methionine by accepting a methyl group from the FH_4 pool via vitamin B_{12}.

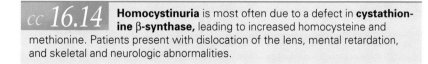

cc 16.13 Elevated levels of serum **homocysteine** have been correlated with an increased risk of coronary artery disease.

- **Homocysteine** can also react with serine to form **cystathionine**. The cleavage of cystathionine produces cysteine, NH_4^+, and α-ketobutyrate, which is converted to propionyl CoA.

cc 16.14 **Homocystinuria** is most often due to a defect in **cystathionine β-synthase,** leading to increased homocysteine and methionine. Patients present with dislocation of the lens, mental retardation, and skeletal and neurologic abnormalities.

(4) **Valine and isoleucine,** two of the three branched chain amino acids, form succinyl CoA (see Figure 16-9).

- Degradation of all three branched chain amino acids begins with a **transamination**, followed by an **oxidative decarboxylation** catalyzed by the branched chain α-ketoacid dehydrogenase complex (Figure 16-10). This enzyme, like pyruvate dehydrogenase and α-ketoglutarate dehydrogenase, requires thiamine pyrophosphate, lipoic acid, CoA, flavin adenine dinucleotide (FAD), and NAD⁺.
- **Valine** is eventually converted to succinyl CoA via propionyl CoA and methylmalonyl CoA.
- **Isoleucine** also forms succinyl CoA after two of its carbons are released as acetyl CoA.

> cc *16.15* In **maple syrup urine disease,** the enzyme complex that decarboxylates the transamination products of the **branched chain amino acids** (the α-ketoacid dehydrogenase) is defective (see Figure 16-10). Valine, isoleucine, and leucine accumulate. **Urine has the odor of maple syrup. Mental retardation** and **poor myelination** of nerves occur. Dietary restrictions are difficult to implement because three essential amino acids are required.

  d. Amino acids that form fumarate
  (1) Three amino acids (**phenylalanine, tyrosine,** and **aspartate**) are converted to fumarate (see Figure 16-8A).

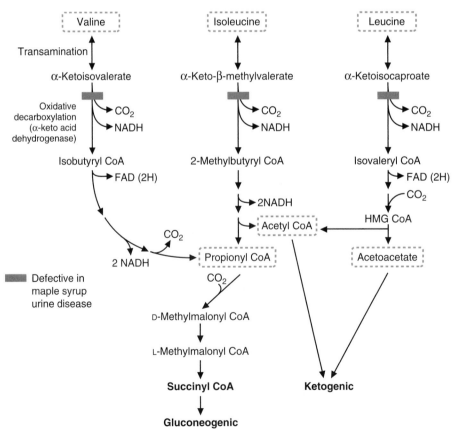

Figure 16-10 Degradation of branched chain amino acids. Valine forms propionyl coenzyme A (CoA). Isoleucine forms propionyl CoA. Leucine forms acetoacetate and acetyl CoA. FAD = flavin adenine dinucleotide.

(2) **Phenylalanine** is converted to **tyrosine** by phenylalanine hydroxylase in a reaction requiring tetrahydrobiopterin and O_2 (Figure 16-11).

> *cc* **16.16**   In **phenylketonuria** (PKU), the conversion of phenylalanine to tyrosine is defective due to defects in **phenylalanine hydroxylase.** A variant, nonclassical PKU, is a result of a defective enzyme in **tetrahydrobiopterin synthesis.** Phenylalanine accumulates in both disorders and is converted to compounds such as the phenylketones, which give the **urine a musty odor. Mental retardation** occurs. PKU is treated by restriction of phenylalanine in the diet.

(3) **Tyrosine**, which is obtained from the diet or by hydroxylation of phenylalanine, is converted to homogentisic acid. The aromatic ring is opened and cleaved, forming **fumarate** and **acetoacetate.**

> *cc* **16.17**   In **alcaptonuria, homogentisic acid,** which is a product of phenylalanine and tyrosine metabolism, accumulates because **homogentisate oxidase** is defective (see Figure 16-11). Homogentisic acid autooxidizes, and the products polymerize, **forming dark-colored pigments,** which accumulate in various tissues and are sometimes associated with a **degenerative arthritis.**

(4) **Aspartate** is converted to fumarate via reactions of the **urea cycle** and the **purine nucleotide cycle.** Aspartate reacts with IMP to form AMP and fumarate in the purine nucleotide cycle.

e. **Amino acids that form oxaloacetate** (see Figure 16-8A)

  (1) **Aspartate** is transaminated to form oxaloacetate.

  (2) **Asparagine** loses its amide nitrogen as NH_4^+, forming aspartate in a reaction catalyzed by asparaginase.

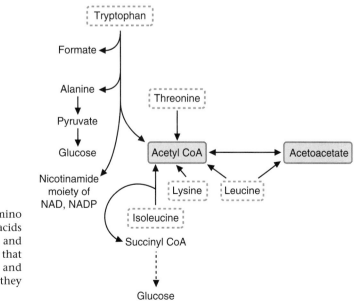

Figure 16-11   Ketogenic amino acids. Some of these amino acids (tryptophan, phenylalanine, and tyrosine) also contain carbons that can form glucose. Leucine and lysine are strictly ketogenic; they do not form glucose.

cc 16.18 In **acute lymphocytic leukemia** (ALL), the malignant cells are **unable to produce asparagine. To prevent proliferation, a recombinantly** produced **asparaginase** (converting asparagine to aspartate) is used to deplete circulating levels of asparagine.

4. *Amino acids that are converted to acetyl CoA or acetoacetate* (see Figure 16-11)
   a. Four amino acids (**lysine, threonine, isoleucine,** and **tryptophan**) can form acetyl CoA.
   b. **Phenylalanine** and **tyrosine** form acetoacetate.
   c. **Leucine** is degraded to form both acetyl CoA and acetoacetate.

cc 16.19 **Isovaleric acidemia** results from a defect in **isovaleryl CoA dehydrogenase,** preventing the degradation of isovaleryl CoA during the **degradation of leucine.** The defect results in **neuromuscular irritability** and **mental retardation.** The patient has a distinctive odor of "**sweaty feet.**" Limiting the intake of leucine helps limit the progression of symptoms.

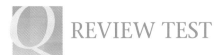# REVIEW TEST

*Directions: Each of the numbered questions or incomplete statements in this section is followed by answers or by completions of the statement. Select the **one** lettered answer or completion that is **best** in each case.*

1. Multiple carboxylase deficiency will lead to the excretion of which of the following?

(A) Vitamin B_{12}
(B) Biotin
(C) Propionic acid
(D) Methylmalonic acid
(E) Succinic acid

2. In the synthesis of cysteine, the carbon atoms (nearest precursor) are provided by which of the following?

(A) Aspartic acid
(B) Methionine
(C) Oxaloacetic acid
(D) Serine
(E) Homocysteine

3. When a large amount of leucine is metabolized by muscle, the release of alanine from muscle increases. Why?

(A) Carbon skeleton of leucine is converted to alanine.
(B) Carbon skeleton of leucine is converted to pyruvate.
(C) Leucine carbon skeleton is converted to glutamate, which in turn is metabolized by the tricarboxylic acid (TCA) cycle to oxaloacetate (OAA): OAA →→→ alanine.
(D) Nitrogen of leucine is transaminated directly to pyruvate (formed in glycolysis).
(E) Nitrogen of leucine is transaminated first to form glutamate and then transferred by transamination to pyruvate (formed in glycolysis).

4. Oral contraceptives are known to lower blood levels of folate and vitamin B_6. Which of the following conversion processes might be directly affected?

(A) Citrulline to arginine in the urea cycle
(B) Valine to succinyl CoA

(C) Glutamate to glutamine by glutamine synthase
(D) Propionyl CoA to methylmalonyl CoA
(E) Phenylalanine to tyrosine

5. Which of the following is the correct enzyme–genetic defect disease pair?

(A) Argininosuccinate synthetase–citrullinemia
(B) Arginase–argininosuccinate aciduria
(C) Ornithine transcarbamylase–congenital hyperammonemia type I
(D) Argininosuccinate lyase–arginemia
(E) Carbamoyl phosphate synthetase–congenital hyperammonemia type II

6. Which of the following is a common compound shared by the TCA cycle and the urea cycle?

(A) α-Ketoglutarate
(B) Succinyl coenzyme A (CoA)
(C) Oxaloacetate
(D) Fumarate
(E) Arginine

7. Which of the following enzymes requires adenosine triphosphate (ATP) to mediate its reactions?

(A) Argininosuccinate lyase
(B) Argininosuccinate synthetase
(C) Arginase
(D) Glutaminase
(E) Ornithine transcarbamoylase

8. Which of the following is the common nitrogen acceptor for all reactions involving transaminase?

(A) α-Ketoglutarate
(B) α-Ketobutyrate
(C) Pyruvate
(D) Oxaloacetate
(E) Acetoacetate

9. Which of the following best describes glutamate?

(A) It is produced in a transamination reaction in which aspartate reacts with oxaloacetate.

(B) It undergoes a series of reactions in which it cyclizes to produce histidine.

(C) It can be converted to arginine by a series of reactions, some of which require urea cycle enzymes.

(D) It is produced by the action of glutamate dehydrogenase, an enzyme that requires NH_4^+ and flavin adenine dinucleotide (FAD).

(E) Glutamate dehydrogenase converts proline to glutamate.

10. In mammals and birds, the cysteinyl and methionyl sulfur is predominantly excreted in what form?

(A) Cystathionine

(B) Inorganic sulfate

(C) Homocystine

(D) Homocysteine

(E) *S*-adenosyl homocysteine

11. A 5-year-old, mentally retarded child is seen by an ophthalmologist due to "blurry vision." Ocular examination demonstrates bilateral lens dislocations. On further work-up, imaging is significant for osteoporosis, and a urine analysis is remarkable for an accumulation of homocysteine. Serum analysis would most likely show an elevation of which of the following substances?

(A) Cystathionine

(B) Valine

(C) Phenylalanine

(D) Tyrosine

(E) Methionine

12. A 3-month-old child is being evaluated due to vomiting and an episode of convulsions. Physical exam was remarkable for hepatomegaly. Serum lab results demonstrated hyperammonemia. A deficiency in which of the following enzymes would most likely cause an elevation of blood ammonia levels?

(A) Carbamoyl phosphate synthetase II

(B) Glutaminase

(C) Argininosuccinase lyase

(D) Glutamate dehydrogenase

(E) Urease

13. A 48-year-old man, who was diagnosed with human immunodeficiency virus (HIV), has been struggling with acquired immunodeficiency syndrome (AIDS) for the past 2 years. He is now cachectic and having a difficult time obtaining any caloric intake, yet he refuses to take a nasogastric or gastric feeding tube. Because his muscles and organs are metabolically active, which of the following amino acids will produce both glucose and ketone bodies as an energy source?

(A) Alanine

(B) Tyrosine

(C) Proline

(D) Glycine

(E) Leucine

14. A 55-year-old man suffers from cirrhosis of the liver. Toxins such as ammonia are not properly metabolized by the liver and can now damage structures such as the brain. Which of the following amino acids covalently binds ammonia and transports and stores it in a nontoxic form?

(A) Aspartate

(B) Glutamate

(C) Serine

(D) Cysteine

(E) Histidine

15. In a 39-year-old woman who just gave birth, chorionic villus sampling was performed, and a battery of genetic panels was assessed on the newborn. One marker indicated a defective cystathionine β-synthase. Which of the following compounds would you most likely expect to be elevated in the blood of the infant at birth if the mother was not treated properly?

(A) Glutarate

(B) Methionine

(C) Valine

(D) Threonine

(E) Glutamate

16. A 27-year-old, semiprofessional tennis player seeks advice from a hospital-based nutritionist concerning his diet supplements. His coach had given him amino acid supplements consisting of phenylalanine and tyrosine. The rationale was that these precursors to several neurotransmitters will "help his brain focus" on his game. In reality, the excess amino acids are used for energy, with a poor and eclectic diet. The phenylalanine will, upon metabolism, enter the TCA cycle as which of the following?

(A) Oxaloacetate
(B) Citrate
(C) α-Ketoglutarate
(D) Fumarate
(E) Succinyl CoA

17. A 2-year-old girl was seen in the emergency room for vomiting and tremors. The elevated plasma ammonium ion concentration was 195 μM (normal, 11–50 μM). Metabolic screens of serum and urine were ordered and were remarkable for an elevation in the amino acid arginine in serum. You conclude that this patient may have a defect in which of the following enzymes?

(A) Carbamoyl phosphate synthetase I
(B) Carbamoyl phosphate synthetase II
(C) Ornithine transcarbamoylase
(D) Arginase
(E) Argininosuccinate lyase

18. A 23-year-old, Golden Gloves boxing contender presents with assorted metabolic disorders, most notably ketosis. During the history and physical exam, he describes his training regimen, which is modeled after the Rocky films and involves consuming a dozen raw eggs a day for protein. Raw eggs contain a 70-kD protein called avidin, with an extremely high affinity for a cofactor required by propionyl CoA carboxylase, pyruvate carboxylase, and acetyl CoA carboxylase. The patient is deficient in which of the following cofactors?

(A) Tetrahydrobiopterin
(B) Tetrahydrofolate
(C) Biotin
(D) Cobalamine
(E) Pyridoxal phosphate

19. A new test is developed that can non-radioactively "label" compounds in the human body. As a physician with a background in the new field of metabolomics, you assess a 21-year-old with classical phenylketonuria (PKU). Phenylalanine is fed with a label in the phenyl ring. In the urine, in which of the following compounds would you expect to find the greatest amount of label?

(A) Tyrosine
(B) Tryptophan
(C) Epinephrine
(D) Phenylketone
(E) Acetate

20. During a medical rotation, a medical student volunteered for a respiratory physiology exam that determines basal metabolic rate and the respiratory quotient. She followed the protocol for a resting individual in the postabsorptive state. Which of the following amino acids would be found in the highest concentration in serum?

(A) Alanine and glutamine
(B) Arginine and ornithine
(C) Glutamate and aspartate
(D) Branched chain amino acid
(E) Hydrophobic amino acids

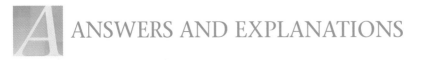

1–C. The carboxylases are involved in transfers of CO_2 primarily from propionyl co-enzyme A (CoA) to methylmalonyl CoA, thus multiple carboxylase deficiency would increase excretion of the substrate propionyl CoA. Methylmalonate is a product in a reaction catalyzed by a carboxylase. Biotin is only a cofactor and not a product of the carboxylases, and vitamin B_{12} is a cofactor from methylmalonyl CoA to succinyl CoA, which then feeds to the tricarboxylic acid (TCA) cycle.

2–D. This question refers to the precursor of the carbon atoms of cysteine that are provided by serine. Homocysteine, a direct precursor, only supplies sulfur. These two molecules form cystathionine. Methionine is the precursor to homocysteine. Aspartate and oxaloacetate are involved in transamination and do not directly affect cysteine synthesis.

3–E. Leucine is ketogenic, so it forms glucose. The only way for a part of the skeleton nitrogen to enter glycolysis is by transamination to an intermediate (glutamate) that can then be transferred (to pyruvate). The nitrogen cannot be transaminated to pyruvate since leucine does not enter glycolysis. The carbons will not be converted to alanine, pyruvate, or glutamate going to the TCA cycle.

4–B. Folate and vitamin B_6 (pyridoxine, a precursor of pyridoxal phosphate [PLP]) are cofactors. There are many steps going from valine to succinyl CoA requiring transamination (PLP). The conversion of citrulline to arginine does not require cofactors. Glutamate to glutamine uses adenosine triphosphate (ATP) and fixes ammonia. Propionyl CoA to methylmalonyl CoA requires biotin. Phenylalanine to tyrosine requires tetrahydrobiopterin (not tetrahydrofolate).

5–A. Defective argininosuccinate synthetase yields citrullinemia. Defective arginase yields mild hyperammonemia. Ornithine transcarbamylase and carbamoyl phosphate synthetase yield congenital hyperammonemia types II and I, respectively. Defective argininosuccinate lyase yields hyperammonemia.

6–D. Fumarate is in both the urea and TCA cycles. α-Ketoglutarate, succinyl CoA, and oxaloacetate (OAA) are only in the TCA cycle. Arginine is only in the urea cycle.

7–B. Argininosuccinate synthetase requires ATP. All of the other enzymes listed do not require energy and are exergonic reactions; remember, ΔG is negative.

8–A. All transaminases all have α-ketoglutarate as the common nitrogen acceptor. Oxaloacetate is a common nitrogen donor. Serine is deaminated to pyruvate, and threonine is deaminated to α-ketobutyrate. Other amino acids are converted to acetoacetate.

9–C. Glutamate can be reduced to glutamate semialdehyde and then transaminated to form ornithine, which can be converted to arginine via enzymes of the urea cycle. Glutamate semialdehyde cyclizes to form proline. (Histidine cannot be synthesized in humans.) Aspartate and α-ketoglutarate undergo a transamination reaction that produces oxaloacetate and glutamate. The reaction catalyzed by glutamate dehydrogenase requires NADH or NADPH; it produces glutamate from α-ketoglutarate and NH_4^+.

10–B. In the degradation of cysteine and its precursor methionine, the sulfur is converted to inorganic sulfate and excreted. Homocysteine, its oxidized form homocystine, and cystathionine are precursors of cysteine. S-adenosyl homocysteine is formed by the demethylation of *S*-adenosylmethionine (SAM) and is covered in Chapter 17.

11–E. The child has homocystinuria, a deficiency of cystathionine synthetase. This enzyme is in the pathway responsible for metabolism of sulfur-containing amino acids and normally catalyzes the conversion of homocysteine to cystathionine. When the enzyme is defective, homocysteine (normally a degradation product of methionine) is remethylated by a salvage pathway, resulting in the resynthesis of methionine. The methionine levels in the plasma are elevated as a result. The clinical characteristics are mental retardation, osteoporosis, and dislocation of the ocular lens.

12–C. There are two major types of hyperammonemia: acquired and hereditary. The hereditary type can result from deficiencies of any of the five enzymes of the urea cycle, although argininosuccinase lyase deficiency was the first reported. The rest of the choices are enzymes that produce ammonia, except for carbamoyl phosphate synthetase II, which is a cytosolic enzyme involved in pyrimidine synthesis.

13–B. The three amino acids that contain a six-membered ring are both ketogenic and glucogenic: tyrosine, phenylalanine, and tryptophan. Leucine is ketogenic; and alanine, proline, and glycine are only glucogenic.

14–B. Glutamate and ammonia form glutamine, as catalyzed by glutamine synthetase at the cost of 1 ATP. Cysteine is not directly involved with ammonia. Aspartate and ammonia both donate a nitrogen to form urea (along with ammonia). Histidine and serine are deaminated, forming ammonia. Central nervous system dysfunction due to high ammonia–level hepatic encephalopathy results in a sequelae of symptoms such as asterixis, confusion, and coma.

15–B. The molecular defect involved with cystathionine β-synthase is homocystinuria, leading to increased homocysteine and methionine. Glutamate is involved in another pathway, and glutarate is a distractor. Valine and threonine are "downstream" of the cystathionine and are not increased by blocking the step.

16–D. It is true (see Chapter 17) that tyrosine and phenylalanine are precursors to synthesize neurotransmitters, but excess amino acid intake leads to degradation. First, phenylalanine can be converted directly to tyrosine and, through homogentisic acid, enters the TCA cycle as fumarate. Asp and Asn enter through OAA; Glu directly feeds into α-ketoglutarate; and Val, Thr, Ile, and Met enter via propionyl CoA to succinyl CoA (see Table 16-1 for amino acid abbreviations).

17–D. This is another case of hyperammonemia. The presence of elevated arginine indicates that the block is the conversion to the next step. Arginase converts arginine to ornithine. Arginosuccinate lyase is the step to synthesize to arginine. Ornithine transcarbamoylase converts ornithine to citrulline, and the carbamoyl phosphate synthetases are involved in the beginning of the urea cycle.

18–C. The cofactor required for propionyl CoA carboxylase, pyruvate carboxylase, and acetyl-CoA carboxylase is biotin. Avidin binds extremely tightly (hence the name <u>avid</u>in) to biotin, which can not be used by various enzymes as a cofactor, so their many substrates build up. None of these enzymes use other cofactors, and avidin does not bind to them.

19–D. Phenylketonuria (PKU) is a defect in phenylalanine hydroxylase, resulting in a block in the conversion of phenylalanine to tyrosine. Phenylalanine accumulates in both disorders and is converted to phenylketones. Tyrosine is the product whose formation is blocked, and epinephrine, a product of tyrosine, would not be made or "labeled." Acetate and tryptophan are very far downstream from tyrosine.

20–A. Because the postabsorptive state (after a meal) is being referred to, we are referring to amino acid synthesis. Essential amino acids that are not synthesized are not being referred to, therefore choices B, D, and E cannot be correct. Regarding choice C (glutamate and aspartate), although nonessential, these amino acids are the key elements involved in transamination, mediating transfer of nitrogen groups from one amino acid to another amino acid, so they are never in high concentrations themselves, but in flux.

Products Derived from Amino Acids

I. Special Products Derived from Amino Acids

A. Creatine (Figure 17-1)

    1. **Creatine** is produced from glycine, arginine, and *S*-adenosylmethionine (SAM). Glycine combines with arginine to form ornithine and guanidinoacetate, which is methylated by SAM to form creatine.

    2. **Creatine** travels from the liver to other tissues where it is converted to **creatine phosphate.** Adenosine triphosphate (ATP) phosphorylates creatine to form creatine phosphate in a reaction catalyzed by **creatine kinase (CK).**

> *cc 17.1* There are two different subunits of CK, the M (muscle) subunit and the B (brain) subunit. These subunits function as dimers as MM, MB, or BB. Heart tissue has predominately **CK-MB,** which is released into the serum with **myocardial infarction** (MI), becoming **elevated within hours of an MI** and remaining elevated for at least 2 days.

        a. Muscle and brain contain large amounts of creatine phosphate.

        b. **Creatine phosphate** provides a small reservoir of high-energy phosphate that readily regenerates ATP from adenosine diphosphate (ADP). It plays a particularly important role during the early stages of exercise in muscle, where the largest quantities of creatine phosphate are found.

        c. Creatine also transports high-energy phosphate from mitochondria to actomyosin fibers.

    3. Creatine phosphate spontaneously cyclizes, forming **creatinine**, which is **excreted by the kidney.**

> *cc 17.2* The amount of **creatinine** excreted per day depends on **body muscle mass** and **kidney function** and is constant at about 15 millimoles for the average person. In cases of kidney failure, creatinine rises, as does the blood urea nitrogen (BUN).

B. Glutathione (GSH) (Figure 17-2)

    1. *Structure*

        a. GSH is a tripeptide.

        b. It is synthesized from glutamate, cysteine, and glycine.

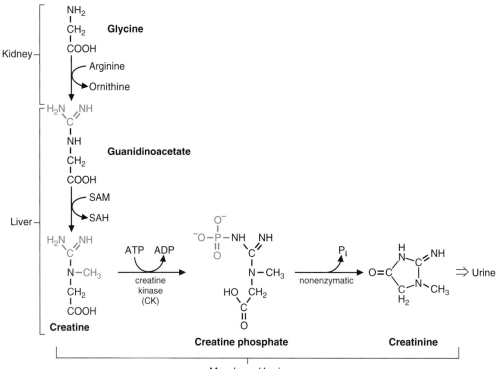

Figure 17-1 The synthesis of creatine phosphate and its spontaneous (nonenzymatic) conversion to creatinine. ADP = adenosine diphosphate; ATP = adenosine triphosphate; P_i = inorganic phosphate; SAH = S-adenosylhomocysteine; SAM = S-adenosylmethionine.

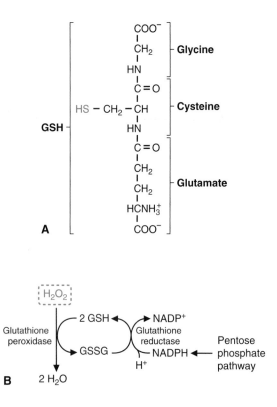

Figure 17-2 Glutathione (GSH) and the redox cycle. **(A)** The structure of glutathione. **(B)** The oxidation of glutathione by the oxidizing agent hydrogen peroxide (H_2O_2) and regeneration of reduced glutathione (GSSG).

2. *Function*

a. Involved in the transport of amino acids across the cell membranes (the γ-**glutamyl cycle**).

b. Aids in the rearrangement of protein disulfide bonds under **oxidizing conditions** and **detoxification reactions** (see Figure 17-2B).

(1) The sulfhydryl groups of GSH are used to reduce oxidized proteins, resulting in the 2 molecules of GSH disulfide bonded together as **GSSG.**

(2) GSSG is reduced back to 2 molecules of GSH through the action of **glutathione reductase**, an NADPH-requiring enzyme.

> *cc 17.3* **Acetaminophen** is the drug that is most commonly ingested in overdoses. **Glutathione** plays a major role in detoxifying this potential hepatotoxic and lethal agent. As stores of GSH dwindle, the patient moves from malaise and vomiting to **jaundice**, gastrointestinal bleed, **encephalopathy,** and finally **death.** *N*-**Acetylcysteine (NAC)** is a medication that replenishes levels of GSH during acetaminophen toxicity.

C. Nitric Oxide (NO) (Figure 17-3)

1. *Synthesis*

a. Liberated in the conversion of L-arginine to citrulline

b. The enzyme **nitric oxide synthase (NOS)** is a complex enzyme requiring NADPH, flavin adenine dinucleotide (FAD), flavin mononucleotide (FMN), and tetrahydrobiopterin (BH₄).

c. NOS is found in three major isoforms.

(1) Neuronal NOS (nNOS or NOS-1).

(2) Macrophage or inducible NOS (iNOS or NOS-2).

(3) Endothelial NOS (eNOS or NOS-3).

2. *Function*

a. **iNOS** is important in **macrophages** for creating NO for the generation of free radicals, which are **bactericidal.**

b. NO stimulates the influx of Ca^{2+} into vascular endothelial cells, with the activation of **cyclic guanosine monophosphate** (cGMP) resulting in relaxation of vascular smooth muscle (NO is also known as **endothelium-derived relaxation factor [EDRF]**).

> *cc 17.4* Numerous pharmacologic agents known as **nitrates** (i.e., **nitroglycerine, nitroprusside,** and **isosorbide dinitrate**) release NO once they are in the blood stream and are used in the **control of blood pressure** in select patients.

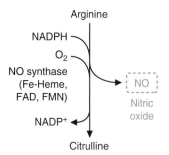

Figure 17-3 Nitric oxide synthase synthesizes the free radical nitric oxide. FAD = flavin adenine dinucleotide; Fe-Heme = iron hemoglobin; FMN = flavin mononucleotide.

D.   Products formed by amino acid decarboxylations

1. Amines are produced by decarboxylation of amino acids in reactions that use pyridoxal phosphate (PLP) as a cofactor.
2. γ-Aminobutyric acid (**GABA**), an inhibitory neurotransmitter, is produced by decarboxylation of **glutamate** (Figure 17-4).

> *cc* **17.5**   GABA promotes **neuron inhibition** by promoting entry of chloride into the neuron. Numerous pharmacologic agents (i.e., benzodiazepines, topiramate, lamotrigine, and tiagabine) **stimulate GABA** activity in the **treatment of seizures** and other hyperspastic disorders.

3. **Histamine** is produced by decarboxylation of **histidine**.
   a. Histamine causes vasodilation and bronchoconstriction.
   b. In the stomach, it stimulates the secretion of hydrochloric acid (HCl).

> *cc* **17.6**   Histidine binds to **H1 receptors** in the stomach, stimulating the release of gastric acid. Pharmacologic blockers of H1 receptors are used in the treatment of **gastric reflux. H2 receptors** are located on basophils and stimulate their degranulation during the allergic response. H2 receptor blockers are used to treat **allergic conditions.**

4. The initial step in **ceramide** formation involves the condensation of **palmitoyl coenzyme A (CoA)** with **serine,** which undergoes a simultaneous decarboxylation. Ceramide forms the sphingolipids (e.g., sphingomyelin, cerebrosides, and gangliosides).
5. The production of **serotonin** from tryptophan and of **dopamine** from tyrosine involves decarboxylations of amino acids.

E.   Products derived from tryptophan

1. **Serotonin, melatonin,** and the nicotinamide moiety of **NAD** and **NADP** are formed from tryptophan (Figure 17-5).

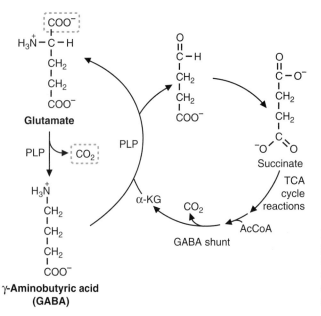

Figure 17-4   The decarboxylation of glutamate to form γ-aminobutyric acid (GABA). AcCoA = acetyl coenzyme A; α-KG = α-ketoglutarate; PLP = pyridoxal phosphate; TCA = tricarboxylic acid.

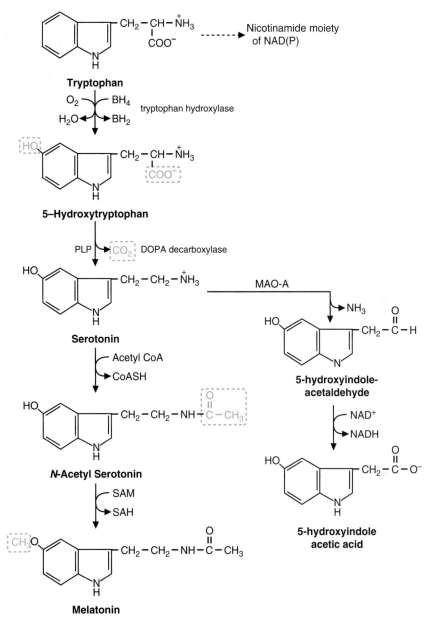

Figure 17-5   Synthesis and inactivation of serotonin biosynthesis. CoA = coenzyme A; dopa = dihydroxyphenylalanine; MAO-A = monoamine oxidase-A; PLP = pyridoxal phosphate; SAH = S-adenosylhomocysteine; SAM = S-adenosylmethionine.

2. **Tryptophan** is hydroxylated in a **BH$_4$**-requiring reaction similar to the hydroxylation of phenylalanine. The product, 5-hydroxytryptophan, is decarboxylated to form **serotonin**.

cc 17.7   **Serotonin** is an important stimulatory neurotransmitter involved in mood. **Selective serotonin reuptake inhibitors** (SSRIs) promote serotonin's actions and are first-line agents in **the treatment of depression**.

> *cc 17.8* **Carcinoid tumors** overproduce the neurotransmitter **serotonin,** with the accumulation of the primary metabolite 5-hydroxyindole acetic acid **(5-HIAA).** When these tumors metastasize to the liver, they cause **carcinoid syndrome,** which is characterized by diarrhea, flushing, wheezing, and cardiac valve damage.

3. **Serotonin** undergoes acetylation by acetyl CoA and methylation by SAM to form **melatonin** in the pineal gland.
4. Tryptophan can be converted to the nicotinamide moiety of **NAD** and **NADP** (see Figure 17-5), although the major precursor of nicotinamide is the vitamin niacin (nicotinic acid). Thus, to a limited extent, tryptophan can spare the dietary requirement for niacin.

F. Products derived from phenylalanine and tyrosine

1. *Phenylalanine* can be hydroxylated to form **tyrosine** in a reaction that requires **BH₄**. Tyrosine can be hydroxylated to form **dopa** (3,4-dihydroxyphenylalanine) (Figure 17-6).
2. *Thyroid hormones* (Figure 17-7)
   a. The follicular cells of the thyroid gland produce the protein **thyroglobulin,** which is secreted into the colloid.
   b. **Iodine,** which is concentrated in the follicular cells by a pump in the cell membrane, is oxidized by a peroxidase. Iodination of **tyrosine residues** in thyroglobulin produces monoiodotyrosine (MIT) and diiodotyrosine (DIT), which undergo **coupling reactions** to produce 3,5,3'-triiodothyronine (T_3) and 3,5,3',5'-tetraiodothyronine (T_4), which is also known as thyroxine.

> *cc 17.9* Agents used in the treatment of **hyperthyroidism** (i.e., **Graves disease**), such as **propylthiouracil** and **methimazole,** inhibit the iodination of tyrosine residues as well as the coupling reaction.

   c. Thyroid-stimulating hormone (**TSH**) stimulates **pinocytosis** of thyroglobulin, and **lysosomal proteases** cleave peptide bonds, releasing free T_3 and T_4 from thyroglobulin. These hormones enter the blood.
3. *Melanins,* which are pigments in skin and hair, are formed by polymerization of oxidation products (quinones) of **dopa.** In this case, dopa is formed by hydroxylation of tyrosine by an enzyme that uses copper rather than BH₄.

> *cc 17.10* **Albinism** results from a **defect in the conversion of tyrosine to melanin,** with partial or full absence of this pigment in the **hair, skin, and/or eye.** The disorder results from a deficiency of the enzyme **tyrosinase** (which converts tyrosine to melanin), or in defects in **tyrosine transport.** Lack of melanin **increases the risk** of developing **skin cancer.**

4. *The catecholamines* (dopamine, norepinephrine, and epinephrine) are derived from tyrosine in a series of reactions (see Figure 17-6).
   a. **Synthesis of the catecholamines**
      (1) Phenylalanine forms tyrosine, which forms **dopa.** In this case, both of these hydroxylation reactions require **BH₄**.
      (2) Decarboxylation of dopa forms the neurotransmitter **dopamine.**

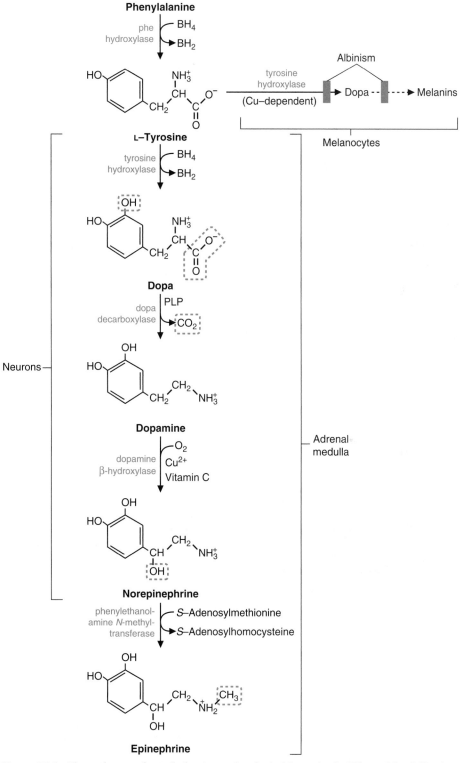

Figure 17-6   The pathways of catecholamine and melanin biosynthesis. BH_2 = oxidized dihydrobiopterin; BH_4 = tetrahydrobiopterin; Cu = copper; dopa = dihydroxyphenylalanine.

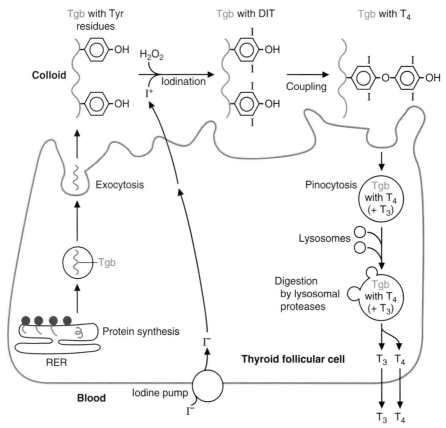

Figure 17-7 The synthesis of thyroid hormones. DIT = diiodotyrosine; H_2O_2 = hydrogen peroxide; RER = rough endoplasmic reticulum; T_3 = triiodothyronine; T_4 = tetraiodothyronine; Tgb = thyroglobulin; Tyr = tyrosine.

> *cc* **17.11** In **Parkinson disease,** dopamine levels are decreased because of a deficiency in conversion of dopa to dopamine. The common characteristics are **tremors,** difficulty initiating voluntary movement, a **masked face** with a staring expression, and a **shuffling gait. Infantile forms** of the disease have been found to be due to defects in **tyrosine hydrolyase.**

    (3) Hydroxylation of dopamine by an enzyme that requires copper and vitamin C yields the neurotransmitter **norepinephrine.**

    (4) Methylation of norepinephrine in the adrenal medulla by SAM forms the hormone **epinephrine.**

  b. Inactivation of the catecholamines

    (1) The catecholamines are inactivated by monoamine oxidase (**MAO**), which produces ammonium ion (NH_4^+) and hydrogen peroxide (H_2O_2) and converts the catecholamine to an aldehyde, and by catecholamine O-methyltransferase (**COMT**), which methylates the 3-hydroxy group.

> *cc* **17.12** Inhibition of **MAO** and **COMT** are both approaches in the treatment of neuropsychiatric disorders such as depression and **Parkinson disease.**

(2) The major urinary excretory product of the deaminated, methylated catecholamines is **VMA** (vanillylmandelic acid, or 3-methoxy-4-hydroxymandelic acid).

> *cc 17.13* Patients with **pheochromocytomas** overproduce adrenally synthesized catecholamines and have increased levels of **VMA**; urinary levels of VMA are used to diagnosis these tumors.

II.   Tetrahydrofolate and *S*-Adenosylmethionine

A.   Tetrahydrofolate

1. *The nature of tetrahydrofolate (FH₄) and its derivatives*
   a. **FH₄** cannot be synthesized in the body.
      (1) It is produced from the vitamin folate.
      (2) **NADPH** and **dihydrofolate reductase** convert folate to dihydrofolate (FH₂), which undergoes a second reduction by the same enzyme to form **FH₄** (Figure 17-8A).

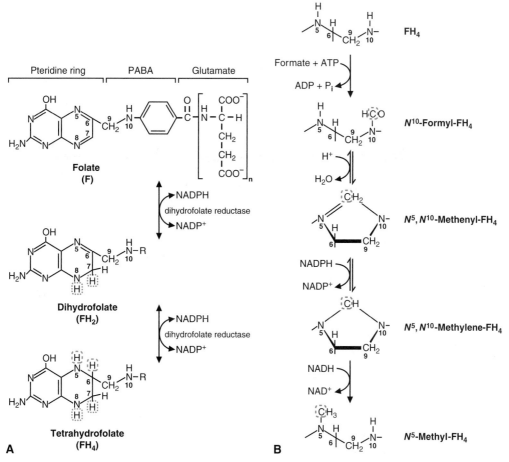

Figure 17-8   Tetrahydrofolate (FH₄). **(A)** Reduction of folate by dihydrofolate reductase. **(B)** The 1-carbon groups carried by FH₄. The 1-carbon groups are indicated by *dashed boxes*. Only atoms 5, 6, 9, and 10 of FH₄ are shown. The remainder of the structure is shown in **A**. ADP = adenosine diphosphate; ATP = adenosine triphosphate; PABA = para-aminobenzoic acid; P$_i$ = inorganic phosphate.

   b. The **1-carbon groups** of FH$_4$ can be oxidized and reduced (Figure 17-8B). The most reduced form, N^5-methyl-FH$_4$, cannot be reoxidized under physiologic conditions.
2. *Sources of 1-carbon groups carried by FH$_4$*
   a. Serine, glycine, formaldehyde, histidine, and formate transfer 1-carbon groups to FH$_4$ (Figure 17-9, *top*).
   b. **Serine, glycine,** and **formaldehyde** produce N^5,N^{10}-methylene-FH$_4$.
      (1) **Serine** transfers a 1-carbon group to FH$_4$ and is converted to glycine in a reversible reaction. Because serine can be derived from glucose, this 1-carbon group can be obtained from dietary carbohydrate.
      (2) When **glycine** transfers a 1-carbon unit to FH$_4$, NH$_4^+$ and CO$_2$ are produced.
      (3) **Formaldehyde,** which can be produced from the –N–CH$_3$ of epinephrine, forms N^5,N^{10}-methylene-FH$_4$.
   c. **Histidine** is degraded to formiminoglutamate (FIGLU). The formimino group reacts with FH$_4$, releasing NH$_4^+$ and producing glutamate and N^5,N^{10}-methylene-FH$_4$.
   d. **Formate,** which can be derived from tryptophan, produces N^{10}-formyl-FH$_4$.
3. *Recipients of 1-carbon groups*
   a. The 1-carbon groups that FH$_4$ receives are transferred to various compounds (see Figure 17-9, *bottom*).
   b. **Purines precursors** obtain carbons 2 and 8 from FH$_4$. Purines are required for DNA and RNA synthesis.
   c. **Deoxyuridine monophosphate (dUMP)** forms thymidine monophosphate (dTMP) by accepting a 1-carbon group from FH$_4$ (Figure 17-10). This reaction produces the **thymine** required for **DNA synthesis.**
      (1) The methylene group is reduced to a methyl group in this reaction, and FH$_4$ is oxidized to FH$_2$.
      (2) FH$_2$ is reduced to FH$_4$ in the NADPH-requiring reaction catalyzed by **dihydrofolate reductase.**

> *cc* **17.14** **Methotrexate** is a structural analog of folic acid that inhibits **dihydrofolate reductase.** It functions primarily by **inhibiting purine synthesis** and, therefore, slows down cell proliferation as in **cancer** or autoimmune diseases like **rheumatoid arthritis.**

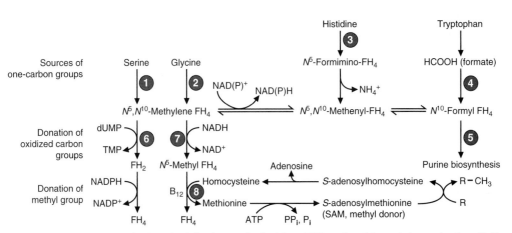

Figure 17-9 The sources of carbon (1–4) for the tetrahydrofolate (FH$_4$) pool and the recipients of carbon (5–8) from the pool. ATP = adenosine triphosphate; dUMP = deoxyuridine monophosphate; FH$_2$ = dihydrofolate; P$_i$ = inorganic phosphate; PP$_i$ = inorganic pyrophosphate; SAH = S-adenosylhomocysteine; SAM = S-adenosylmethionine; TMP = thymidine monophosphate.

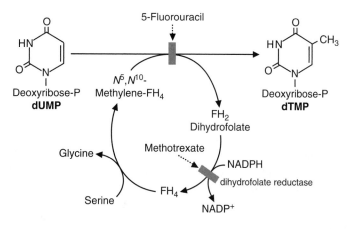

Figure 17-10 The transfer of a 1-carbon unit from serine to deoxyuridine monophosphate (dUMP) to form deoxythymidine monophosphate (dTMP). Tetrahydrofolate (FH$_4$) is oxidized to dihydrofolate (FH$_2$) in this reaction. FH$_2$ is reduced to FH$_4$ by dihydrofolate reductase. The carbon group that is transferred is indicated by *dashed boxes. Rectangles* indicate the steps at which the antimetabolites methotrexate and 5-fluorouracil (5-FU) act.

> *cc* **17.15** **Trimethoprim** is a **folate analog** that binds specifically to **bacterial dihydrofolate reductase.** It is a potent antibacterial compound often used in conjunction with **sulfonamides,** which also inhibit the same pathway in bacteria.

    d. Glycine obtains a 1-carbon group from FH$_4$ to form **serine.**

    e. Vitamin B$_{12}$ obtains a methyl group from 5-methyl-FH$_4$. The methyl group is transferred from methyl-B$_{12}$ to homocysteine to form **methionine** (see Figure 17-9, *bottom*). This is the only fate of 5-methyl-FH$_4$.

B. S-Adenosylmethionine (SAM)

    1. SAM is synthesized from **methionine** and **ATP.**

    2. Methyl groups are supplied by SAM for the following conversions (see Figure 17-9, *bottom*):

        a. Guanidinoacetate to **creatine**

        b. Phosphatidylethanolamine to **phosphatidylcholine**

        c. Norepinephrine to **epinephrine**

        d. Acetylserotonin to **melatonin**

        e. Polynucleotides to methylated polynucleotides

    3. When SAM transfers its methyl group to an acceptor, *S*-adenosylhomocysteine (SAH) is produced.

    4. SAH releases adenosine to form homocysteine, which obtains a methyl group from vitamin B$_{12}$ to form methionine. Methionine reacts with ATP to regenerate SAM (see Figure 17-9, *bottom*).

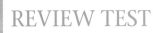

REVIEW TEST

*Directions: Each of the numbered questions or incomplete statements in this section is followed by answers or by completions of the statement. Select the **one** lettered answer or completion that is **best** in each case.*

1. Tetrahydrobiopterin (BH_4) is required in which of the following reactions?

(A) Norepinephrine synthesis
(B) Serotonin synthesis
(C) Dopamine formation from dopa
(D) Phenylalanine synthesis
(E) Melatonin synthesis from its direct precursor

2. The biosynthetic pathway involves both BH_4 and a pyridoxal phosphate (PLP)-dependent decarboxylation reaction to form which of the following?

(A) Histamine
(B) γ-Aminobutyric acid (GABA)
(C) Creatine
(D) Epinephrine
(E) Carnitine

3. A dietary deficiency in tryptophan will do which of the following?

(A) Have no detrimental effect since tryptophan is not an essential amino acid
(B) Have a detrimental effect on the biosynthesis of melatonin
(C) Have a detrimental effect on the biosynthesis of norepinephrine
(D) Have a detrimental effect on the biosynthesis of glutathione
(E) Have a detrimental effect on the biosynthesis of histamine

4. Concerning 1-carbon metabolism, which of the following occurs?

(A) BH_4 takes part in the biosynthesis of epinephrine by transferring a methyl group to the amine nitrogen.
(B) Biotin is the cofactor in the addition of a methyl group to make creatine.
(C) Vitamin B_{12} transfers a methyl group to the amine nitrogen during synthesis of epinephrine.

(D) Serine is the major source of 1-carbon units for folate-dependent reactions.
(E) N^5-formyl-tetrahydrofolate is the cofactor adding a methyl group to vanillylmandelic acid.

5. S-adenosylmethionine (SAM) is required for which of the following reactions?

(A) Ceramide formation from palmitoyl CoA
(B) Thymine production
(C) Creatine from guanidinoacetate
(D) Histamine from histidine
(E) Norepinephrine from dopamine

6. Which of the following compounds is a recipient of the 1-carbon groups that tetrahydrofolate receives and transfers?

(A) Serine
(B) Formaldehyde
(C) Glycine
(D) Formiminoglutamate (FIGLU)
(E) Formate

7. 5-Fluorouracil (5-FU) is an effective chemotherapeutic agent because it interferes with DNA synthesis by directly inhibiting which of the following reactions?

(A) Dihydrofolate (FH_2) → tetrahydrofolate (FH_4)
(B) Deoxyuridine monophosphate (dUMP) → thymidine monophosphate (dTMP)
(C) Glutamine + phosphoribosyl 1-pyrophosphate (PRPP) → phosphoribosylamine
(D) Methyl B_{12} → vitamin B_{12}
(E) Vitamin B_{12} → methyl B_{12}

8. Which amino acid can be converted to the nonadenine dinucleotide portion of NAD?

(A) Histidine
(B) Tyrosine

(C) Tryptophan
(D) Phenylalanine
(E) Arginine

9. Which of the following is a compound formed from both a hydroxylation with an enzyme requiring vitamin C and subsequent methylation?

(A) Histamine
(B) Epinephrine
(C) GABA
(D) Carnitine
(E) Creatinine

10. Which of the following sentences best describes glutathione (GSH)?

(A) It is known as GSH because it is the tripeptide glutamate, serine, and histidine.
(B) GSH can be reduced and binds to cysteines but not through disulfide bonds.
(C) Protein disulfide isomerase can make dimers of glutathione.
(D) GSH is involved in amino acid transport via the γ-glutamyl cycle.
(E) GSH is comprised of glutamate, cysteine, and histidine.

11. A 56-year-old man with longstanding, poorly controlled diabetes visits his primary care physician for a follow-up after a recent hospitalization. The patient experienced an episode of acute renal failure while in the hospital, and his creatinine level rose to 3.4 (normal, 0.7–1.5). Creatinine, a marker of kidney function, is produced from which of the following precursors?

(A) Glutamine, aspartic acid, and CO_2
(B) Glutamine, cysteine, and glycine
(C) Serine and palmityl coenzyme A (CoA)
(D) Glycine and succinyl CoA
(E) Glycine, arginine, and
S-adenosylmethionine

12. A 75-year-old man experiences sever chest pain radiating down his left arm. He calls 911 and is transferred to the emergency room where an electrocardiogram (ECG) indicates that he had a myocardial infarc-

tion. Serum levels of creatine kinase (specifically CK-MB) are found to be elevated. What is the biologic role of the normal product of this enzyme?

(A) An intracellular antioxidant
(B) A storage form of high-energy phosphate
(C) Acts as an inhibitory neurotransmitter
(D) Stimulates the release of hydrochloric acid (HCl) from the stomach
(E) A bactericidal product released from macrophages

13. A 16-year-old girl is found by her parents on the bathroom floor unconscious with an empty bottle of acetaminophen in the toilet. She is rushed to the hospital where she is given several doses of N-acetylcysteine. Acetaminophen overdose is potentially life threatening because it depletes cellular stores of which substance?

(A) Nitric oxide
(B) Histamine
(C) Creatinine
(D) Glutathione
(E) Serotonin

14. A 43-year-old man with a long history of poorly controlled hypertension presents to the emergency room with a severe headache. His blood pressure is found to be dramatically elevated at 250/148 mm Hg. Which of the following products, derived from amino acids, might bring down his dangerously high blood pressure?

(A) Melanin
(B) Nitric oxide
(C) GABA
(D) Dopamine
(E) Serotonin

15. A 56-year-old woman develops diarrhea, flushing, wheezing, and a heart murmur. A computed tomography (CT) scan of the abdomen demonstrates a mass in the ileum along with multiple masses in the liver suspicious for metastasis. A biopsy of a liver mass reveals a diagnosis of a carcinoid tumor. The patient has elevated levels of the serotonin metabolite, 5-hydroxyindole

acetic acid (5-HIAA). Serotonin is normally produced from which amino acid precursor?

(A) Tyrosine
(B) Arginine
(C) Histidine
(D) Glycine
(E) Tryptophan

16. A couple of African-American descent gives birth to a boy after an otherwise uneventful pregnancy. The child is exceptionally fair-skinned and has almost white hair. Further exam reveals red pupils. A postnatal screen is likely to confirm the deficiency of which of the following enzymes?

(A) Peroxidase
(B) Inducible nitric oxide synthase (iNOS)
(C) Glutathione reductase
(D) Tyrosinase
(E) *S*-Adenosylmethionine

17. A 40-year-old woman complains of decreased energy, significant weight gain, and cold intolerance. She is seen by her family physician, who has labs drawn that indicate she has a decreased level of thyroid hormone. Which of the following is a precursor to thyroid hormone?

(A) Melanin
(B) Dopa
(C) Tryptophan
(D) Tyrosine
(E) Niacin

18. A 59-year-old woman develops a shuffling gait and a pill-rolling tremor. She is referred to a neurologist for evaluation. After a thorough workup, a diagnosis of Parkinson disease is made, and the patient is placed on a monoamine oxidase inhibitor (MAOI). The drug, in this case, is given to decrease the degradation of which of the following?

(A) Serotonin
(B) Nicotinamide
(C) 5-HIAA
(D) Endothelium-derived relaxation factor (EDRF)
(E) Dopamine

19. A 12-year-old boy develops convulsions. After running an electroencephalogram (EEG), a neurologist determines that the child has epilepsy. He his started on a benzodiazepine, which promotes the activity of GABA. GABA is derived from the amino acid glutamate via which of the following biochemical reactions?

(A) Deamination
(B) Decarboxylation
(C) Hydroxylation
(D) Iodination
(E) Methylation

20. A 63-year-old woman reports a long history of joint pain. Her fingers are severely deformed secondary to rheumatoid arthritis. Upon visiting a rheumatologist, she is started on methotrexate. This drug inhibits which of the following conversions?

(A) Dopamine to norepinephrine
(B) Tyrosine to dopa
(C) Folate to dihydrofolate
(D) Histamine to formiminoglutamate (FIGLU)
(E) Norepinephrine to vanillylmandelic acid

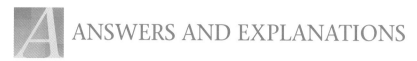

ANSWERS AND EXPLANATIONS

1–B. Tetrahydrobiopterin (BH_4) is required for serotonin synthesis via tryptophan → 5-hydroxytryptophan and decarboxylation to serotonin. Biosynthesis of epinephrine requires S-adenosylmethionine (SAM). Dopamine from dihydroxyphenylalanine (dopa) is a decarboxylation (although synthesis of dopa requires BH_4). Phenylalanine is not synthesized; it is an essential amino acid (conversion to tyrosine uses BH_4). Melatonin from serotonin requires acetylation by acetyl coenzyme A (CoA) and methylation by SAM.

2–D. Epinephrine synthesis requires both BH_4 and a pyridoxal phosphate (PLP)-dependent decarboxylation from phenylalanine → tyrosine → dopa → dopamine → epinephrine. Both histidine → histamine and glutamate → γ-aminobutyric acid (GABA) require PLP for decarboxylation (but not BH_4). Creatine is produced from glycine, arginine, and SAM.

3–B. A tryptophan deficiency will adversely affect synthesis of melatonin because it is a precursor for this compound. Tryptophan is an essential amino acid but is not a precursor for norepinephrine (tyrosine is the precursor), glutathione (a tripeptide synthesized from glutamate, cysteine, and glycine), or histamine (histidine is the precursor).

4–D. For folate-dependent reactions, serine supplies 1-carbon units. The biosynthesis of epinephrine and the addition of a methyl group to form creatine is mediated by S-adenosylmethionine (SAM). Catecholamine O-methyltransferase (COMT) methylates catecholamines to inactivate them via the action of monoamine oxidase.

5–C. SAM is required to convert guanidinoacetate → creatine. Folate is required for thymine synthesis. Palmitoyl CoA is condensed with serine → ceramide via decarboxylation. Histidine → histamine via decarboxylation. Epinephrine → norepinephrine requires vitamin C and copper.

6–C. Glycine obtains a 1-carbon group from tetrahydrofolate (FH_4) to form serine (it can also donate a 1-carbon group). Serine donates to glycine, and formaldehyde donates to N^5,N^{10}-methylene-FH_4. The formimino group of formiminoglutamate (FIGLU) reacts with FH_4, forming N^5,N^{10}-methylenyl-FH_4; formate forms serine N^5,N^{10}-formyl-FH_4.

7–B. Methotrexate inhibits the reaction of dihydrofolate (FH_2) → tetrahydrofolate (FH_4), which is mediated by dihydrofolate reductase. 5-FU inhibits the reaction of deoxyuridine monophosphate (dUMP) → thymidine monophosphate (dTMP). The remaining reactions are not directly affected by 5-FU. Glutamine to create phosphoribosylamine is the first step in purine biosynthesis. Methyl B_{12} → vitamin B_{12} provides the methyl group for the biosynthesis of methionine from homocysteine; and the reverse reaction does not occur in the cell because there is no demethylation for the reaction.

8–C. Tryptophan can be converted (although not the major precursor) to the nicotinamide moiety of NAD. All of the other choices can be made into bioactive products, although these are predominantly amino acid neurotransmitters.

9–B. Epinephrine forms when dopamine is hydroxylated by an enzyme that requires copper and vitamin C, to form norepinephrine, which is subsequently methylated. Histamine is derived by decarboxylation of histidine. GABA is decarboxylated glutamate. Creatinine is formed by a SAM methylation, and carnitine is an acyl group acceptor.

10–D. Glutathione (GSH) is involved in the transport of amino acids across the cell membranes via the γ-glutamyl cycle. GSH is a tripeptide synthesized from glutamate, cysteine, and glycine. GSH can dimerize by glutathione reductase and can rearrange protein disulfide bonds.

11–E. Creatinine is formed from the cyclization of creatine phosphate, which is formed from glycine, arginine, and SAM. Glutamine, aspartic acid, and CO_2 are involved in the synthesis of pyrimidines. Glutamine, cysteine, and glycine form the antioxidant molecule glutathione. Serine and palmityl CoA form ceramide. Glycine and succinyl CoA are the precursors to the formation of heme.

12–B. Creatine kinase phosphorylates creatine to form creatine kinase, a source of high-energy phosphate in muscle cells. Glutathione functions as an intracellular antioxidant. GABA is an example of an inhibitory neurotransmitter. Histamine, which is derived from histidine, stimulates the release of hydrochloric acid (HCl) from the stomach. Nitric oxide is one of the bactericidal substances (free radicals) released from macrophages.

13–D. Glutathione plays an important role in detoxifying acetaminophen. As cellular stores of glutathione are depleted, hepatocytes are damaged, resulting in jaundice and encephalopathy. Nitric oxide is an important vasodilator. Histamine mediates HCl release from the stomach as well as bronchoconstriction of the lungs. Creatine is a storage form of high-energy phosphate when phosphorylated. Serotonin is a neurotransmitter involved in mood and depression.

14–B. Nitric oxide, also referred to as endothelium-derived relaxing factor (EDRF), relaxes the smooth muscle of blood vessels and thus lowers blood pressure. Melanin is derived from tyrosine and is the major skin pigment. GABA is an inhibitory neurotransmitter, whereas both dopamine and serotonin are normally stimulatory neurotransmitters involved in affecting mood.

15–E. Serotonin, which is overproduced in carcinoid syndrome, is an indolamine neurotransmitter derived from tryptophan. Tyrosine is the precursor to the catecholamine neurotransmitters, including dopamine, norepinephrine, and epinephrine. Nitric oxide, an important vasodilator, is derived from arginine. Histidine forms histamine, which is an important inflammatory mediator. Glycine can function as an inhibitory neurotransmitter.

16–D. Albinism results from a defect in the enzyme tyrosinase, which is important in the conversion of tyrosine to melanin. Peroxidase is important in the formation of thyroid hormone. Glutathione reductase is an NADPH-requiring enzyme involved in regenerating oxidized glutathione. SAM is a methyl donor for numerous 1-carbon donor reactions.

17–D. Thyroid hormone is an iodinated molecule produced by several complex reactions in the follicular cells of the thyroid and the colloid from tyrosine. Melanin and dopamine are also synthesized from the amino acid tyrosine. Tryptophan serves as the precursor for serotonin, as well as niacin.

18–E. Parkinson disease results from a relative deficiency of dopamine. Monoamine oxidase (MAO) and catecholamine O-methyltransferase (COMT) are both enzymes that degrade catecholamines such as dopamine, epinephrine, and norepinephrine. MAOs can also degrade serotonin, resulting ultimately in the formation of 5-HIAA. Nicotinamide can be synthesized from tryptophan. EDRF is a short-acting substance that rapidly degrades spontaneously.

19–B. Decarboxylation of glutamate results in the formation of the inhibitory neurotransmitter GABA. Hydroxylation of tyrosine forms dopa. Thyroid hormone requires iodination of tyrosine molecules. Methylation of norepinephrine forms the adrenal hormone epinephrine. A deaminated metabolite of catecholamines is vanillylmandelic acid, which is excreted in the urine.

20–C. Methotrexate inhibits the enzyme dihydrofolate reductase, which is the enzyme that converts folate to dihydrofolate and, subsequently, dihydrofolate tetrahydrofolate. Dopamine β-hydroxylase converts dopamine to norepinephrine. Tyrosine hydroxylase is the enzyme that converts tyrosine to dopa. Histamine is degraded to FIGLU. Norepinephrine is deaminated and methylated by the sequential action of MAO and COMT.

Nucleotide and Porphyrin Metabolism

I. Purine and Pyrimidine Metabolism

A. Purine synthesis (Figure 18-1, *left*)

1. The **purine base** is synthesized on the **ribose moiety.**
   a. 5′-Phosphoribosyl-1′-pyrophosphate (**PRPP**) is the activated substrate in the synthesis of purine and pyrimidine synthesis. PRPP is formed from adenosine triphosphate (ATP), and ribose is formed by **PRPP synthetase.**

   > *cc* **18.1** **Overactivity of PRPP synthetase,** due to a lack of feedback inhibition, is an X-linked disorder resulting in **overproduction of nucleotides.** The condition leads to increased degradation as well, resulting in **hyperuricemia, gout,** and kidney stones.

   b. **PRPP** provides the ribose moiety, reacting with **glutamine** to form phosphoribosylamine.
      (1) This first step in purine biosynthesis produces N9 of the purine ring.
      (2) It is inhibited by adenosine monophosphate (AMP) and guanosine monophosphate (GMP).
   c. A **glycine** molecule is added to the growing purine precursor.
      (1) Then C8 is added by **methenyl tetrahydrofolate**
      (2) N3 is added by **glutamine.**
      (3) C6 is added by CO_2.
      (4) N1 is added by **aspartate.**
      (5) Finally C2 is added by **formyl tetrahydrofolate** (see Figure 18-1, *bottom*).
   d. **Inosine monophosphate (IMP),** which contains the base hypoxanthine, is generated.
      (1) IMP is cleaved in the liver.
      (2) Its free base, or nucleoside, travels to various tissues where it is reconverted to the nucleotide.

2. **IMP** is the **precursor** of both **AMP** and **GMP.**
   a. In the formation of **GMP,** IMP is converted first to xanthosine monophosphate by the enzyme **IMP dehydrogenase** and finally to GMP by the action of GMP synthetase.

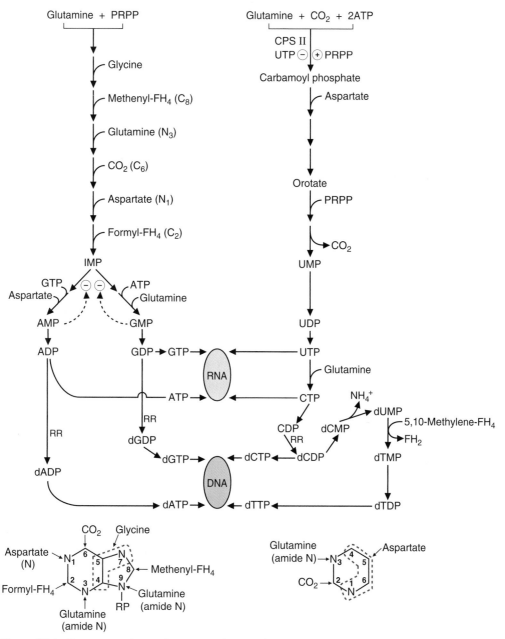

Figure 18-1 De novo synthesis of purines and pyrimidines. Ribonucleotide reductase (RR) catalyzes the reduction of the ribose moiety in adenosine diphosphate (ADP), guanosine diphosphate (GDP), and cytidine diphosphate (CDP) to deoxyribose. The source of each of the atoms is indicated in the boxes at the bottom of the figure. In hereditary orotic aciduria, the enzymes converting orotate to uridine monophosphate (UMP) are defective. AMP = adenosine monophosphate; CPS II = carbamoyl phosphate synthetase II; d before the phosphates = deoxy; FH_4 = tetrahydrofolate; GMP = guanosine monophosphate; GTP = guanosine triphosphate; IMP = inosine monophosphate; PRPP = 5'-phosphoribosyl-1'-pyrophosphate; TMP = thymidine monophosphate; TTP = thymidine triphosphate; UTP = uridine monophosphate.

> *cc* **18.2** **Mycophenolic acid** is a powerful immunosuppressant and a reversible inhibitor of **IMP dehydrogenase.** The drug limits the formation of nucleic acids in activated and **proliferating immune cells** and is used in treating **autoimmune disease** as well as to prevent **transplant rejection.**

   b. In the formation of **AMP**, IMP is converted first to adenylosuccinate by the enzyme **adenylosuccinate synthetase** and finally to AMP by the action of adenylosuccinase.
   c. By feedback inhibition, each product regulates its own synthesis from the IMP branch point and also inhibits the initial step in the pathway.
   d. AMP and GMP can be phosphorylated to the triphosphate level.
   e. ATP and guanosine triphosphate (GTP) can be used for energy-requiring processes or for **RNA synthesis.**
3. **Reduction of the ribose moiety to deoxyribose** occurs at the diphosphate level and is catalyzed by **ribonucleotide reductase,** which requires the protein thioredoxin.
4. After the diphosphates are phosphorylated, deoxyadenosine triphosphate (dATP) and deoxyguanosine triphosphate (dGTP) can be used for **DNA synthesis.**

> *cc* **18.3** The antineoplastic agent **hydroxyurea** is an inhibitor of **ribonucleotide reductase.** It is used in the treatment of **chronic myelogenous leukemia,** polycythemia vera, and essential thrombocytosis.

5. **Purine bases** can be salvaged by **reacting with PRPP** to re-form nucleotides (Figure 18-2). The purine-salvage enzymes are hypoxanthine-guanine phosphoribosyl transferase (**HGPRT**) and adenine phosphoribosyl transferase (**APRT**).

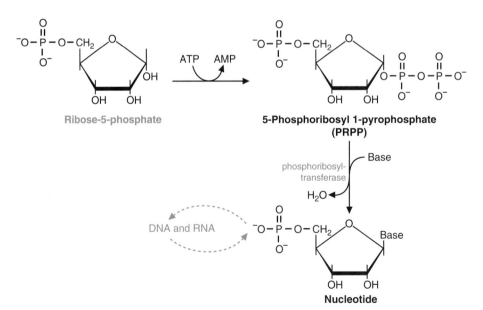

Figure 18-2 Salvage of the purine bases. Salvage of guanine, adenine, and hypoxanthine occurs in reactions catalyzed by phosphoribosyl transferase. AMP = adenosine monophosphate; ATP = adenosine triphosphate.

cc *18.4* **Lesch-Nyhan syndrome** is caused by a **defective HGPRT.** Purine bases cannot be salvaged (i.e., reconverted to nucleotides). The purines are converted instead to **uric acid,** which increases in the blood. **Mental retardation** and **self-mutilation** are characteristics of the disease.

cc *18.5* Autosomal recessive mutations in **APRT** result in the inability of cells to salvage the purine base adenine. Patients develop **nephrolithiasis** with **renal colic, hematuria, recurrent urinary tract infections,** and **dysuria.**

B. **Purine degradation** (Figure 18-3)

1. In the degradation of the purine nucleotides, **phosphate** and **ribose** are removed first; then the nitrogenous base is oxidized.

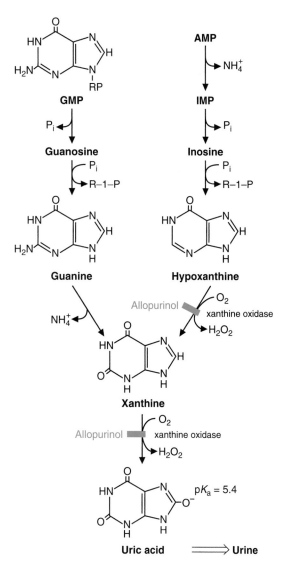

Figure 18-3 Purine degradation. Allopurinol (AP), which inhibits xanthine oxidase, is used to treat gout. Gout occurs when uric acid crystals precipitate in joints because of an increased concentration in the blood. AMP = adenosine monophosphate; GMP = guanosine monophosphate; H_2O_2 = hydrogen peroxide; IMP = inosine monophosphate; P = phosphate; R-1-P = ribose 1-phosphate.

2. *Degradation of GMP* (see Figure 18-3, *left*)
   a. GMP is degraded to guanosine by the removal of the phosphate by a 5′ nucleotidase.
   b. Guanosine is degraded to guanine and ribose 1-phosphate by **purine nucleoside phosphorylase (PNP).**

> *cc* **18.6** Deficiency of **PNP** results in accumulation of both **dATP and dGTP** in lymphoid tissue, which is **toxic to immune cells.** Patients present with **decreased numbers of T cells** and **lymphopenia.** Neurologic symptoms, including **mental retardation** and muscle spasticity, and **autoimmune disease** are present.

   c. **Guanine** is then converted to xanthine.
3. **Degradation of AMP** (see Figure 18-3, *right*)
   a. AMP is degraded to adenosine by the removal of the phosphate by a 5′ nucleotidase.
   b. Adenosine is converted to inosine by the enzyme **adenosine deaminase (ADA).**

> *cc* **18.7** **ADA deficiency** leads to **severe combined immunodeficiency (SCID).** As in PNP deficiency, both **dATP and dGTP** accumulate. ADA deficiency results in a **T-, B-,** and **natural killer (NK)**–cell deficiency with marked lymphopenia.

   c. Degradation of inosine by **PNP** produces hypoxanthine and ribose 1-phosphate.
   d. Hypoxanthine is oxidized to xanthine by xanthine oxidase; this enzyme requires molybdenum.
4. **Xanthine** is oxidized to **uric acid** by xanthine oxidase.

> *cc* **18.8** **Allopurinol,** the inhibitor of **xanthine oxidase,** is used in the treatment of gout. More recently, **febuxostat,** a novel **nonpurine analog** inhibitor of xanthine oxidase, has been used.

5. **Uric acid,** which is not very water soluble, is **excreted** by the **kidneys.**

> *cc* **18.9** **Gout** results from accumulation of **uric acid** with the formation of uric acid crystals in the joints, especially the **first metatarsal phalangeal joint (podagra).** This results in a **painful arthritis** that is treated with multiple agents like allopurinol.

C. **Pyrimidine synthesis** (see Figure 18-1, *right*)

1. The **pyrimidine base** is synthesized prior to addition of the ribose moiety.
   a. In the first reaction, **glutamine** reacts with CO_2 and 2 ATP to form **carbamoyl phosphate.**
      (1) This reaction is analogous to the first reaction of the urea cycle.
      (2) However, for pyrimidine synthesis, glutamine provides the nitrogen, and the reaction occurs in the cytosol, where it is catalyzed by **carbamoyl phosphate synthetase II,** which is inhibited by uridine triphosphate (UTP).
   b. An **aspartate** molecule adds to carbamoyl phosphate. The molecule closes to yield a ring, which is oxidized, forming orotate.
   c. **Orotate reacts with PRPP,** producing orotidine 5′-phosphate (OMP), which is decarboxylated to form uridine monophosphate (UMP). Both reactions are catalyzed by **UMP synthase,** which functions both as orotate phosphoribosyl transferase and OMP decarboxylase.

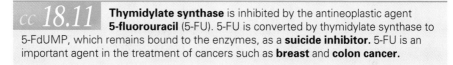

cc 18.10 In **hereditary orotic aciduria,** orotic acid is excreted in the urine because **UMP synthase is defective.** Pyrimidines cannot be synthesized, and therefore, **growth retardation occurs.** Oral administration of uridine bypasses the metabolic block and provides a source of pyrimidines.

2. **UMP is phosphorylated to UTP,** which obtains an amino group from glutamine to form cytidine triphosphate (CTP). UTP and CTP are used for **RNA** synthesis.
3. The ribose moiety of cytidine diphosphate (CDP is reduced to **deoxyribose,** forming deoxycytidine diphosphate (dCDP). **Ribonucleotide reductase** is the enzyme.
   a. dCDP is deaminated and dephosphorylated to form **deoxyuridine monophosphate (dUMP).**
   b. dUMP is converted to **thymidine monophosphate (dTMP)** by **thymidylate synthase,** which requires methylene tetrahydrofolate.

cc 18.11 **Thymidylate synthase** is inhibited by the antineoplastic agent **5-fluorouracil** (5-FU). 5-FU is converted by thymidylate synthase to 5-FdUMP, which remains bound to the enzymes, as a **suicide inhibitor.** 5-FU is an important agent in the treatment of cancers such as **breast** and **colon cancer.**

   c. Phosphorylations produce dCTP and deoxythymidine triphosphate (dTTP), which are precursors of **DNA.**

D. Pyrimidine degradation.   In pyrimidine degradation, the carbons produce CO_2, and the nitrogens produce urea.

II. Heme Metabolism

A. Heme consists of a **porphyrin ring** coordinated with **iron** and is found mainly in **hemoglobin** but is also present in **myoglobin** and the **cytochromes.**

B. Heme synthesis (Figure 18-4)

1. In the first step of heme synthesis, **glycine** and **succinyl coenzyme A (CoA)** condense to form δ-aminolevulinic acid (δ-ALA). **Pyridoxal phosphate** is the cofactor for **δ-aminolevulinic acid synthase.** Glycine is decarboxylated in this reaction.
2. **Heme regulates** its own **production** by repressing the synthesis of δ-ALA synthase in the liver.
3. Two molecules of δ-ALA condense to form the pyrrole porphobilinogen. This condensation reaction is mediated by **δ-aminolevulinic acid dehydrogenase.**

cc 18.12 **δ-ALA dehydrogenase** is inhibited by heavy metal ions such as **lead.** This inhibition results in the **anemia** seen in patients with lead poisoning. Accumulation of lead leads to **abdominal pain** and **encephalopathy** with cognitive and motor impairment.

4. Four **porphobilinogens** form the first in a series of porphyrins; these are hydroxymethylbilane, uroporphyrinogen III, coproporphyrinogen III, and protoporphyrinogen IX.
5. The **porphyrins** are altered by decarboxylation and oxidation, and protoporphyrin IX is formed.

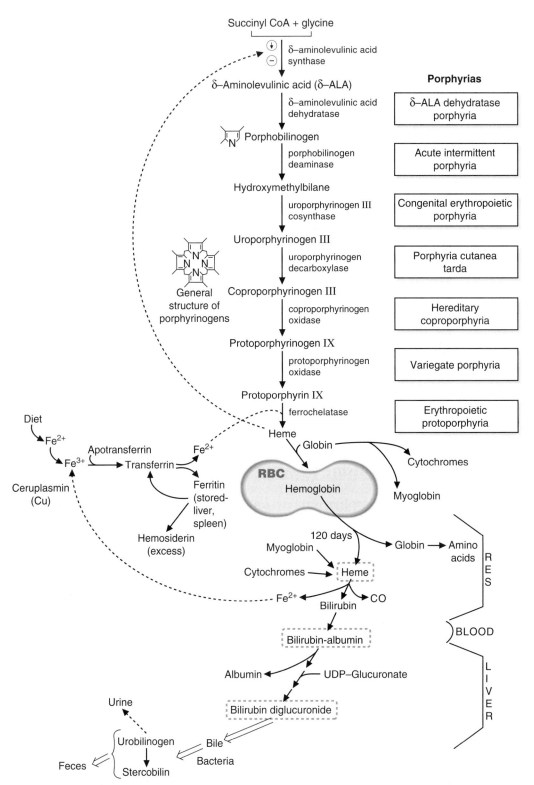

Figure 18-4 Hemoglobin synthesis and degradation. Regulation of heme synthesis occurs by repression of the synthesis of the enzyme δ-aminolevulinic acid (δ-ALA) synthase, by inhibition of this enzyme by heme in the liver, and by induction of this enzyme by erythropoietin in bone marrow. Bilirubin is converted to urobilinogens and stercobilins by bacterial flora in the intestine. PLP = pyridoxal phosphate; RBC = red blood cell; RES = reticuloendothelial system; ⊕ = repression of enzyme synthesis; ⊖ = inhibition.

6. **Protoporphyrin IX** binds **iron (Fe^{2+})**, forming **heme.**
   a. **Iron** obtained from the diet is transported via **transferrin** and is stored as **ferritin** in the liver and spleen (see Figure 18-4, *left*).
   b. **Vitamin C** increases the uptake of iron from the intestinal tract.
   c. **Ceruloplasmin**, a protein that contains copper, is involved in the oxidation of iron.
   d. **Excess iron** is stored as **hemosiderin.**
7. **Erythropoietin** induces heme synthesis in bone marrow.

> **cc 18.13**   **Erythropoietin,** which is produced by **recombinant DNA technology,** is used in the management of **anemia resulting from kidney failure, hemolytic anemia,** or **anemia associated with chemotherapy.**

8. **Heme stimulates** synthesis of the protein **globin** by maintaining the translational initiation complex on the ribosome in its active state (see Figure 18-4, *middle*).
9. Defects in the biosynthesis of heme result in a group of disorders known as **porphyrias** (see Table 18-1).

C. Heme degradation (see Figure 18-4, *middle*)

1. After **red blood cells,** which contain hemoglobin, reach their lifespan of about 120 days, they are **phagocytosed** by cells of the reticuloendothelial system.

TABLE 18-1	*Porphyrias*		
	Disease	Enzyme Deficiency	Clinical Consequence
cc 18.14	δ-ALA dehydrogenase porphyria	δ-ALA dehydrogenase	**Autosomal recessive** disorder characterized by acute attacks of **abdominal pain** and **neuropathy.**
cc 18.15	Acute intermittent porphyria	Hydroxymethylbilane synthase (porphobilinogen deaminase)	**Autosomal dominant** disorder with **periodic attacks** of **abdominal colic,** peripheral **neuropathy, psychiatric disorders,** and tachycardia. Attacks are **precipitated by drugs** such as gonadal steroids, **barbiturates,** and alcohol.
cc 18.16	Congenital erythropoietic porphyria	Uroporphyrinogen III cosynthase	**Autosomal recessive** disorder with **photosensitivity.** Sometimes it is almost immediate and **so severe** that the infant may scream when put in sunlight, with erythema, swelling, and **blistering occurring on exposed sites.** The patient may also have **hemolytic anemia** and **splenomegaly.**

(continued)

	Disease	Enzyme Deficiency	Clinical Consequence
cc **18.17**	Porphyria cutanea tarda	Uroporphyrinogen decarboxylase	This **autosomal dominant** disorder is the most common porphyria. It results in **photosensitivity** with vesicles and bullae on skin of exposed areas.
cc **18.18**	Hereditary coproporphyria	Coproporphyrinogen oxidase	An **autosomal dominant** disorder that presents with photosensitivity and **neurovisceral symptoms**, like colic.
cc **18.19**	Variegate porphyria	Protoporphyrinogen oxidase	An **autosomal dominant** disorder that presents with **photosensitivity** along with **neurologic symptoms** and **developmental delay** in children.
cc **18.20**	Erythropoietic protoporphyria	Ferrochelatase	**Autosomal dominant** disorder characterized by **photosensitivity** with skin lesions after brief sun exposure. Patients may also have **gallstones** and **mild liver dysfunction**.

TABLE 18-1 *Porphyrias (Continued)*

δ-ALA = δ-aminolevulinic acid.

(1) Globin is released and converted to amino acids.
(2) Heme is degraded to **bilirubin**, which is excreted in the bile.

> *cc* **18.21** **Jaundice** results from a deficiency in the liver's ability to conjugate and/or transport bilirubin. Jaundice refers to the **yellow color** of **skin and eyes** that results from the deposition of bilirubin. Causes include **hemolytic anemia,** primary **liver disease, obstruction of the biliary system,** and **congenital deficiencies** of the enzymes responsible for the **metabolism of bilirubin**.

2. **Heme** is oxidized and cleaved to produce carbon monoxide and biliverdin, a green pigment.
3. **Iron** is released, oxidized, and returned by transferrin to the iron stores of the body.
4. **Bilirubin,** which is produced by reduction of biliverdin, is carried by the protein albumin to the liver.
5. In the liver, bilirubin reacts with **UDP-glucuronate** to form bilirubin monoglucuronide, which is converted to the diglucuronide.

> *cc* **18.22** **Crigler-Najjar syndrome** results from a **deficiency of bilirubin uridine diphosphate gluconyl transferase** (UDP-GT). **Type I** results from a **complete absence of the gene,** with severe hyperbilirubinemia that accumulates in the brain of affected newborns, causing a toxic encephalopathy (kernicterus). **Type II,** a benign form, results from a mutation causing a **partial deficiency** of the gene.

cc *18.23*   **Gilbert syndrome** is a relatively **common** and benign disorder (2–10% of the population) that results from decreased activity of UDP-GT. Occasional bouts of mild jaundice with increased physiologic stress occur during hemolysis or hepatocellular injury.

6. Formation of the diglucuronide increases the solubility of the pigment, and **bilirubin diglucuronide** is **secreted** into the **bile.**
7. **Bacteria** in the intestine convert bilirubin to **urobilins** and **stercobilins,** which give feces its brown color.

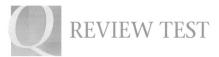

REVIEW TEST

Directions: Each of the numbered questions or incomplete statements in this section is followed by answers or by completions of the statement. Select the **one** lettered answer or completion that is **best** in each case.

1. The conversion of inosine monophosphate (IMP):

(A) To adenosine monophosphate (AMP) is inhibited by guanosine monophosphate (GMP).
(B) To AMP requires uridine monophosphate (UMP).
(C) To GMP requires the GMP kinase.
(D) To GMP requires adenosine triphosphate (ATP).
(E) To guanosine diphosphate (GDP) requires ribonucleotide reductase.

2. Which of the following is converted directly to heme in a single enzymatic reaction?

(A) Biliverdin
(B) Bilirubin diglucuronide
(C) Uroporphyrinogen I
(D) Protoporphyrin IX (III)
(E) Coproporphyrinogen III

3. Comparing reactions to the de novo synthesis of the pyrimidine and purine heterocyclic rings indicates which of the following?

(A) Glycine is used for neither.
(B) Aspartate is used for neither.
(C) Aspartate is used for both.
(D) Aspartate is used only for the pyrimidine ring.
(E) Carbomyl phosphate synthesized from ATP, CO_2, and ammonia is used for synthesis of the pyrimidine ring.

4. For the heme biosynthetic pathway, which of the following is directly required?

(A) Alanine
(B) Iron (Fe^{2+})
(C) Diglucuronides
(D) Carbon monoxide
(E) Acetyl coenzyme A (CoA)

5. Which of the following compounds is used for purine and pyrimidine synthesis?

(A) Orotic acid
(B) IMP
(C) Nucleoside phosphorylase
(D) Sodium urate
(E) Phosphoribosyl pyrophosphate (PRPP)

6. Which of the following is the committed step for de novo purine ring synthesis?

(A) Phosphorylation of ribose 5-phosphate
(B) Phosphorylation of hypoxanthine
(C) A reaction involving glutamine + PRPP
(D) A reaction requiring ATP
(E) The formation of carbamoyl phosphate

7. Which of the following compounds is the direct precursor for the heme nitrogen atoms?

(A) Glucose
(B) Glycine
(C) Succinyl CoA
(D) Alanine
(E) Pyridoxal phosphate

8. Which of the following statements about heme and iron metabolism is correct?

(A) Iron is stored in the liver as transferrin.
(B) Iron (as Fe^{3+}) is inserted into protoporphyrin IX in the last step of heme synthesis.
(C) δ-Aminolevulinic acid (δ-ALA) synthase catalyzes the regulated and rate-limiting step in heme biosynthesis.
(D) The major route for bilirubin excretion is via the urine.
(E) The iron produced by heme degradation is excreted in the feces.

9. Excessive degradation of AMP and GMP would result in increased urinary excretion of which of the following?

(A) Creatinine
(B) Urea
(C) Uric acid

(D) Thiamine
(E) Thymine

10. Which of the following statements best describes bilirubin?

(A) It is made more soluble in the liver by attachment of residues of glucose.
(B) It is excreted mainly in the urine.
(C) It is produced by oxidation of heme, with loss of carbon monoxide.
(D) It contains iron in the Fe^{2+} state.
(E) It contains iron in the Fe^{3+} state.

11. A 56-year-old diabetic with end-stage renal disease receives a kidney transplant from his son. His nephrologist is concerned for the possibility of transplant rejection and puts the patient on mycophenolic acid, which inhibits which important enzyme in the synthesis of nucleotides?

(A) PRPP
(B) IMP dehydrogenase
(C) Adenylosuccinate synthase
(D) Ribonucleotide reductase
(E) Adenylosuccinase

12. A physician evaluates a 32-year-old patient for fatigue. The patient is found to have an elevated white blood cell count and an enlarged spleen. A referral to an oncologist results in a diagnosis of chronic myelogenous leukemia. Treatment with hydroxyurea, a ribonucleotide reductase inhibitor, is begun. The normal function of this enzyme is to do which of the following?

(A) Form PRPP from adenosine diphosphate (ADP) and ribose
(B) Convert xanthine to uric acid
(C) Form carbonyl phosphate from glutamine, CO_2, and 2 ATP
(D) Convert ribose to deoxyribose
(E) Degrade guanosine to guanine and ribose 1-phosphate

13. A 4-day-old infant develops severe jaundice and is transferred to the neonatal intensive care unit for aggressive phototherapy. He is found to have complete lack of uridine diphosphate gluconyl transferase. Which of the following disorders does the infant have?

(A) Crigler-Najjar syndrome
(B) Gilbert syndrome
(C) Dubin-Johnson syndrome
(D) Hereditary orotic aciduria
(E) Gout

14. A 3-year-old boy is brought to the emergency room with abdominal pain, mental status changes, and fatigue. On history, the physician finds that the patient lives in an older house and has been sucking on the paint chips that have crumbled in the window sills. The doctor suspects lead poisoning. Lead typically interferes with which of the following enzymes?

(A) Cytochrome oxidase
(B) Protoporphyrinogen oxidase
(C) UMP synthase
(D) δ-ALA dehydrogenase
(E) Porphobilinogen deaminase

15. A child is noted to have recurrent respiratory infections that necessitate hospitalization. His lab tests demonstrate a decrease in T cells, B cells, and natural killer cells and decreased antibodies. He is found to have severe combined immunodeficiency. The enzyme that is defective in this disorder is important in which of the following processes?

(A) Conversion of ribonucleotides to deoxyribonucleotides
(B) Formation of AMP
(C) Degradation of deoxyadenosine triphosphate (dATP)
(D) Synthesis of UMP
(E) Conversion of deoxyuridine monophosphate (dUMP) to thymidine monophosphate (dTMP)

16. A 7-year-old boy suffers from mental retardation and self-mutilation (e.g., biting through lip) and has an increased susceptibility to gout. These symptoms are characteristic of Lesch-Nyhan syndrome, which is due to a mutation in which of the following?

(A) Salvage pathway for pyrimidines
(B) De novo biosynthesis of purines
(C) Xanthine oxidase

(D) Salvage pathway for purines
(E) De novo biosynthesis of pyrimidines

17. A 58-year-old man is awoken by a throbbing ache in his great toe. He has suffered these symptoms before, usually after indulging in a rich meal. On exam, he is noted to have an angry inflamed great toe; also of note are several small nodules on the antihelix of his ear. Inhibition of which of the following proteins might prevent further occurrences of this man's ailments?

(A) Carbamoyl phosphate synthetase II
(B) Hypoxanthine-guanine phosphoribosyl transferase (HGPRT)
(C) PRPP synthetase
(D) Xanthine oxidase
(E) Orotate phosphoribosyl transferase

18. An 8-year-old boy sees a dermatologist because he has developed vesicles and bullae on his face and arms that appeared after a week-long trip to Florida. His father has a similar condition. A diagnosis of porphyria cutanea tarda is confirmed by finding elevated levels of porphyrins in his serum, urine, and stool. His disease is due to a deficiency of which of the following enzymes?

(A) δ-ALA dehydrogenase
(B) Porphobilinogen deaminase
(C) Uroporphyrinogen III cosynthase
(D) Ferrochelatase
(E) Uroporphyrinogen decarboxylase

19. A 17-year-old young woman, who recently began taking birth control pills, presents to the emergency room with cramping abdominal pain, anxiety, paranoia, and hallucinations. A surgical evaluation, including ultrasound and computed tomography (CT) scan, fails to demonstrate an acute abdominal process. A urinalysis reveals an increase in urine porphyrins. Which of the following is the most likely?

(A) Congenital erythropoietic porphyria
(B) Variegate porphyria
(C) Porphyria cutanea tarda
(D) Acute intermittent porphyria
(E) Erythropoietic protoporphyria

20. An otherwise healthy 19-year-old man recovering from a respiratory infection sees his family physician. His exam is unremarkable except for a slight degree of yellow discoloration to his skin and eyes. Labs are ordered that reveal a mild increase in unconjugated bilirubin but no other abnormalities. Which of the following is the most likely diagnosis in this patient?

(A) Crigler-Najjar syndrome, type I
(B) Crigler-Najjar syndrome, type II
(C) Gilbert syndrome
(D) Lead poisoning
(E) Erythropoietin deficiency

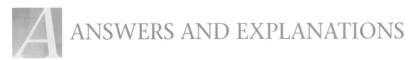

ANSWERS AND EXPLANATIONS

1–D. The conversion of inosine monophosphate (IMP) to guanosine monophosphate (GMP) requires adenosine triphosphate (ATP). The conversion of IMP to adenosine monophosphate (AMP) is inhibited by AMP, requires guanosine triphosphate (GTP), and requires AMP kinase. Conversion of guanosine diphosphate (GDP) to its deoxy form (dGDP) requires ribonucleotide reductase.

2–D. During heme synthesis, protoporphyrin IX binds iron, forming heme in a single step. Biliverdin and bilirubin diglucuronide are heme degradation products. The other choices are "upstream" in the pathway to heme synthesis, so this requires multiple steps.

3–C. Aspartate is used for de novo synthesis of **both** the pyrimidine and purine heterocyclic rings. Glycine is used for purine ring biosynthesis. Carbomyl phosphate uses ATP, CO_2, and glutamine for pyrimidine ring synthesis.

4–B. Iron (Fe^{2+}) is directly required for heme biosynthesis. Succinyl coenzyme A (CoA) and glycine conjugate are required for the first step (not acetyl CoA and alanine). Diglucuronides and carbon monoxide are degradation products.

5–E. Synthesis of both purine and pyrimidine uses phosphoribosyl pyrophosphate (PRPP). Orotate (orotic acid) is used only in pyrimidine synthesis, and IMP is used only for purine synthesis. Sodium urate and nucleoside phosphorylase are both involved in purine degradation.

6–C. The committed step for de novo purine ring synthesis involves glutamine and PRPP. The precursor to PRPP is formed from ATP and ribose 5-phosphate, not the rate-limiting step. Hypoxanthine is involved in purine degradation, and carbamoyl phosphate is involved in pyrimidine synthesis.

7–B. Glycine is the source for heme nitrogens by condensation with succinyl CoA to form δ-aminolevulinic acid (δ-ALA). Two molecules of δ-ALA condense to form the pyrrole porphobilinogen. Succinyl CoA supplies carbon atoms (there are no nitrogens in the molecule). Pyridoxal phosphate (PLP) is an enzyme cofactor. Alanine and glucose have no function in this context.

8–C. The first and rate-limiting step in heme biosynthesis involves condensation of glycine and succinyl CoA to form δ-ALA. Iron is stored as ferritin and transported in the blood in transferrin. In the Fe^{2+} (not Fe^{3+}) state, it is inserted into protoporphyrin IX to form heme. Heme degradation forms bilirubin (excreted mainly via the intestine), and iron is returned to the body's iron stores and not excreted.

9–C. The purine bases adenine (A) and guanine (G) in the monophosphate form are oxidized to uric acid, not urea, which is excreted in the urine. Excessive production of uric acid or hyperuricemia can result in the condition known as gout. Thymine is a pyrimidine, and thiamine is a vitamin.

10–C. Bilirubin is produced by oxidation of heme after its iron is released; carbon monoxide is produced in this reaction. Bilirubin diglucuronide, which contains two glucuronic acid (not glucose) residues, is excreted into the bile by the liver.

11–B. Mycophenolic acid, a potent immunosuppressant, is an inhibitor of IMP dehydrogenase, which normally converts IMP to xanthosine monophosphate. PRPP synthase catalyses the initial step in nucleotide metabolism, forming PRPP from ATP and ribose. Adenylosuccinate synthase and adenylosuccinase are sequential enzymes in the synthesis of AMP.

12–D. Ribonucleotide reductase converts ribose diphosphates to deoxyribose diphosphates for the use in DNA synthesis. Again, PRPP synthase forms PRPP from ATP and ribose. Xanthine oxidase converts xanthine to uric acid. Carbonyl phosphate is synthesized by carbonyl phosphate synthetase from glutamate, CO_2, and 2 ATP. Purine nucleoside phosphorylase degrades guanosine to guanine and ribose 1-phosphate.

13–A. Crigler-Najjar type I results from a complete lack of uridine diphosphate glucosyl transferase and is a lethal condition. Gilbert syndrome is a mild defect in bilirubin conjugation that is usually asymptomatic, although it is due to a subtle defect in the same enzyme. Dubin-Johnson syndrome is a transport defect in bilirubin and does not involve conjugation. Hereditary orotic aciduria results form a defect in pyrimidine synthesis. Gout results from hyperuricemia and not hyperbilirubinemia.

14–D. Lead inhibits hemoglobin synthesis by inhibiting δ-ALA dehydrogenase. Cytochrome oxidase is an enzyme of the electron transport chain inhibited by cyanide and carbon monoxide. Protoporphyrinogen oxidase is deficient in variegate porphyria. UMP synthase is defective in the genetic condition of hereditary orotic aciduria. Patients with acute intermittent porphyria have a deficiency of porphobilinogen deaminase.

15–C. The enzyme deficiency in severe combined immunodeficiency (SCID) is likely adenosine deaminase, which normally degrades adenosine to inosine. The conversion of ribonucleotides to deoxyribonucleotides is performed by ribonucleotide reductase. AMP is formed from IMP through the action of adenylosuccinate synthetase, followed by the action of adenylosuccinate. UMP synthase is an important enzyme in the formation of UMP and, subsequently, cytidine triphosphate (CTP) and thymidine triphosphate (TTP). The conversion of deoxyuridine monophosphate (dUMP) to thymidine monophosphate (dTMP) is mediated by thymidylate synthase.

16–D. Lesch-Nyhan syndrome results from a defect in hypoxanthine-guanine phosphoribosyl transferase (HGPRT). The "salvage" pathway of purines being reconverted to nucleotides is blocked. PRPP synthetase is an important enzyme in de novo biosynthesis of purines, the overactivity of which can cause gout. Xanthine oxidase is important in the degradation of purines, the inhibition of which is a treatment for gout. Carbamoyl phosphate synthase is an enzyme involved in pyrimidine biosynthesis.

17–D. Gout is caused by either the increased production or reduced excretion of uric acid, leading to the deposition of urate crystals. Allopurinol, a xanthine oxidase inhibitor, decreases the production of urate from hypoxanthine and xanthine. Carbamoyl phosphate synthase is an enzyme in pyrimidine biosynthesis. HGPRT is an enzyme in the pathway for purine salvage. Orotate phosphoribosyl transferase is important in the synthesis of pyrimidines. PRPP synthetase is an important enzyme in the biosynthesis of purines; overactivity can cause gout.

18–E. Cutanea tarda is the most common of the porphyrias and results from a deficiency of uroporphyrinogen decarboxylase. Deficiency of δ-ALA dehydrogenase results in δ-ALA dehydrogenase porphyria. Acute intermittent porphyria is due to a deficiency of porphobilinogen deaminase (also known as hydroxymethylbilane synthase). Deficiency of uroporphyrinogen III cosynthase results in congenital erythropoietic porphyria. Finally, ferrochelatase deficiency results in erythropoietic protoporphyria.

19–D. Acute intermittent porphyria is an autosomal dominant disease resulting from the deficiency of porphobilinogen deaminase (also known as hydroxymethylbilane synthase). Often these intermittent attacks are provoked by drugs such as gonadal steroids, barbiturates, or alcohol. The other choices, including congenital erythropoietic porphyria, porphyria cutanea tarda, variegate porphyria, and erythropoietic protoporphyria, are considered erythropoietic porphyries, which are characterized by photosensitivity and rarely exhibit abdominal pain.

20–C. This patient has Gilbert syndrome, which is a common disorder that manifests with mild jaundice as a result of decreased bilirubin uridine diphosphate gluconyl transferase (UDP-GT) activity. Crigler-Najjar syndrome also results from a deficiency of the same enzyme, although it is far rarer and, in the case of type I disease, is lethal. Lead poisoning would lead to anemia, not jaundice. Erythropoietin deficiency is seen in patients with renal failure because erythropoietin is normally produced by the kidney.

Integrative Metabolism and Nutrition

I. Dietary Requirements

A. The **Recommended Daily Allowance (RDA)** is the average daily dietary intake level that is sufficient to meet the nutritional requirement of nearly all individuals.

1. Based on a **Food Pyramid** (Figure 19-1), the distribution of food intake is allocated as demonstrated.
2. The average daily caloric energy requirement for an adult is **2000 kcal/day**.
3. The Food Pyramid has recently been changed to reflect current nutritional data. It now also recommends **exercise** as a component of the Pyramid.

> *cc 19.1*   Anorexia nervosa is characterized by **self-induced weight loss.** Individuals frequently affected include young, affluent, white women, who in spite of an emaciated appearance, often claim to be "fat." It is partially a behavioral problem; those afflicted are obsessed with losing weight.

> *cc 19.2*   People with bulimia suffer from binges of **overeating** followed by **self-induced vomiting** to avoid gaining weight.

B. Carbohydrates

1. **Carbohydrates** should constitute between **45–65%** of daily caloric intake.
2. Dietary carbohydrates should be limited in simple sugars and starches.
3. Consuming a high-fiber diet provides bulk without the addition of significant calories
4. Addition of refined sugars to the diet adds calories without the addition of nutrients.

C. Lipids

1. **Fat** should constitute 30% or less of the total calories—10% each of polyunsaturated, monounsaturated, and saturated fatty acids.
2. **Cholesterol** intake should be no more than 300 mg/day.
3. **Essential fatty acids** are the precursors of the polyunsaturated fatty acids required for the **synthesis of** prostaglandins and other **eicosanoids. Linoleic** and α-**linolenic acids** are the major dietary sources.

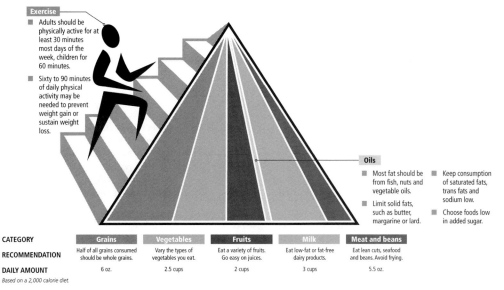

Figure 19-1 The new Food Pyramid.

D. Protein

1. The recommended protein intake is 0.8 g/kg body weight per day.

2. *Essential amino acids*

a. **Nine** amino acids cannot be synthesized in the body and, therefore, must be present in the diet in order for protein synthesis to occur. The essential amino acids are **histidine, isoleucine, leucine, lysine, methionine, phenylalanine, threonine, tryptophan,** and **valine.**

b. Only a small amount of **histidine** is required in the diet; however, **larger amounts** are required for **growth** (e.g., children, pregnant women, people recovering from injuries).

c. Because **arginine** can be synthesized only in limited amounts, it is required in the diet for **growth.**

> **cc 19.3** Kwashiorkor commonly occurs in children in third-world countries where the **diet,** which is **adequate in calories,** is **low in protein.** A deficiency of dietary protein causes a decrease in protein synthesis that eventually affects the regeneration of intestinal epithelial cells, and thus, the problem is further compounded by **malabsorption.** Hepatomegaly and a **distended abdomen** are often observed.

> **cc 19.4** **Marasmus** results from a **diet deficient** in both **protein and calories.** Persistent starvation ultimately results in death.

E. Water-soluble vitamins   (Table 19-1)

• Vitamins and minerals are required in the diet. Many serve as cofactors for enzymes.

1. *Thiamine pyrophosphate* (see Figure 7-5A)

a. Thiamine pyrophosphate is involved in the **decarboxylation of α-keto acids.**

TABLE 19-1 *Water-Soluble Vitamin Deficiencies*

	Vitamin	Biochemical Function	Clinical Consequence of Vitamin Deficiency
cc 19.5	Thiamine (B₁)	Cofactor for pyruvate and α-ketoglutarate dehydrogenase	**Beriberi:** High-output **heart failure** (wet beriberi) and **peripheral neuropathy** (dry beriberi). **Wernicke-Korsakoff syndrome:** Deficiency state seen in chronic **alcoholics** manifesting with **ataxia, ophthalmoplegia,** confusion, and **confabulation.**
cc 19.6	Riboflavin (B₂)	Precursor to the coenzymes flavin mononucleotide (**FMN**) and flavin adenine dinucleotide (**FAD**)	Deficiency is rare in developed countries because **grain and cereal products are fortified with riboflavin.** Deficiency is associated with atrophy of the tongue (**glossitis**), fissures of the corner of the mouth (**cheilosis**), dermatitis, and corneal ulceration.
cc 19.7	Niacin (B₃)	Required for the production of **NAD⁺** and **NADP⁺** as well as numerous **dehydrogenases**	Deficiency results in **pellagra,** which is characterized by **diarrhea, dementia,** and **dermatitis.** Deficiency can result from use of the antituberculoid medication **isoniazid, Hartnup disease,** or **carcinoid syndrome.**
cc 19.8	Pyridoxine (B₆)	Required for several **transaminase** and **decarboxylation reactions**	The most severe symptoms are due to the requirement of pyridoxine for the **decarboxylation of glutamic acid to the inhibitory neurotransmitter GABA,** resulting in **seizures.** Deficiency can be associated with **isoniazid** or penicillamine use.
cc 19.9	Biotin	Required for some **carboxylation reactions**	Deficiency is rare because biotin is **synthesized by gastrointestinal bacteria,** although deficiency may be associated with long-term antibiotic use. Deficiency is also associated with the **consumption of raw eggs,** which contain **avidin,** a molecule that binds and inhibits the absorption of biotin.

TABLE 19-1	*Water-Soluble Vitamin Deficiencies (Continued)*

	Vitamin	Biochemical Function	Clinical Consequence of Vitamin Deficiency
CC 19.10	Cobalamine (B_{12})	Required by **methylmalonyl CoA mutase** and **methionine synthetase**	Deficiency is associated with the **lack of intrinsic factor**, produced by **parietal cells of the stomach**. Deficiency results in a block in **purine and thymidine biosynthesis**, resulting in **megaloblastic anemia** and **subacute combined degeneration** of the spinal cord. It also causes a **deficiency of folate.**
CC 19.11	Folate	Reduced by dihydrofolate reductase to THF (tetrahydrofolate), which functions as a **1-carbon donor** in many biosynthetic pathways	Lack of folate results in **impaired dTMP synthesis** with **arrest of DNA synthesis** seen mostly in rapidly dividing cells, like hematopoietic cells, resulting in **megaloblastic anemia. Pregnant patients** require more folate because deficiency can result in **neurotubule defects**, such as **spina bifida**, in the developing fetus.
CC 19.12	Vitamin C	**Hydroxylation of proline residues in collagen** and aids in iron absorption	Deficiency can result in **scurvy**, which is characterized by **easy bruising, muscular fatigue, soft swollen gums, hemorrhage**, and anemia.

   b. The α-carbon of the α-keto acid becomes covalently attached to thiamine pyrophosphate, and the carboxyl group is released as CO_2.

   c. Thiamine pyrophosphate is also the cofactor for the **transketolase** of the pentose-phosphate pathway.

   d. Thiamine pyrophosphate is formed from ATP and the vitamin **thiamine**.

  2. *Lipoic acid* (see Figure 7-6)

   a. Lipoic acid oxidizes the keto group of the decarboxylated α-ketoacid

   b. After an α-ketoacid is decarboxylated, the remainder of the compound is oxidized as it is transferred from thiamine pyrophosphate to lipoic acid, which is reduced in the reaction.

   c. The oxidized compound, which forms a thioester with lipoate, is then transferred to the sulfur of coenzyme A.

   d. Because there is a limited amount of lipoate in the cell, reduced lipoate must be reoxidized so that it can be reused in these types of reactions. It is reoxidized by flavin adenine dinucleotide (FAD), which becomes reduced to $FADH_2$ and is subsequently reoxidized by NAD^+.

   e. Lipoic acid is not derived from a vitamin.

3. *NADPH* (the reduced form of NADP$^+$)
   a. NADPH provides reducing equivalents for the synthesis of **fatty acids** and other compounds and for the reduction of **glutathione.**
   b. NADP$^+$ is identical to NAD$^+$ except that it contains an additional phosphate group (see Figure 8-1).

4. *Biotin*
   a. Biotin is involved in the **carboxylation** of **pyruvate** (which forms oxaloacetate), **acetyl CoA** (which forms malonyl CoA), and **propionyl CoA** (which forms methylmalonyl CoA).
   b. The vitamin biotin is covalently linked to a lysyl residue of the enzyme (see Figure 7-5B).

5. *Pyridoxal phosphate* (Figure 19-2A)
   a. **Pyridoxal phosphate**, an aldehyde, interacts with an amino acid to form a Schiff base. Various products can be generated, depending on the enzyme.
   b. Amino acids are **transaminated, decarboxylated,** or **deaminated** in pyridoxal phosphate–requiring reactions.
   c. Pyridoxal phosphate is derived from **vitamin B$_6$** (pyridoxine).

6. *Tetrahydrofolate* (see Figure 17-8)
   a. Tetrahydrofolate **transfers 1-carbon units** (that are more reduced than CO$_2$) from compounds such as serine to compounds such as dUMP (to form dTMP). Tetrahydrofolate is synthesized from the **vitamin folate.**

7. *Vitamin B$_{12}$* (Figure 19-3)
   a. **Sources of vitamin B$_{12}$**
      (1) Vitamin B$_{12}$ is produced by microorganisms but not by plants.
      (2) Animals obtain vitamin B$_{12}$ from their intestinal flora, from bacteria in their food supply, or by consuming the tissues of other animals.
      (3) **Intrinsic factor**, produced by gastric parietal cells, is required for absorption of vitamin B$_{12}$ by the intestine.
      (4) Vitamin B$_{12}$ is stored and efficiently recycled in the body.
   b. **Functions of vitamin B$_{12}$**
      • Vitamin B$_{12}$ contains **cobalt** in a corrin ring that resembles a porphyrin.
      (1) **Vitamin B$_{12}$** is the cofactor for methylmalonyl CoA mutase, which catalyzes the rearrangement of **methylmalonyl CoA to succinyl CoA.**
      This reaction is involved in the production of succinyl CoA from valine, isoleucine, threonine, methionine, and thymine and the propionyl CoA formed by oxidation of fatty acids with an odd number of carbons.

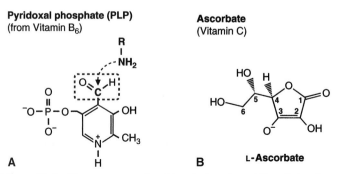

Figure 19-2 The structures of pyridoxal phosphate (**A**) and ascorbate (**B**). *Arrows* indicate the reactive sites.

BOOK STORES INTERNATIO
12 EAST 13TH DRIVE
HUNTINGTON, NY 11743

Merchant ID: 000000000653771
Term ID: 01173595
451209567994

Sale

VISA

XXXXXXXXXXXXX6012

Entry Method: Swiped

Apprvd: Online   Batch#: 000140

03/18/08   15:04:44

Inv #: 000019   Ac   Code: 084283

Total: $ 99.72

Customer Copy

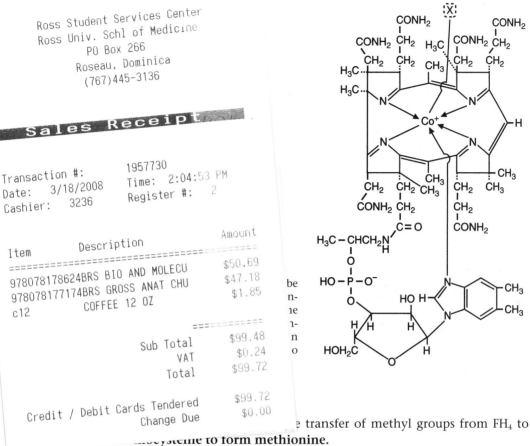

transfer of methyl groups from FH_4 to ...cysteine to form methionine.

8. *Vitamin C* (ascorbic acid) (Figure 19-2B)
   a. It is involved in **hydroxylation reactions**, such as the hydroxylation of prolyl residues in the precursor of collagen.
   b. It functions in the **absorption of iron**.
   c. It is an **antioxidant**.

F. **Fat-soluble vitamins**   (Figure 19-4 and Table 19-2)

1. **Vitamin K** is involved in the activation of precursors of prothrombin and other **clotting factors** by carboxylation of glutamate residues.
2. **Vitamin A** is necessary for the light reactions of **vision**, for normal **growth** and **reproduction**, and for differentiation and maintenance of **epithelial tissues**.
   a. Δ^{11}-*cis*-Retinal binds to the protein opsin, forming rhodopsin. Light causes Δ^{11}-*cis*-retinal in rhodopsin to be converted to all-trans-retinal, which dissociates from opsin, causing changes that allow light to be perceived by the brain.
   b. Retinoic acid, the most oxidized form of vitamin A, acts like a steroid hormone.
3. **Vitamin E** serves as an **antioxidant**.
   a. It prevents free radicals from oxidizing compounds such as polyunsaturated fatty acids.
   b. A major consequence is that the integrity of membranes, which contain fatty acid residues in phospholipids, is maintained.

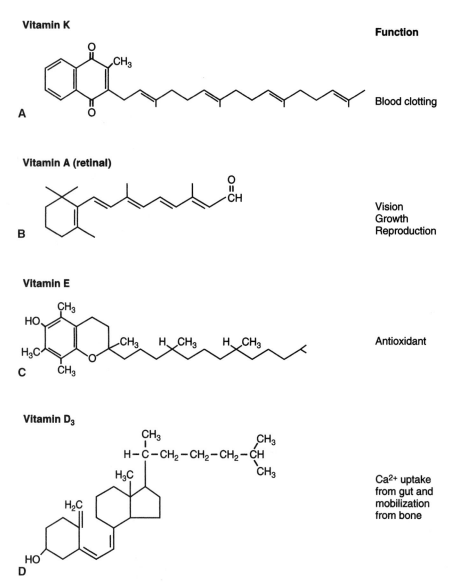

Figure 19-4   The fat-soluble vitamins.

   4. Vitamin D (as 1,25-dihydroxycholecalciferol) is involved in **calcium metabolism.**

G.   Minerals required in large amounts include **calcium and phosphate,** which serve as structural components of bone. Minerals required in trace amounts include **iron,** which is a component of heme (Table 19-3).

II.   Metabolism During the Fed or Absorptive State (Figure 19-5)

A.   The fate of glucose in the liver

   1. Liver cells either oxidize glucose or convert it to glycogen and triacylglycerols.

TABLE 19-2	*Lipid-Soluble Vitamin Deficiencies*	
	Vitamin	**Biochemical Function**	**Clinical Consequence of Vitamin Deficiency**
cc *19.13*	Vitamin A	Required for **growth and differentiation**; required for the production of the light-absorbing vision protein **rhodopsin**	Deficiency results in **night blindness**, dry eyes leading to **corneal damage**, urinary stones.
cc *19.14*	Vitamin D	**Regulation of gene expression** for the **absorption of calcium** from the gastrointestinal tract	**Rickets** results in **children** as a result of **defective bone mineralization** with a "squared" head, deformity of the chest, abnormalities of the spine, and **bowing of the legs**. In **adults**, osteomalacia can occur, with **weakening of bone** and an increased incidence of gross **fracture**.
cc *19.15*	Vitamin E	Functions as an **antioxidant** and free radical scavenger	Deficiency states are rare; however, they may contribute to the development of **atherosclerosis** and **cardiovascular disease**.
cc *19.16*	Vitamin K	Required for the γ-carboxylation of coagulation factors II, VII, IX, and X	Deficiency is seen in **newborns** because vitamin K is **produced by the yet undeveloped gastrointestinal flora**, resulting in **hemorrhage and bleeding diathesis**. The blood thinner **warfarin**, which is used to treat **blood clots**, **antagonizes** the vitamin's actions.

2. **Glucose** is **oxidized** to CO_2 and H_2O to meet the immediate energy needs of the liver.

3. **Excess glucose** is **stored** in the liver as **glycogen**, which is used during periods of fasting to maintain blood glucose.

4. **Excess glucose** can be **converted to fatty acids** and a **glycerol** moiety, which combine to form **triacylglycerols**, which are released from the liver into the blood as **very low–density lipoproteins (VLDL)**.

B. The fate of glucose in other tissues

1. The **brain**, which depends on glucose for its energy, **oxidizes glucose to CO_2 and H_2O**, producing ATP.

2. **Red blood cells**, lacking mitochondria, oxidize glucose to **pyruvate** and **lactate**, which are released into the blood.

Table 19-3	*Important Mineral Deficiencies*		
	Mineral	Biochemical Function	Clinical Consequence of Mineral Deficiency
cc 19.17	Copper	Component of many oxidases in oxidative metabolism, neurotransmitter synthesis, and collagen synthesis	Deficiency results in muscle weakness, neurologic defects, and abnormal collagen cross linking.
cc 19.18	Iodine	Essential component of thyroid hormone	Deficiency results in Goiter and hypothyroidism and is uncommon in developed countries with the advent of iodized salt.
cc 19.19	Iron	Essential component of hemoglobin, as well as other metalloenzymes	Deficiency results in defective hemoglobin production and the development of hypochromic, microcytic anemia.
cc 19.20	Selenium	Component of glutathione peroxidase	Deficiency results in cardiomyopathy (Keshan disease).
cc 19.21	Zinc	Component of many oxidases	Deficiency results in growth retardation and impaired wound healing.

3. **Muscle cells** take up glucose by a **transport** process that is **stimulated by insulin.** They **oxidize glucose** to CO_2 and H_2O to generate ATP for contraction, and they also **store** glucose as **glycogen** for use during contraction.

4. **Adipose cells** take up glucose by a **transport** process that is **stimulated by insulin.** These cells oxidize glucose to produce energy and convert it to the glycerol moiety used to produce triacylglycerol stores.

C. The fate of lipoproteins in the fed state

1. The triacylglycerols of **chylomicrons** (produced from dietary fat) and **VLDL** (produced from glucose by the liver) are **digested** in capillaries by **lipoprotein lipase** to form fatty acids and glycerol.

2. The **fatty acids** are taken up by **adipose tissue**, converted to **triacylglycerols**, and stored.

D. The fate of amino acids in the fed state.   Amino acids from dietary proteins enter cells and are:

1. Used for **protein synthesis** (which occurs on ribosomes and requires mRNA). Proteins are constantly being synthesized and degraded.

2. Used to make **nitrogenous compounds** such as heme, creatine phosphate, epinephrine, and the bases of DNA and RNA.

3. Oxidized to generate **ATP**.

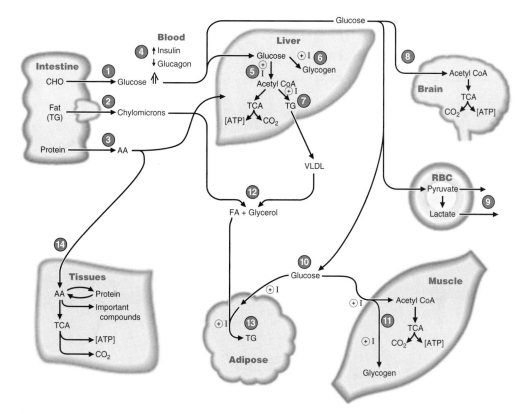

Figure 19-5   The fed state. The *circled numbers* serve as a guide, indicating the approximate order in which the processes begin to occur. AA = amino acid; ATP = adenosine triphosphate; CoA, coenzyme A; FA = fatty acid; I = insulin; RBC = red blood cells; TCA = tricarboxylic acid; TG = triacylglycerols; VLDL = very low–density lipoprotein; ⊕ = stimulated by.

III.   Fasting (Figure 19-6)

A.   **The liver during fasting**

   1. The liver produces **glucose** and **ketone bodies** that are released into the blood and serve as sources of energy for other tissues.
   2. *Production of glucose by the liver*
      a. The liver has the major responsibility for **maintaining blood glucose levels.** Glucose is required particularly by tissues such as the brain and red blood cells. The brain oxidizes glucose to CO_2 and H_2O, while red blood cells oxidize glucose to pyruvate and lactate.
      b. Glycogenolysis
         (1) About 2–3 hours after a meal, the liver begins to break down its glycogen stores by the process of glycogenolysis, and glucose is released into the blood.
         (2) Glucose is taken up by tissues and oxidized.
      c. **Gluconeogenesis**
         (1) After about 4–6 hours of fasting, the **liver** begins the process of gluconeogenesis. Within 30 hours, liver glycogen stores are depleted, leaving gluconeogenesis as the major process responsible for maintaining blood glucose.
         (2) **Carbon sources** for gluconeogenesis are:
            (a) **Lactate** produced by tissues like red blood cells or exercising muscle

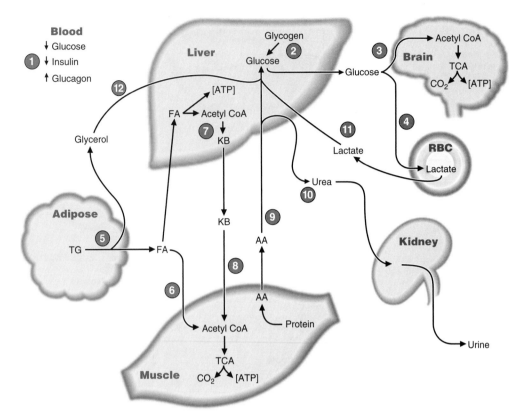

Figure 19-6 The fasting (basal) state. This state occurs after an overnight (12-hour) fast. The *circled numbers* serve as a guide, indicating the approximate order in which the processes begin to occur. KB = ketone bodies. For other abbreviations, see Figure 19-5.

(b) **Glycerol** from breakdown of triacylglycerols in adipose tissue
(c) **Amino acids**, particularly alanine, from muscle protein
(d) **Propionate** from oxidation of odd-chain fatty acids (minor source)

3. Production of ketone bodies by the liver
    a. As glucagon levels rise, adipose tissue breaks down its **triacylglycerol stores** into fatty acids and glycerol, which are released into the blood.
    b. Through the process of **β-oxidation**, the liver converts the fatty acids to acetyl coenzyme A (CoA).
    c. **Acetyl CoA** is used by the liver for the synthesis of the ketone bodies, **acetoacetate and β-hydroxybutyrate.** The liver cannot oxidize ketone bodies and releases them into the blood.

B. Adipose tissue during fasting

1. As glucagon levels rise, adipose **triacylglycerol stores** are **mobilized.** The liver converts the fatty acids to ketone bodies and the glycerol to glucose.
2. Tissues such as muscle oxidize the fatty acids to CO_2 and H_2O.

C. Muscle during fasting

1. *Degradation of muscle protein*

   a. During fasting, muscle protein is degraded, producing amino acids that are partially metabolized by muscle and released into the blood, mainly as **alanine** and **glutamine.**

   b. Tissues, such as **gut** and **kidney**, metabolize the glutamine.

   c. The products (mainly **alanine**) travel to the **liver** where the carbons are converted to glucose or ketone bodies and the nitrogen is converted to urea.

  2. *Oxidation of fatty acids and ketone bodies*

   a. During **fasting**, muscle oxidizes fatty acids released from adipose tissue and ketone bodies produced by the liver.

   b. During **exercise**, muscle can also use its own glycogen stores as well as glucose, fatty acids, and ketone bodies from the blood.

IV.   Prolonged Fasting (Starvation)

A.   Metabolic changes in starvation   (Figure 19-7). When the body enters the **starved state**, after **3–5 days of fasting**, changes occur in the use of fuel stores.

  1. Muscle decreases its use of ketone bodies and oxidizes fatty acids as its primary energy source.

  2. Because of decreased use by muscle, **blood ketone body levels rise.**

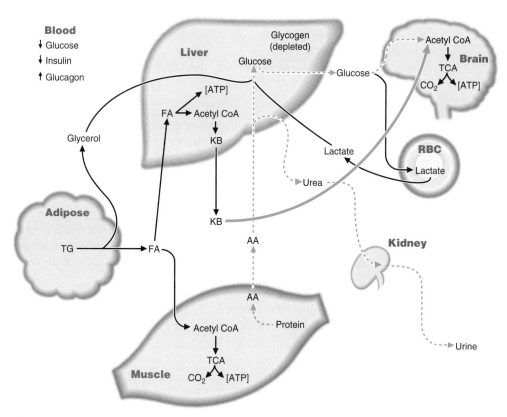

Figure 19-7   The starved state. This state occurs after 3–5 days of fasting. Dashed lines indicate processes that have decreased, and the heavy solid line indicates a process that has increased relative to the fasting state. For abbreviations, see Figures 19-5 and 19-6.

3. The **brain** then takes up and **oxidizes ketone bodies** to derive energy. Conse-quently, the brain decreases its use of glucose, although glucose is still a major fuel for the brain.

4. Liver **gluconeogenesis decreases.**

5. **Muscle protein is spared** (i.e., less muscle protein is degraded to provide amino acids for gluconeogenesis).

6. Because of decreased conversion of amino acids to glucose, **less urea is produced** from amino acid nitrogen in starvation than after an overnight fast.

B. **Fat: the primary fuel**

1. The body uses its fat stores as its primary source of energy during starvation, con-serving functional protein.

2. Overall, fats are quantitatively the most important fuel in the body.

3. The length of time that a person can survive without food depends mainly on the amount of fat stored in adipose tissue.

V. Biochemical Functions of Tissues

A. **Stomach**

1. Chief cells produce the proteolytic enzyme **pepsin** as its inactive precursor pepsino-gen. Pepsin digests proteins.

2. Parietal cells produce hydrochloric acid (**HCl**) and **intrinsic factor.**

   a. **HCl** causes pepsinogen (the precursor of pepsin) to cleave itself (autocataly-sis), producing **pepsin.**

   b. **Intrinsic factor** binds dietary **vitamin B_{12}** and aids in its absorption.

B. **Gallbladder**

1. **Bile salts,** synthesized in the liver from cholesterol, pass through the gallbladder into the intestine, where they aid in lipid digestion.

2. **Bilirubin diglucuronide,** produced in the liver from bilirubin (the excretory product of heme degradation), passes through the gallbladder into the intestine.

C. **Pancreas**

1. The pancreas **produces bicarbonate (HCO_3^-),** which neutralizes stomach acid as it enters the intestinal lumen. The subsequent increase in pH in the lumen allows more extensive **ionization of bile salts** (so they serve as better detergents) and increases the **activity of digestive enzymes.**

2. The pancreas produces **digestive enzymes** (e.g., trypsin, chymotrypsin, the car-boxypeptidases, elastase, α-amylase, lipase).

3. The B (or β) cells of the endocrine pancreas produce **insulin** (the hormone that stimulates the storage of fuels in the fed state), and the A (or α) cells produce **glucagon** (the hormone that stimulates the release of stored fuels during fasting).

D. **Intestine**

1. **Enzymes** from the **exocrine pancreas digest food** in the intestinal lumen.

2. **Digestive enzymes** are bound to the brush borders of **intestinal epithelial cells** (aminopeptidases, di- and tripeptidases, lactase, sucrase, maltases, and isomaltases).

3. **Absorption** of digestive products occurs through intestinal epithelial cells.
4. Intestinal epithelial cells produce **chylomicrons** from the digestive products of dietary fat (fatty acids and 2-monoacylglycerols) and secrete the chylomicrons into the lymph.
5. Most **bile salts** are **resorbed** in the ileum and **recycled** by the liver. Only **5% are excreted** in the feces. This excretion of bile salts, along with cholesterol secreted by the liver into the gut via the gallbladder, is the major means by which the body disposes of the cholesterol ring system (sterol nucleus).

E. **Liver**

1. **Functions** of the liver include the following.
   a. Storage of **glycogen** produced from dietary carbohydrate.
   b. Synthesis of very low–density lipoprotein (**VLDL**), mainly from dietary carbohydrate.
   c. Production of high-density lipoprotein (**HDL**), which transfers C_{II} and E apoproteins to chylomicrons and VLDL, converts cholesterol to cholesterol esters (via the lecithin-cholesterol acyl transferase or LCAT reaction), and reduces blood cholesterol levels by participating in the process by which cholesterol and cholesterol esters are transported from tissues to the liver.
   d. **Maintenance of blood glucose** during fasting via glycogenolysis and gluconeogenesis.
   e. Production of **urea** from nitrogen derived, in part, from amino acids as they are being converted to glucose (via gluconeogenesis) during fasting.
   f. Production of **ketone bodies** from fatty acids derived from lipolysis of adipose triacylglycerols during fasting.
   g. Synthesis of **cholesterol** (which is also made in other tissues).
   h. Conversion of cholesterol to **bile salts.**
   i. Production of many **blood proteins** (e.g., albumin, blood clotting proteins).
   j. **Production of purines** and **pyrimidines,** which are transported to other tissues via red blood cells.
   k. **Degradation of purines** (to uric acid) and **pyrimidines** (to CO_2, H_2O, and urea).
   l. **Oxidation of drugs** and other **toxic compounds** via the cytochrome P450 system.
   m. **Conjugation of bilirubin** and excretion of bilirubin diglucuronide into the bile.
   n. **Oxidation of alcohol** via alcohol and acetaldehyde dehydrogenases and the microsomal ethanol oxidizing system (MEOS).
   o. Synthesis of **creatine** (from guanidinoacetate), which is used to produce creatine phosphate, mainly in muscle and brain.
   p. Conversion of **dietary fructose** to glycolytic intermediates.
2. **If liver cell function is compromised** (e.g., in viral hepatitis or alcoholic cirrhosis), then the following occurs.
   a. NH_4^+, which is **toxic** (particularly to the central nervous system), **increases** in the blood.
   b. The blood urea nitrogen (**BUN**) level **decreases** because the liver has a decreased capacity to produce urea.
   c. **Blood glucose decreases** because of decreased glycogenolysis and gluconeogenesis.
   d. Blood **cholesterol** levels **decrease.**
   e. Production of **bile salts decreases.**
   f. **Bilirubin** levels **increase** in the body (causing jaundice).

    g. Lysis of damaged liver cells allows **enzymes** to **leak** into the blood.

    h. Chronic liver problems result in **decreased protein synthesis.**

        (1) Serum proteins (e.g., albumin) decrease.

        (2) VLDL production decreases because of decreased apoprotein B-100, and triacylglycerols accumulate in the liver. A fatty liver results.

  3. Specific diseases that affect the liver are as follows.

    a. Glycogen storage diseases

    b. Alcoholism

        (1) Oxidation of ethanol **produces NADH** by reactions that occur in the liver.

        (2) Ingestion of ethanol without food intake results in high [NADH]/[NAD$^+$], which can cause:

            (a) Increased conversion of pyruvate to lactate, producing a **lactic acidosis.**

            (b) Inhibition of gluconeogenesis, leading to **hypoglycemia.**

            (c) Increased levels of glycerol 3-phosphate, which combines with fatty acids from adipose triacylglycerols to form VLDL. Increased VLDL levels in the blood produce a **hyperlipidemia.**

        (3) In **chronic alcoholism, protein synthesis decreases** in the liver. Thus, VLDL secretion decreases, leading to a **fatty liver** (the accumulation of triacylglycerol).

    c. Diabetes mellitus (DM)

        (1) Low insulin levels (type 1) or insensitivity to insulin (type 2) results in increased glycogenolysis and gluconeogenesis, which contribute to the **elevated blood glucose levels.**

        (2) Increased ketone body production can lead to **diabetic ketoacidosis (DKA)** particularly in type 1 DM. Ketone body synthesis increases because of increased release of fatty acids from adipose triacylglycerols.

F. Brain

  1. Glucose is the major fuel for the brain.

  2. The brain can use **ketone bodies** but only **after 3–5 days of fasting when blood ketone body levels are elevated.**

  3. The brain needs energy to **think** (i.e., memory involves RNA synthesis), conduct **nerve impulses,** synthesize **neurotransmitters,** etc.

    a. Abrupt decreases in blood glucose can result in **coma** from **lack of ATP.**

    b. Very elevated blood glucose levels can cause a **hyperosmolar coma.**

    c. Synthesis of some neurotransmitters (e.g., GABA, serotonin, dopamine) involves decarboxylation of amino acids and requires pyridoxal phosphate (from vitamin B$_6$).

G. Red blood cells

  1. Red blood cells **lack mitochondria,** so they have no TCA cycle, β-oxidation of fatty acids, electron transport chain, and other pathways that occur in mitochondria.

  2. Glucose is the **major fuel** for red blood cells. Glucose is converted to pyruvate and lactate.

  3. Red blood cells **carry bases** and **nucleosides** from the liver to other tissues.

  4. The major function of red blood cells is to **carry O$_2$** from the lungs to the tissues and to aid in the **return of CO$_2$** from the tissues to the lungs.

H. Adipose tissue

  1. The **major fuel** of adipose tissue is **glucose.**

2. **Insulin** stimulates the **transport of glucose** into adipose cells.
3. The function of adipose tissue is to **store triacylglycerol** in the fed state and release it (via **lipolysis**) during fasting.
   a. **In the fed state**, insulin stimulates the synthesis and secretion of lipoprotein lipase (LPL), which degrades the triacylglycerols of chylomicrons and VLDL in the capillaries. Fatty acids from these lipoproteins enter adipose cells and are converted to triacylglycerols and stored. Glucose provides the glycerol moiety. (Glycerol is not used because adipose cells lack glycerol kinase.)
   b. **During fasting**, hormone-sensitive lipase (phosphorylated and activated via a cAMP-mediated mechanism) initiates lipolysis in adipose cells.
   c. **In diabetes mellitus**, low insulin levels (type 1) or insulin resistance (type 2) results in decreased degradation of the triacylglycerols of chylomicrons and VLDL (because of decreased LPL).

I. Muscle

1. Muscle uses **all fuels** that are available (glycogen stores and fatty acids, glucose, ketone bodies, lactate, and amino acids from the blood) to obtain energy for contraction.
2. During fasting, muscle protein is degraded to provide **amino acids** (particularly alanine) for **gluconeogenesis.**
3. **Creatine phosphate** transports high-energy phosphate from the mitochondria to actinomyosin fibers and provides ATP for muscle contraction.
4. **Creatinine** is produced nonenzymatically from creatine phosphate, and a **constant amount** (dependent on body muscle mass) is released into the blood each day and excreted by the kidneys.
5. **Muscle glycogen phosphorylase** differs from liver phosphorylase but catalyzes the same reaction (glycogen + P_i ↔ glucose 1-phosphate).
6. **Insulin** stimulates the **transport of glucose** into muscle cells.

J. Heart

1. The heart is a specialized muscle that uses **all fuels** from the blood.
2. The muscle-brain **(MB) isozyme** of creatine kinase (CK) is found in heart muscle. Its release can be used to monitor a heart attack.
3. *Heart disease*
   a. **Atherosclerotic plaques** can occlude blood vessels, blocking the flow of nutrients and O_2. Muscle tissue beyond the block suffers from a lack of energy and can die. When the amount of functional cardiac muscle tissue that remains is insufficient to pump blood through the body at a normal rate, **heart failure** occurs.
   b. **High blood cholesterol** levels are associated with increased risk of a heart attack (or a stroke, which is caused by a similar process in the brain). Cholesterol is carried in the blood lipoproteins and is elevated in a group of conditions known as the **hyperlipidemias.**

K. Kidney

1. The kidney **excretes substances** from the body via the urine, including **urea** (produced by the urea cycle in the liver), **uric acid** (from purine degradation), **creatinine** (from creatine phosphate), NH_4^4 (from glutamine via glutaminase), H_2SO_4 (produced from the sulfur of cysteine and methionine), and **phosphoric acid.**

2. Daily **creatinine** excretion is **constant** and depends on body muscle mass. It is used as a measure of kidney function (the creatinine clearance rate).

3. **Glutaminase** action increases during **acidosis** and produces NH_3, which enters the urine and reacts with H^+ to form NH_4^+. NH_4^+ buffers the urine and removes acid (H^+) from the body.

4. **Uric acid** excretion is inhibited by lead (Pb) and metabolic acids (ketone bodies and lactic acid). High blood uric acid can result in **gout.** Gout can be caused either by increased production or by decreased excretion of uric acid.

5. **Kidney dysfunction** can lead to increased BUN, creatinine, and uric acid in the blood and decreased levels of these compounds in the urine.

6. During ketoacidosis, **ketone bodies** are excreted by the kidney, and during lactic acidosis, **lactic acid** is excreted.

7. Elevated blood glucose (over 180 mg/dL) in diabetes mellitus results in **excretion of glucose** in the urine.

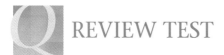 REVIEW TEST

Directions: Each of the numbered questions or incomplete statements in this section is followed by answers or by completions of the statement. Select the **one** lettered answer or completion that is **best** in each case.

1. Which of the following amino acids is essential in the human diet?

(A) Serine
(B) Lysine
(C) Glutamate
(D) Tyrosine
(E) Cysteine

2. After fasting for 12 hours, a student consumes a large bag of pretzels. This meal will:

(A) replenish liver glycogen stores.
(B) increase the rate of gluconeogenesis.
(C) reduce the rate at which fatty acids are converted to adipose triacylglycerols.
(D) increase blood glucagon levels.
(E) result in glucose being oxidized to lactate by the brain and to CO_2 and H_2O by red blood cells.

3. Which of the following would be observed in a person who is resting after an overnight fast?

(A) Liver glycogen stores are completely depleted.
(B) Liver gluconeogenesis is not an important process.
(C) Muscle glycogen stores are used to maintain blood glucose.
(D) Fatty acids are released from adipose triacylglycerol stores.
(E) The liver is oxidizing ketone bodies to CO_2 and H_2O.

4. Which of the following would be observed in a person after 1 week of starvation?

(A) The brain uses glucose and ketone bodies as fuel sources.
(B) Liver glycogen stores are only partially depleted due to an increase in gluconeogenesis.
(C) Nitrogen balance is maintained because muscle protein releases

amino acids to compensate for the lack of dietary protein.
(D) Fatty acids from adipose stores are the major source of fuel for red blood cells.

5. When compared with his state after an overnight fast, a person who fasts for 1 week will have:

(A) higher levels of blood glucose.
(B) less muscle protein.
(C) more adipose tissue.
(D) lower levels of ketone bodies in the blood.

6. Which of the following compounds can be synthesized in humans?

(A) Riboflavin
(B) Linoleic acid
(C) Leucine
(D) Thiamine
(E) Niacin

7. In which of the following tissues is glucose the major fuel in prolonged fasting?

(A) Muscle
(B) Brain
(C) Liver
(D) Red blood cells
(E) Kidney

8. Which of the following vitamins is required for the synthesis of NAD^+?

(A) Riboflavin
(B) Pantothenic acid
(C) Niacin
(D) Vitamin B_6

9. Which of the following vitamins is required for the synthesis of flavin adenine dinucleotide (FAD)?

(A) Riboflavin
(B) Pantothenic acid

(C) Niacin
(D) Vitamin B_6

10. Which of the following vitamins is required for the synthesis of coenzyme A?

(A) Riboflavin
(B) Pantothenic acid
(C) Niacin
(D) Vitamin B_6

11. Which of the following vitamins is required for the synthesis of flavin mononucleotide (FMN)?

(A) Riboflavin
(B) Pantothenic acid
(C) Niacin
(D) Vitamin B_6

12. Which of the following vitamins is required for the synthesis of pyridoxal phosphate?

(A) Riboflavin
(B) Pantothenic acid
(C) Niacin
(D) Vitamin B_6

13. Which of the following processes is affected by vitamin A deficiency?

(A) Blood clotting
(B) Calcium metabolism
(C) Collagen synthesis
(D) Vision

14. Which of the following processes is affected by vitamin C deficiency?

(A) Blood clotting
(B) Calcium metabolism
(C) Collagen synthesis
(D) Vision

15. Which of the following processes is affected by vitamin D deficiency?

(A) Blood clotting
(B) Calcium metabolism
(C) Collagen synthesis
(D) Vision

16. Which of the following processes is affected by vitamin K deficiency?

(A) Blood clotting
(B) Calcium metabolism

(C) Collagen synthesis
(D) Vision

17. A 57-year-old male with chronic pancreatitis, secondary to alcoholism, is admitted to the hospital for treatment. Given his pancreatitis, which of the following vitamin deficiencies is of concern?

(A) Vitamin B_{12} (cobalamine)
(B) Folic acid
(C) Vitamin B_2 (riboflavin)
(D) Vitamin B_6 (pyridoxine)
(E) Vitamin D

18. A 54-year-old Native-American living on an Indian reservation in southwest Arizona presents to the clinic with impaired memory, diarrhea, and a rash on the face, neck, and dorsum of the hands. It is likely that this patient has a deficiency of which vitamin?

(A) Vitamin B_3 (niacin)
(B) Homocysteine
(C) Folic acid
(D) Vitamin C
(E) Vitamin E

19. A 32-year-old female presents to the physician with extreme fatigue and neurologic complaints. On exam, it is found that she has decreased positional and vibrational sense, and her complete blood count reveals megaloblastic anemia. She relates a history of gastric resection 4 years ago for severe stomach ulcers. She is likely suffering a deficiency of what essential vitamin?

(A) Vitamin C
(B) Vitamin D
(C) Vitamin K
(D) Vitamin B_{12} (cobalamine)
(E) Folate

20. A postpartum woman from a rural Appalachian community recently gave birth to a baby boy with the aid of a midwife at home. She now brings the baby to the hospital because of continued bleeding and oozing from the umbilical stump. It is likely that this bleeding diathesis is secondary to a deficiency of which vitamin?

(A) Vitamin A
(B) Vitamin E

(C) Vitamin D
(D) Vitamin K
(E) Folic acid

21. A 75-year-old chronic alcoholic presents to emergency room after being found on the railroad tracks passed out. On examination, he is found to have a distended abdomen that is equivalent in size to a full-term pregnant woman's belly. Which of the following functions of the liver has been compromised to cause this finding?

(A) Lipid metabolism
(B) Albumin synthesis
(C) Estrogen metabolism
(D) Alcohol detoxification
(E) Decreased production of coagulation factors

22. A 45-year-old male alcoholic walks into the emergency room with a clumsy, wide-based gait and appears confused. On physical exam, nystagmus is pronounced. A blood gas demonstrates a metabolic acidosis, while serum analysis gives a blood alcohol level of 0.13. This patient should most probably be treated with IV fluids containing which of the following?

(A) Thiamin
(B) Riboflavin
(C) Niacin
(D) Pantothenic acid
(E) Biotin

23. A fourth-year medical student does an international rotation in Subsaharan Africa. While immunizing children against polio, he sees hundreds of malnourished children in refugee camps with bloated-appearing abdomens. He learns that they are severely protein deficient because they are fed a diet of cornmeal that is provided by international relief agencies. These children likely suffer from which of the following?

(A) Marasmus
(B) Anorexia nervosa
(C) Bulimia

(D) Kwashiorkor
(E) Cachexia

24. A 42-year-old male has been in the intensive care unit following a motor vehicle accident. He sustained numerous long bone fractures and has been bedridden for 2 months. He has begun to develop ulcers on the dependent areas of his body. A nutritionist was consulted. The nutritionist recommended supplementation of which of the following to aid in wound healing?

(A) Copper
(B) Iodine
(C) Iron
(D) Selenium
(E) Zinc

25. A 23-year-old body builder visits his physician with complaints of fatigue, depression, insomnia, hair loss, and dry skin. He tells the physician he has been "bulking up" for an upcoming competition, and his meals consist mostly of eight raw eggs along with low-fat milk. The physician suspects biotin deficiency given the patient's diet and symptoms. Which of the following is biotin required for?

(A) The formation of *cis*-retinol
(B) Transfer of 1-carbon units
(C) Hydroxylation reactions
(D) Carboxylation of pyruvate
(E) Decarboxylation of α-ketoacids

26. A 26-year-old female meets with her family physician to discuss family planning. She is interested in starting a family soon and is looking for advice on what nutritional supplements would be beneficial during pregnancy. The physician suggests which two supplements as the most important?

(A) Selenium and vitamin K
(B) Copper and riboflavin
(C) Iron and folate
(D) Vitamin C and vitamin D
(E) Vitamin A and biotin

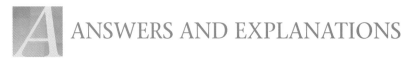
ANSWERS AND EXPLANATIONS

1–B. Lysine cannot be synthesized and must be obtained in the diet. Serine and glutamate can be synthesized from glucose. Cysteine can be synthesized from serine, obtaining its sulfur from methionine. Tyrosine is produced from phenylalanine.

2–A. After a meal of carbohydrates, glycogen is stored in the liver and in muscle, and triacylglycerols are stored in adipose tissue. The level of glucagon in the blood decreases, and gluconeogenesis decreases. The brain oxidizes glucose to CO_2 and H_2O, while the red blood cells produce lactate.

3–D. During fasting, fatty acids are released from adipose tissue and oxidized by other cells. Liver glycogen is not depleted until about after 30 hours of fasting. After an overnight fast, both glycogenolysis and gluconeogenesis by the liver help maintain blood glucose. Muscle glycogen stores are not used to maintain blood glucose. The liver produces ketone bodies but does not oxidize them.

4–A. After 3–5 days of starvation, the brain begins to use ketone bodies, in addition to glucose, as a fuel source. Glycogen stores in the liver are depleted during the first 30 hours of fasting. Inadequate protein in the diet results in negative nitrogen balance. Red blood cells cannot oxidize fatty acids because they do not have mitochondria.

5–B. If a person who has fasted overnight continues to fast for 1 week, muscle protein will continue to decrease because it is being converted to blood glucose. However, it will not decrease at as rapid a rate as with a briefer fast because the brain is using ketone bodies and, therefore, less glucose. The person's blood glucose levels will decrease only slightly because initially glycogenolysis and then gluconeogenesis by the liver act to maintain blood glucose levels. Adipose tissue will decrease as triacylglycerol is mobilized. Fatty acids from adipose tissue will be converted to ketone bodies in the liver. Blood ketone body levels will rise, and ketone bodies will be used by the brain.

6–E. Although niacin is a vitamin, it can be synthesized to a limited extent from tryptophan.

7–D. Red blood cells use glucose (via glycolysis) as their only energy source because they do not have an active tricarboxylic acid (TCA) cycle; they lack mitochondria. The other tissues have mitochondria and can use other fuels.

8–C. NAD⁺ contains niacin.

9–A. FAD contains riboflavin.

10–B. Coenzyme A contains pantothenic acid.

11–A. FMN contains riboflavin.

12–D. Pyridoxal phosphate contains vitamin B_6.

13–D. Vitamin A is required for formation of the visual pigments.

14–C. Vitamin C is required for the hydroxylation of proline and lysine residues in the precursor of collagen. Defective collagen formation results in scurvy, which is characterized by bleeding gums.

15–B. Vitamin D stimulates calcium uptake from the intestine and resorption from bone and urine.

16–A. Vitamin K is required for blood clotting.

17–E. Although it is true that alcoholics are often malnourished and deficient in many vitamins, the question focuses on the deficiencies associated with pancreatitis. The function of the exocrine pancreas is necessary for the absorption of fat-soluble vitamins, and vitamin D is the only vitamin listed that is fat soluble; the other vitamins listed are water soluble.

18–A. The patient presents with the classic presentation of pellagra, or niacin deficiency, with diarrhea, dementia, and dermatitis. Niacin is synthesized from the essential amino acid tryptophan, which is particularly deficient in corn-based diets. Decreased homocysteine, an amino acid, has been associated with cardiovascular disease. Folic acid deficiency often manifests with anemia. Vitamin C deficiency results in scurvy. Vitamin E deficiency is rare and can result in neurologic symptoms.

19–D. Both folate and vitamin B_{12} deficiency lead to a megaloblastic anemia secondary to a reduction in DNA synthesis. Only vitamin B_{12} deficiency causes neurologic dysfunction associated with damage to the dorsal spinal columns. The history of gastric resection is consistent with a deficiency of intrinsic factor required for reabsorption of vitamin B_{12} in the terminal ileum.

20–D. Deficiency of vitamin K results in abnormal bleeding because it is required for γ-carboxylation of clotting factors II, VII, IX, and X. Because newborns have inadequate intestinal flora, which is the primary source of vitamin K, they often have such a deficiency. Vitamin A deficiency results in vision changes and defects in epithelial cell function. Vitamin D deficiency in children results in rickets. Folic acid deficiency during early embryogenesis can result in neural tube defects.

21–B. Accumulation of fluid in the peritoneum, termed ascites, is caused by increased back pressure into capillaries and decreased albumin. Albumin is the primary protein that maintains oncotic pressure within the vessels and is synthesized by the liver. Defects in lipoprotein synthesis will indeed lead to accumulation of lipids in liver cells, leading to fatty liver. The liver is also responsible for the metabolism of estrogens, a failure of which leads to hyperestrogenism. The body actually becomes more capable of metabolizing alcohol in chronic alcoholics. The liver produces coagulation factors, and in severe liver disease, bleeding diathesis can result.

22–A. Wernicke encephalopathy, with the classic triad of ataxia, confusion, and ophthalmoplegia (and nystagmus), is due to thiamine deficiency. Thiamine is an essential coenzyme in carbohydrate metabolism including the pentose-phosphate pathway (transketolase) and the tricarboxylic acid cycle (pyruvate decarboxylase and α-ketoglutarate). Riboflavin deficiency is possible in malnourished alcoholics, causing cheilosis, glossitis, and corneal changes. Niacin deficiency causes diarrhea, dementia, and dermatitis. Deficiencies of pantothenic acid and biotin are rare.

23–D. Protein deficiency, as in kwashiorkor, results in a deficiency of visceral proteins including those in the blood that normally provide oncotic pressure to retain fluid within vessels. As such, patients with kwashiorkor have abdominal bloating secondary to edema. Marasmus is a deficiency of calories and protein; the children in this question are presumably receiving carbohydrate calories through the cornmeal. Anorexia nervosa and bulimia are disorders of self-induced weight loss that are mostly found in developed countries. Cachexia is weight loss associated with cancer.

24–E. Zinc is a trace element that aids in wound healing and is often given as a nutritional supplement, along with vitamin C, in such a setting. Iodine is required for thyroid hormone synthesis, and deficiency is rarely a problem in the Western world. Copper is required for collagen synthesis, and deficiency is quite rare without an inborn error in copper metabolism. Selenium deficiency results in cardiomyopathy (Keshan disease) and is most common in China.

25–D. Biotin deficiency is rare except in cases of parenteral feeding or in cases of excess consumption of raw eggs, as the egg protein avidin binds biotin and inhibits its absorption. Biotin is a required cofactor for the carboxylation of pyruvate, acetyl CoA, and propionyl CoA. Folate is involved in 1-carbon transfer reactions. Vitamin C is important for the hydroxylation of collagen. Vitamin A is required for the production of the light-absorbing protein *cis*-retinol. Finally, thiamine is a cofactor for the decarboxylation of α-ketoacids.

26–C. Pregnancy is a time of increased metabolic demand, and two of the most important supplements are iron, to prevent anemia, and folate, to prevent neurotubule defects in the developing fetus. Copper and selenium are trace elements that are rarely deficient. Riboflavin is often found in grain products. Vitamin C and vitamin D are often obtained appropriately from the diet. Vitamin A derivatives are often teratogenic and, therefore, should be avoided during pregnancy. Vitamin K deficiency is common in newborns, and often, they are supplemented at birth.

Molecular Endocrinology

I. General Mechanisms of Hormone Action

A. **Hormones that bind to cell membrane receptors**

1. *Hormones that activate tyrosine kinases* (Figure 20-1)
   a. **Insulin** binds to a receptor on the cell surface, causing the β subunits of the receptor (that extend through the membrane) to **phosphorylate** themselves on **tyrosine residues** located on the inner surface.
   b. The phosphorylated receptor acts as a **kinase**, phosphorylating an intracellular protein known as **insulin receptor substrate** (IRS).
   c. Phosphorylated IRS then activates other signal transduction proteins, **initiating a sequence of events** that ultimately produce the intracellular effects of insulin.

2. *Hormones that act through cyclic nucleotides* (Figure 20-2)
   a. Epinephrine and certain polypeptide hormones, such as glucagon, bind to **receptors on the external surface** of the cell membrane.
      (1) These hormone-receptor complexes interact with **G proteins** (so-called because they bind guanine nucleotides) (Figure 20-3) and activate **adenylate cyclase, which converts adenosine triphosphate (ATP) to cyclic adenosine monophosphate (cAMP).**
      (2) cAMP activates **protein kinase A,** which subsequently **phosphorylates** certain intracellular proteins, altering their activity.
      (3) The activity of these proteins can be returned to their previous state by **phosphatases** that **dephosphorylate** these proteins. The activity of the phosphatases is controlled by hormones such as insulin, which opposes the action of glucagon.
   b. Some of these hormone-receptor complexes **lower cAMP** levels, either by inhibiting adenylate cyclase or by activating the **phosphodiesterase** that cleaves cAMP to adenosine monophosphate (AMP).

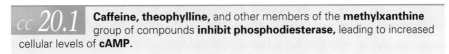

cc 20.1 **Caffeine, theophylline,** and other members of the **methylxanthine** group of compounds **inhibit phosphodiesterase,** leading to increased cellular levels of **cAMP.**

   c. At least one hormone, **atrial natriuretic peptide (ANP),** activates guanylate cyclase, which produces cyclic guanosine monophosphate (cGMP).
      (1) **cGMP** activates **protein kinase G.**
      (2) ANP is released from atrial cells of the heart and produces effects that include increased urine volume, excretion of sodium ions, and vasodilation.

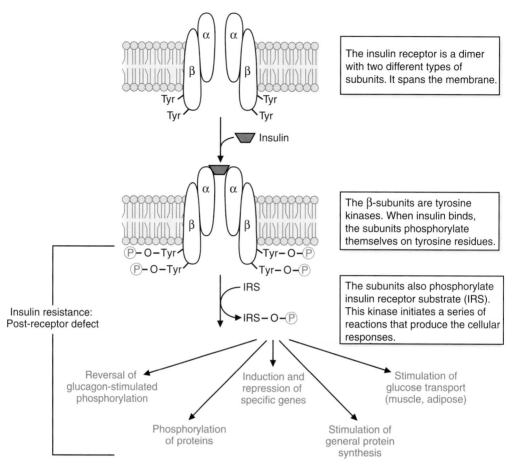

Figure 20-1 The actions of insulin. Insulin resistance or type 2 diabetes mellitus is caused by a post-receptor defect. IRS = insulin receptor substrate; P = phosphate; Tyr = tyrosine.

3. *Hormones that act through calcium (Ca^{2+}) and the phosphatidylinositol bisphosphate (PIP_2) system* (Figure 20-4)
   a. Some hormones (e.g., thyrotropin-releasing hormone [TRH] and oxytocin) interact with G proteins to alter the amount and distribution of calcium ions within the cell and activate **protein kinase C.**
   b. Hormone–G protein complexes **open calcium channels** within the cell membrane, allowing extracellular calcium to move into the cell.
   c. Some complexes **activate phospholipase C**, which cleaves PIP_2 in the cell membrane to produce two messengers, diacylglycerol (DAG) and phosphatidylinositol bisphosphate (PIP_2) (Figure 20-5).
      (1) **DAG activates protein kinase C**, which phosphorylates certain proteins, altering their activity.
      (2) **IP_3 causes Ca^{2+} to be released** from intracellular stores, such as those in the endoplasmic reticulum.
      (3) Ca^{2+}, either directly or complexed with calmodulin, interacts with proteins, altering their activity.

B. **Hormones that bind to intracellular receptors and activate genes** (Figure 20-6)

   1. **Steroid** and **thyroid** hormones, 1,25-dihydroxycholecalciferol (**1,25-DHC**), and **retinoic acid** cross the cell membrane and bind to **intracellular receptors.**

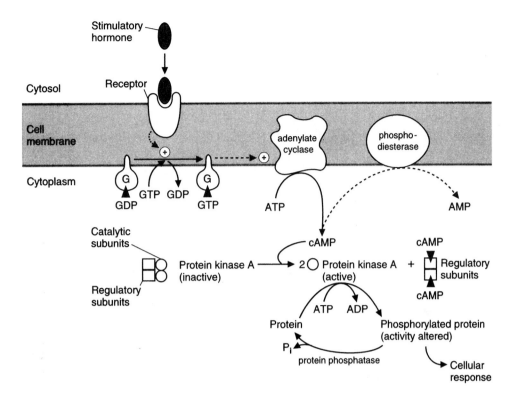

Figure 20-2   The production and action of cyclic adenosine monophosphate (cAMP). G = G proteins (G proteins function when guanosine triphosphate [GTP] is bound); O = free catalytic subunits; ⊟ = regulatory subunits of protein kinase A; ⊕ = stimulates; GDP = guanosine diphosphate.

> *cc* **20.2**   **Androgen insensitivity syndrome** (formerly know as testicular feminization) results in **mutations in the steroid receptor for androgens.**
> This disorder is an **X-linked disease** resulting in the lack of masculinization of genitalia of chromosomally male individuals, giving them the **phenotypic appearance of females.**

2. **Intracellular receptors** contain domains that bind the hormone and domains that bind to **regulatory elements** (i.e., hormone response elements [HRE]) **on DNA** that stimulate or inhibit the synthesis of mRNA (see Figure 20-6). Translation of this messenger RNA (mRNA) produces **proteins** that are responsible for the physiologic effects of the hormone.

II.   Regulation of Hormone Levels

A.   Regulation of hormone synthesis and secretion

1. The **release of hormones** is stimulated either by changes in the environment or physiologic state or by a stimulatory hormone from another tissue that acts on the cells that release the hormone. For example:
   a. A **decrease** in **blood pressure** initiates a sequence of events that ultimately causes the adrenal gland to release **aldosterone.**
   b. In response to **stress**, the hypothalamus releases corticotropin-releasing hormone **(CRH)**, which stimulates the anterior pituitary to release **adrenocorticotropic**

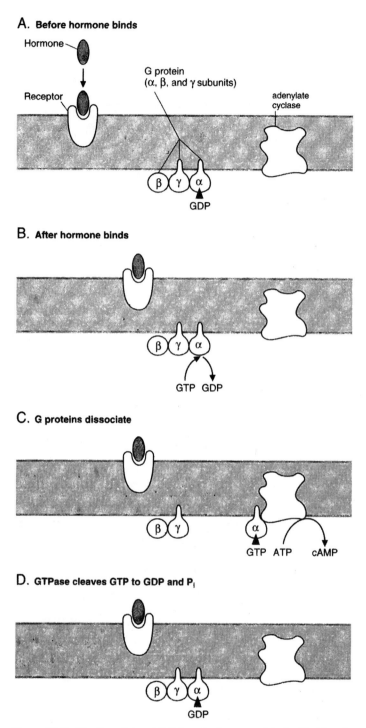

Figure 20-3 The G proteins. **(A)** Before the hormone binds. **(B)** After the hormone binds. Guanosine diphosphate (GDP) on the α subunit of the G proteins is exchanged for guanosine triphosphate (GTP). **(C)** G protein subunits dissociate. The α subunit with GTP activates adenylate cyclase, which converts adenosine triphosphate (ATP) to cyclic adenosine monophosphate (cAMP) **(D)** GTPase cleaves GTP to GDP and inorganic phosphate (P_i); α, β, and γ subunits of the G proteins reassociate. Adenylate cyclase is no longer active.

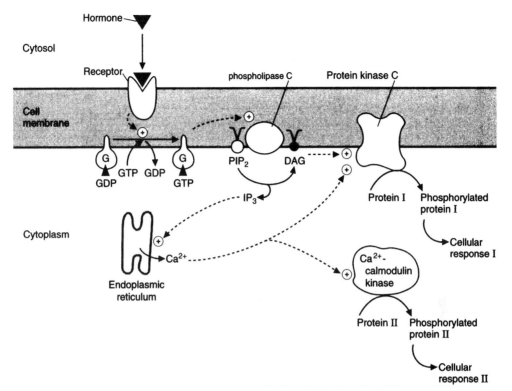

Figure 20-4 Signal transduction involving calcium (Ca^{2+}) and the phosphatidylinositol bisphosphate (PIP_2) system. DAG = diacylglycerol; IP_3 = inositol 1,4,5-trisphosphate; G = G proteins; $\oplus$ = stimulates.

hormone (ACTH). ACTH stimulates the adrenal gland to release **cortisol** (Figure 20-7).

> *cc 20.3* **Cosyntropin test** is used to evaluate **the hypothalamic, pituitary, adrenal (HPA) axis.** Cosyntropin, a synthetic form of ACTH, is administered, and serum cortisol levels are measured at 30 and 60 minutes. Abnormal results suggest **adrenal insufficiency,** requiring the administration of **exogenous corticosteroids.**

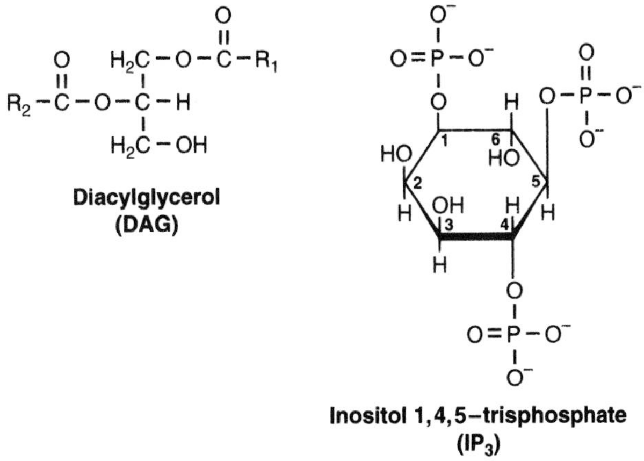

Diacylglycerol (DAG)

Inositol 1,4,5–trisphosphate (IP₃)

Figure 20-5 Structures of diacylglycerol and inositol triphosphate.

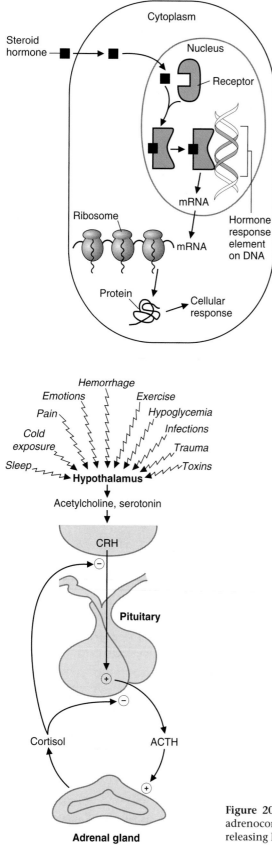

Cytoplasm

Steroid hormone

Nucleus

Receptor

mRNA

Ribosome

mRNA

Hormone response element on DNA

Protein

Cellular response

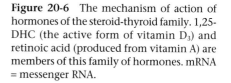

Figure 20-6 The mechanism of action of hormones of the steroid-thyroid family. 1,25-DHC (the active form of vitamin D_3) and retinoic acid (produced from vitamin A) are members of this family of hormones. mRNA = messenger RNA.

Hemorrhage

Emotions Exercise

Pain Hypoglycemia

Cold exposure Infections

Trauma

Sleep Toxins

Hypothalamus

Acetylcholine, serotonin

CRH

Pituitary

Cortisol ACTH

Adrenal gland

Figure 20-7 Hormone feedback regulation. ACTH = adrenocorticotropic hormone; CRH = corticotropin-releasing hormone; $\oplus$ = activates; $\ominus$ = inhibits.

2. The physiologic effect of the hormone or the hormone itself causes a **decrease in the signal** that initially promoted the synthesis and release of the hormone. For example:

   a. **Aldosterone** causes an increased resorption from the kidney tubule of sodium (Na^+) and, consequently, of water, increasing blood pressure.

   b. **Cortisol** feeds back on the hypothalamus and the anterior pituitary, inhibiting the release of CRH and ACTH (see Figure 20-7).

B. Hormone inactivation

   1. After hormones exert their physiologic effects, they are inactivated and excreted or degraded.

   2. Some hormones are converted to compounds that are no longer active and may be readily **excreted** from the body. For example, cortisol, a steroid hormone, is reduced and conjugated with glucuronide or sulfate and excreted in the urine and the feces.

   3. Some hormones, particularly the polypeptides, are taken up by cells via the process of endocytosis and subsequently **degraded by lysosomal enzymes.**

   4. The **receptor**, which is internalized along with the hormone, can either be **degraded** by lysosomal proteases or be **recycled** to the cell membrane.

III. Actions of Specific Hormones

A. **Hypothalamic hormones** (Figure 20-8)

   1. The hypothalamus produces **vasopressin (VP)** and **oxytocin.**

   2. **It also** produces **other hormones** (mainly peptides and polypeptides) that regulate the synthesis and release of hormones from the anterior pituitary.

B. **Hormones of the posterior pituitary** (see Figure 20-8, *top*)

   1. **VP** (also called antidiuretic hormone [ADH]) and **oxytocin** are synthesized in the hypothalamus and travel through nerve axons to the posterior pituitary where they are stored, each complexed with a neurophysin. They are released into the blood in response to the appropriate stimulation.

   2. **VP**, in response to decreased blood volume or increased Na^+ concentration, **stimulates** the **resorption of water** by kidney tubules.

   > *cc 20.4* Overproduction of ADH results in the **syndrome of inappropriate ADH (SIADH).** SIADH manifests with dilutional **hyponatremia, reduced serum osmolarity,** and an inability to dilute the urine. It can be caused by **trauma to the head** or, more likely, from the **ectopic** production of ADH by **lung tumors.**

   3. **Oxytocin promotes** the **ejection of milk** from the mammary gland in response to suckling and the **contraction of the uterus** during childbirth.

C. **Hormones of the anterior pituitary** (see Figure 20-8)

   1. **Prolactin (PRL)**, released in response to prolactin-releasing hormone (PRH) from the hypothalamus caused by suckling of an infant, stimulates the **synthesis of milk proteins** during lactation. Dopamine from the hypothalamus inhibits PRL release.

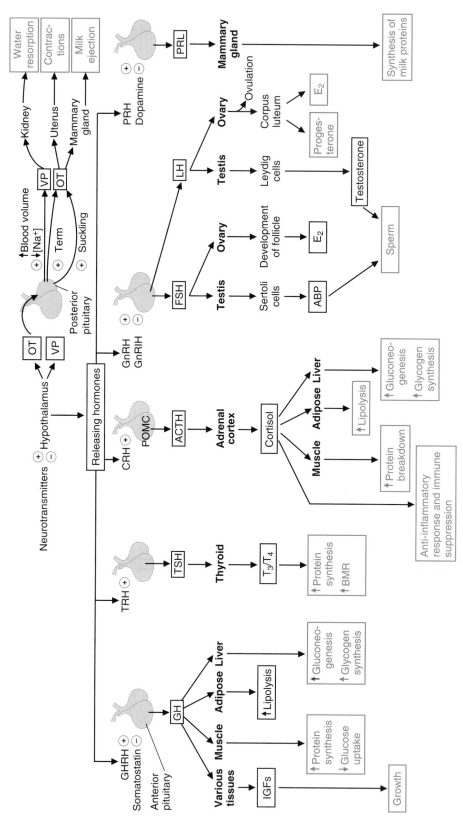

Figure 20-8 The actions of hypothalamic and pituitary hormones on their target cells. BMR = basal metabolic rate. See Table 8-1 for hormone abbreviations.

TABLE 20-1	*Abbreviations for Hormones and Related Compounds*
Abbreviation	**Definition**
ACTH	Adrenocorticotropic hormone
ABP	Androgen binding protein
ADH	Antidiuretic hormone (also known as VP)
ANP	Atrial natriuretic peptide (or atriopeptin)
CRH	Corticotropin-releasing hormone
1,25-DHC	1,25-Dihydroxycholecalciferol
DHEA	Dehydroepiandrosterone
DHT	Dihydrotestosterone
E_2	Estradiol
FSH	Follicle-stimulating hormone
GH	Growth hormone
GRH	Growth hormone–releasing hormone (GHRH)
GnRH	Gonadotropin-releasing hormone
hCG	Human chorionic gonadotropin
IGF	Insulin-like growth factor
LH	Luteinizing hormone
LPH	Lipotropin
MSH	Melanocyte-stimulating hormone
OT	Oxytocin
POMC	Pro-opiomelanocortin
PRH	Prolactin-releasing hormone
PRIH	Prolactin release–inhibiting hormone (PIH)
PRL	Prolactin
PTH	Parathyroid hormone
T_3	Triiodothyronine
T_4	Thyroxine (tetraiodothyronine)
TRH	Thyrotropin-releasing hormone
TSH	Thyroid-stimulating hormone
VP	Vasopressin (also known as ADH)

cc 20.5 The **most common tumor of the pituitary is a prolactinoma.** Patients present with **double vision,** due to compression of the optic chiasm, as well as **amenorrhea** and **galactorrhea.** Hyperprolactinemia can also result from **drugs that inhibit dopamine's action,** including some of the **antipsychotic medications** used for schizophrenia.

2. **Growth hormone (GH)** stimulates the **release of insulin-like growth factors** (IGFs) and **antagonizes** the **effects of insulin on carbohydrate and fat metabolism.** The release of GH is stimulated by growth hormone–releasing hormone (GHRH) and inhibited by somatostatin from the hypothalamus.

3. **Thyroid-stimulating hormone (TSH),** which is produced in response to TRH from the hypothalamus, **stimulates** the release of triiodothyronine (T_3) and tetraiodothyronine (T_4) from the thyroid gland.

cc 20.6 TSH is used to screen patients for thyroid disease. **Elevated levels of TSH** suggest low levels of thyroid hormone, i.e., **hypothyroidism,** whereas **low levels** suggest increased thyroid, i.e., **hyperthyroidism.**

4. **Luteinizing hormone (LH)** and follicle-stimulating hormone (**FSH**) **stimulate** the **gonads** to release hormones that are involved in reproduction. The release of LH

and FSH is stimulated by gonadotropin-releasing hormone (GnRH) and inhibited by GnRIH from the hypothalamus.

5. The protein product of the **pro-opiomelanocortin (POMC)** gene, produced in response to CRH from the hypothalamus, is cleaved to generate a number of polypeptides.

   a. **ACTH** stimulates the production of cortisol and has a permissive effect on the production of aldosterone by the adrenal cortex.

   b. **Lipotropin (LPH)** may be cleaved to form melanocyte-stimulating hormone and endorphins.

   c. **Melanocyte-stimulating hormone (MSH)**, which is part of ACTH and LPH, stimulates the production of the pigment melanin by the melanocytes in the skin.

   d. **Endorphins** produce analgesic effects.

> **cc 20.7**   **Opioids** are pharmacologic agents that mimic the effects of endogenous endorphins. Several opioid derivatives, such as **morphine,** are used for **pain control;** however, they have significant **addictive potential.**

D. Thyroid hormone

1. T_3 is much more active metabolically than T_4.

   a. Although the thyroid secretes some T_3, the majority is produced by **deiodination of T_4**, a process that occurs in nonthyroidal tissue.

   b. During starvation, T_4 is converted to reverse T_3 (rT_3), which is not active.

2. **Thyroid hormone** binds to nuclear receptors and **regulates the expression of many genes.**

3. Thyroid hormone is necessary for **growth, development**, and **maintenance** of almost all tissues of the body. It **stimulates** oxidative metabolism and causes the **basal metabolic rate (BMR)** to increase.

> **cc 20.8**   In patients with hypothyroidism, the stimulatory effect of thyroid hormone on the oxidation of fuels is diminished. As a consequence, the generation of ATP is reduced, causing a sense of **weakness, fatigue,** and **hypokinesis.** The **reduced BMR** is associated with diminished heat production, causing **cold intolerance** and **decreased sweating.** With less demand for the delivery of fuels and oxygen to peripheral tissues, the circulation is slowed, causing a reduction in heart rate and, when far advanced, a reduction in blood pressure.

> **cc 20.9**   When the thyroid gland secretes excessive quantities of thyroid hormone, the rate of oxidation of fuels by muscle and other tissues is increased (i.e., the **BMR** is **increased**). With enhanced oxidative metabolism, heat production is increased, leading to a sense of **heat intolerance** and the need to dissipate heat through **increased sweating.** Thyroid hormone excess raises the tone of the sympathetic (adrenergic) nervous system, **raising the heart rate** and **systolic blood pressure.** In addition, **tremulousness,** a sense of **restlessness,** and **insomnia** often occur. Since stored fuels in muscle and fat tissue are being used at an excessive rate, **weight loss** occurs despite increased caloric intake.

E. Hormones that stimulate growth

1. **Insulin** and **GH** stimulate growth and promote protein synthesis.

2. However, **GH antagonizes** many of the metabolic actions of **insulin**, stimulating gluconeogenesis and promoting lipolysis. The result is that alternative fuels are made available so that muscle protein (i.e., growth) can be preserved.

> ### cc 20.10
> Excessive secretion of GH occurs as a result of a **benign tumor** of the **anterior pituitary gland.** If the hypersecretion begins prior to closure of the growth centers in the long bones, excessive height (**gigantism**) occurs. If hypersecretion begins after the growth centers have closed, the bones grow in bulk and width, leading to a condition called **acromegaly.** Soft tissue overgrowth occurs as well, leading to **organomegaly, thickness of the skin,** and **coarseness of the facial features.**

F. **Hormones that mediate the response to stress**

1. **Glucocorticoids** (particularly cortisol) and **epinephrine** act in concert to supply fuels to the blood so that energy can be produced to combat stressful situations.
2. *Glucocorticoids* (Figure 20-9)
   a. In response to ACTH, the adrenal cortex produces glucocorticoids. **Cortisol** is the major glucocorticoid in humans.
   b. Glucocorticoids have **anti-inflammatory effects.** They induce the synthesis of **lipocortin,** a protein that inhibits phospholipase A_2, the rate-limiting enzyme in prostaglandin, thromboxane, and leukotriene synthesis (see Figure 6-18).
   c. Glucocorticoids **suppress the immune response** by causing the lysis of lymphocytes.
   d. Glucocorticoids **influence metabolism** by causing the movement of fuels from peripheral tissues to the liver, where gluconeogenesis and glycogen synthesis are stimulated (see Figures 20-8 and 20-9).
      (1) **Amino acids** are released from muscle protein.
      (2) **Lipolysis** occurs in adipose tissue.

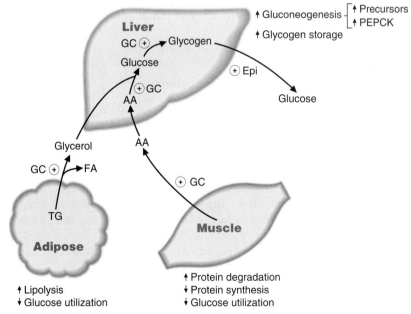

Figure 20-9   The effects of glucocorticoids (GC) on fuel metabolism. Chronic stress causes GC to stimulate the breakdown of fuels in peripheral tissues, and gluconeogenic precursors are converted to glycogen in the liver. Acute stress causes the release of epinephrine (Epi), which stimulates the breakdown of liver glycogen to produce blood glucose as fuel for "fight or flight." Epinephrine also stimulates glycogen breakdown in muscle to produce adenosine triphosphate (ATP) for muscle contraction, and it stimulates lipolysis in adipose tissue and gluconeogenesis in the liver. PEPCK = phosphoenolpyruvate carboxykinase; AA = amino acid; FA = fatty acid.

(3) In addition to providing amino acids and glycerol as carbon sources, **glucocorticoids promote gluconeogenesis** by **inducing** synthesis of the enzyme phosphoenolpyruvate carboxykinase (**PEPCK**).

(4) **Glucose**, which is produced by gluconeogenesis promoted by glucocorticoids, is **stored as glycogen** in the liver.

(5) Glucocorticoids prepare the body during stressful conditions so that fuel stores are ready for the "alarm" reaction mediated by epinephrine.

> *cc* **20.11** **Hypercortisolemia** has an adverse effect on virtually every tissue of the body. Central nervous system effects range from **hyperirritability** to **depression.** The catabolic effect on protein-containing tissues leads to a reduction in the ground substance of bone and, eventually, to **osteoporosis;** loss of muscle protein, which causes **weakness;** and thinning and tearing of dermal and epidermal structures, which is manifest as reddish stripes, or **striae,** over the lower abdomen. Increased vascular fragility also results with **easy bruising.** A suppressive effect on immunocompetence may increase the likelihood of infection. The diabetogenic actions of cortisol may lead to **glucose intolerance** or overt **diabetes mellitus.** A peculiar tendency for the disposition of fat in the face (**moon facies**), posterior neck (**buffalo hump**), thorax, and abdomen, while sparing the distal extremities, causes a distinct **"central obesity."** This constellation of clinical signs and symptoms resulting from chronic hypercortisolemia is referred to as **Cushing syndrome** if the condition is caused by excessive production of **cortisol** by an **adrenal tumor** or by intake of **exogenous glucocorticoids. Cushing disease** refers to hypercortisolemia caused by excessive secretion of **ACTH** by a **pituitary tumor.**

3. *Epinephrine*
   a. Epinephrine increases blood glucose by **stimulating liver glycogenolysis** (see Figure 20-9).
   b. It also **stimulates lipolysis** in adipose tissue and **glycogen degradation in muscle.**
   c. Overall, it makes fuels available for "fight or flight."

G. **Hormones that regulate salt and water balance**

1. In addition to **VP** and **ANP, aldosterone** is involved in regulating salt and water balance.

2. *Synthesis of aldosterone*
   a. **Renin** (produced by the juxtaglomerular cells of the kidney in response to decreased blood pressure, blood volume, or sodium ion concentration) **cleaves angiotensinogen to angiotensin I.**
   b. **Angiotensin I** is **cleaved** to **angiotensin II** by angiotensin converting enzyme (**ACE**), which is made in the lung. Further cleavage to angiotensin III occurs.
   c. **Angiotensin II** acts directly on vascular smooth muscle cells, causing **vasoconstriction,** which increases blood pressure.

> *cc* **20.12** **Angiotensin receptor blockers** (ARBs), such as **losartan,** are used in the management of **hypertension.** They block the effects of angiotensin II, resulting in **vasodilation** and subsequent decreased blood pressure.

   d. **Angiotensin II and III** (and also decreased serum sodium [Na^+] and increased serum potassium [K^+]) **stimulate** the glomerulosa cells of the adrenal cortex to produce and secrete **aldosterone.**

    e. ACTH has a permissive effect (i.e., it maintains cells so that they can respond to angiotensin II).

   3. *Action of aldosterone*

    a. Aldosterone causes the production of proteins in cells of the distal tubule and the collecting ducts of the kidney.

      (1) A **permease** is **produced** that allows Na^+ to enter cells from the lumen.

      (2) **Citrate synthase** is **induced**, which increases the capacity of the tricarboxylic acid (TCA) cycle for the generation of ATP.

      (3) Energy is thus provided to drive the **Na^+-K^+ ATPase pump**, which may also be induced.

    b. Overall, K^+ and hydrogen ions (H^+) are lost; Na^+ is retained; water is resorbed; and blood volume and pressure are increased.

---

cc 20.13 **Primary hyperaldosteronism** is most often the result of an aldosterone secreting tumor of one of the adrenal glands (**Conn syndrome**). This disorder manifests with sodium retention and potassium secretion, with **resultant hypertension** and **hypokalemia.**

---

cc 20.14 A deficiency of adrenocortical secretion of aldosterone is usually accompanied by a reduction in the secretion of other adrenal steroid hormones as well. The loss of adrenocortical steroids is known as **Addison disease.** The mineralocorticoid deficiency leads to a net loss of sodium ions and water in the urine with a reciprocal retention of potassium ions (**hyperkalemia**) and hydrogen ions (**mild metabolic acidosis**). The subsequent contraction of the effective plasma volume may lead to a **reduction in blood pressure.** If volume loss is profound, perfusion of vital tissues, such as the brain, could lead to lightheadedness and possibly loss of consciousness.

  H. **Hormones that control reproduction** (see Figure 20-8, *right*)

   1. The hypothalamus produces **GnRH**, which causes the anterior pituitary to release **FSH** and **LH**, which act on both the **ovary** and the **testis.**

   2. *The action of FSH and LH on the ovary*

    a. **The menstrual cycle**

      (1) Initially, **FSH acts on** the **follicles** to promote maturation of the ovum and to stimulate estradiol (E_2) production and secretion.

      (2) **Estradiol acts on** the uterine **endometrium**, causing it to thicken and vascularize in preparation for implantation of a fertilized egg.

      (3) A **surge of LH** at the midpoint of the menstrual cycle **stimulates** the ripe **follicle to ovulate**, leaving the residual follicle, which forms the **corpus luteum** and **secretes** both **progesterone and estradiol.**

      (4) **Progesterone** causes the endometrium to continue to thicken and vascularize and increase its secretory capacity.

    b. **Events in the absence of fertilization**

      (1) The **corpus luteum regresses** due to declining LH levels. It produces diminishing amounts of progesterone and estradiol.

      (2) Because of the low steroid hormone levels, the cells die, and the degenerating **endometrium is sloughed** into the uterine cavity and excreted (**menstruation**).

      (3) The low levels of estradiol and progesterone cause feedback inhibition to be relieved, and the hypothalamus releases GnRH, initiating a new menstrual cycle.

> *cc 20.15* Combination **oral contraceptive pills** (OCPs) contain **low levels of estrogen and progestin** derivatives, which **reduce both LH and FSH** levels. Decreased levels of these pituitary hormones destroy the **normal cyclicity** of hormones and result in a **failure to ovulate,** thus preventing conception.

c. Events following fertilization

(1) The **corpus luteum is maintained** initially by **human chorionic gonadotropin (hCG)** produced by the cells of the developing embryo (trophoblast).

> *cc 20.16* Over-the-counter **pregnancy tests** detect the presence **of hCG in the urine.** Serum quantitation of hCG levels can be used to differentiate a normal intrauterine pregnancy from an ectopic pregnancy.

(2) Subsequently, the **placenta produces hCG and progesterone.**
(3) After the corpus luteum dies, the **placenta** continues to produce large amounts of **progesterone.**
(4) Near **term,** hCG and, subsequently, **progesterone levels fall.** Fetal cortisol may cause the decline in progesterone.
(5) **Prostaglandin $F_{2\alpha}$ ($PGF_{2\alpha}$)** and **oxytocin** (released from both maternal and fetal pituitaries) stimulate uterine contractions, and the infant is delivered.

> *cc 20.17* **Pitocin** is a synthetic form of **oxytocin** that can be **administered during labor** to **initiate contractions** or augment labor in the event of failure of the normal progression of labor.

3. The action of FSH and LH on the testis

a. **LH stimulates Leydig cells** to produce and secrete testosterone.
b. **FSH** acts on **Sertoli cells** of the seminiferous tubule to promote the synthesis of androgen-binding protein **(ABP).**
c. **ABP binds testosterone** and transports it to the site of spermatogenesis, where **testosterone is converted by 5-α reductase** to the more potent androgen, dihydrotestosterone **(DHT).**

> *cc 20.18* **5-α reductase** is required for **normal male development,** and genetic deficiency of this enzyme results in a **phenotype similar to androgen insensitivity syndrome.** In addition, pharmacologic agents that inhibit this enzyme (i.e., **finasteride**) are used to inhibit some of the effects of DHT in normal men, including **male pattern baldness** and **benign prostatic hyperplasia** (BPH).

d. **Testosterone** plays a role in **spermatogenesis** in the adult male.
(1) Testosterone is responsible for **masculinization** during early development.
(2) At puberty, testosterone promotes **sexual maturation** of the male.

I. Hormones that promote lactation (see Figure 20-8, *far right*)

1. Many hormones are necessary for development of the mammary glands during adolescence.
2. *Preparation of the mammary gland for lactation*
   a. During pregnancy, **prolactin, glucocorticoids, and insulin** are the major hormones responsible for differentiation of mammary alveolar cells into secretory cells capable of producing milk.

      b. PRL stimulates the **synthesis of the milk proteins,** particularly casein and α-lactalbumin.

         (1) **α-Lactalbumin,** the major protein in human milk, serves as a **nutrient.**

         (2) α-Lactalbumin binds to galactosyl transferase, decreasing its K_m for glucose and, thus, **stimulating synthesis** of the milk sugar **lactose.**

      c. Progesterone inhibits milk protein production and secretion during pregnancy.

      d. At term, when progesterone levels fall, the inhibition of milk protein synthesis is relieved.

   3. *Regulation of milk secretion during lactation*

      a. PRL causes milk proteins to be produced and secreted into the alveolar lumen.

      b. Oxytocin causes contraction of the myoepithelial cells surrounding the alveolar cells and the lumen, and **milk is ejected** through the nipple.

      c. The **secretion** of both PRL and oxytocin by the pituitary is stimulated by **suckling** of the infant and by other factors.

J. Hormones involved in growth and differentiation

   1. Retinoids are produced in the body from dietary **vitamin A.** The major dietary source, β-carotene, is cleaved to 2 molecules of retinal.

   2. Retinal (an aldehyde) and **retinol** (an alcohol) are interconverted by oxidation and reduction reactions. **Retinoic acid** is produced by oxidation of retinal and cannot be reduced.

   3. Retinol, the **transport** form, is stored as retinyl esters.

   4. Retinal is a functional component of the reactions of the **visual cycle.**

   5. Retinoic acid is involved in **growth** and also in **differentiation** and **maintenance** of **epithelial tissue.** The functions of **retinoic acid** result from its ability to **activate genes** (i.e., it acts like a steroid hormone).

> *cc 20.19* **Synthetic retinoids** are used in the treatment of **severe acne;** however, they are not to be used in pregnant women due to their **teratogenic effects** on the developing fetus. Exposure to these compounds during development results in central nervous system, **cardiac,** and **craniofacial defects.**

K. Hormones that regulate Ca^{2+} metabolism

   1. Calcium has many important functions. It is involved in blood coagulation, activation of muscle phosphorylase, and secretory processes. It combines with phosphate to form the hydroxyapatite of bone. Parathyroid hormone (**PTH**), **1,25-DHC,** and **calcitonin** are the major regulators of Ca^{2+} metabolism.

   2. PTH, produced in response to low calcium levels, acts to **increase Ca^{2+}** levels in the extracellular fluid.

      a. PTH promotes Ca^{2+} and phosphate mobilization from **bone.**

      b. PTH acts on **renal tubules** to resorb Ca^{2+} and excrete phosphate.

      c. PTH stimulates the **hydroxylation of 25-hydroxycholecalciferol** to form **1,25-DHC,** the active hormone.

> *cc 20.20* Hyperparathyroidism can either be the result of a **tumor of the parathyroid** gland (**primary hyperparathyroidism**) or **renal failure** (**secondary hyperparathyroidism**). Patients can present with **fractures of long bones,** renal **stones,** gastrointestinal disturbance (**groins**), lethargy (**moans**), and weakness.

> *cc 20.21* **Hypoparathyroidism** is most often the result of **trauma** to the parathyroids during **surgical excision of the thyroid.** Patients complain of **neuromuscular excitability** and lethargy.

3. **1,25-DHC** stimulates the synthesis of a protein involved in **Ca²⁺ absorption** by **intestinal** epithelial cells. 1,25-DHC acts synergistically with PTH in **bone resorption** and promotes resorption of Ca^{2+} by **renal tubular cells.**
4. **Calcitonin lowers Ca^{2+}** levels by inhibiting its release from bone and stimulating its excretion in the urine.

L. **Hormones that regulate the utilization of nutrients**

1. *Gut hormones*
   a. **Gastrin** from the gastric antrum and the duodenum stimulates gastric acid and pepsin secretion.

> *cc 20.22* **Gastrinomas,** which are gastrin-secreting endocrine tumors, are associated with **Zollinger-Ellison syndrome.** Hypergastrinemia results in increased hydrochloric acid (HCL) production with resultant **recurrent peptic ulcers.**

   b. **Cholecystokinin (CCK)** from the duodenum and jejunum stimulates contraction of the gallbladder and the secretion of pancreatic enzymes.
   c. **Secretin** from the duodenum and jejunum stimulates the secretion of bicarbonate by the pancreas.
   d. **Gastric inhibitory polypeptide (GIP)** from the small bowel enhances insulin release and inhibits secretion of gastric acid.
   e. **Vasoactive intestinal polypeptide (VIP)** from the pancreas relaxes smooth muscles and stimulates bicarbonate secretion by the pancreas.

> *cc 20.23* **VIPomas** are rare tumors that secrete vasoactive intestinal peptide. This condition is associated with **watery diarrhea, hypokalemia,** and **achlorhydria.**

2. *Insulin and glucagon*
   a. The two major hormones that **regulate fuel metabolism**, insulin and glucagon, are produced by the pancreas.
   b. Their actions are summarized in Table 20-2.

TABLE 20-2	*Actions of Insulin and Glucagon*
Insulin	**Glucagon**
Elevated in the fed state	Elevated during fasting
Promotes the storage of fuels: glycogen and triacylglycerol	Increases the availability of fuels (glucose and fatty acids) in the blood
Stimulates:	*Stimulates:*
Glycogen synthesis in liver and muscle	Glycogen degradation in liver, but *not* in muscle
Triacylglycerol synthesis in liver and conversion to very low–density lipoprotein (VLDL)	Gluconeogenesis
Triacylglycerol storage in adipose tissue	Lipolysis (breakdown of triacylglycerols) in adipose tissue
Glucose transport into muscle and adipose cells	
Protein synthesis and growth	

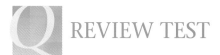

REVIEW TEST

Directions: *Each of the numbered questions or incomplete statements in this section is followed by answers or by completions of the statement. Select the **one** lettered answer or completion that is **best** in each case.*

1. Which of the following statements best describes testosterone?

(A) It is converted to a more active androgen in its target cells.
(B) It acts by binding to receptors on the cell surface.
(C) It is produced from estradiol (E_2).
(D) It stimulates the synthesis of gonadotropin-releasing hormone (GnRH) by the hypothalamus.

2. Which of the following acts to increase the release of Ca^{2+} from the endoplasmic reticulum?

(A) Diacylglycerol (DAG)
(B) Inositol triphosphate (IP_3)
(C) Parathyroid hormone (PTH)
(D) 1,25-Dihydroxycholecalciferol (1,25-DHC)

3. A dietary deficiency of iodine would do which of the following?

(A) Directly affect the synthesis of thyroglobulin on ribosomes
(B) Result in increased secretion of thyroid-stimulating hormone (TSH)
(C) Result in decreased production of thyrotropin-releasing hormone (TRH)
(D) Result in increased heat production

4. GnRH stimulates the release of which of following?

(A) Growth hormone (GH)
(B) Triiodothyronine (T_3) and tetraiodothyronine (T_4)
(C) Prolactin (PRL)
(D) Insulin-like growth factor (IGF)
(E) Luteinizing hormone (LH) and follicle-stimulating hormone (FSH)

5. Which of the following pituitary hormones will **increase** if communication from the hypothalamus is severed?

(A) GH
(B) TSH

(C) PRL
(D) Vasopressin
(E) Cortisol

6. The release of which of the following is inhibited by thyroxine?

(A) LH
(B) PRL
(C) TSH
(D) GH
(E) FSH

7. Which of the following binds to receptors on Leydig cells?

(A) LH
(B) PRL
(C) TSH
(D) GH
(E) FSH

8. Which of the following stimulates production of IGF?

(A) LH
(B) PRL
(C) TSH
(D) GH
(E) FSH

9. Which of the following stimulates the synthesis of milk proteins?

(A) LH
(B) PRL
(C) TSH
(D) GH
(E) FSH

10. Which of the following stimulates the production of progesterone by the corpus luteum?

(A) LH
(B) PRL
(C) TSH
(D) GH
(E) FSH

11. Which of the following stimulates the production of estradiol by the immature ovarian follicle?

(A) LH
(B) PRL
(C) TSH
(D) GH
(E) FSH

12. Action is mediated by a second messenger for which of these steroid hormones?

(A) Cortisol
(B) Aldosterone
(C) Both cortisol and aldosterone
(D) Neither cortisol nor aldosterone

13. Which of the following steroid hormones is synthesized from cholesterol by cells of the adrenal cortex?

(A) Cortisol
(B) Aldosterone
(C) Both cortisol and aldosterone
(D) Neither cortisol nor aldosterone

14. Which of the following steroid hormones has receptors with a DNA binding domain?

(A) Cortisol
(B) Aldosterone
(C) Both cortisol and aldosterone
(D) Neither cortisol nor aldosterone

15. Which of the following steroid hormones is associated with induction of phosphoenolpyruvate carboxykinase (PEPCK)?

(A) Cortisol
(B) Aldosterone
(C) Both cortisol and aldosterone
(D) Neither cortisol nor aldosterone

16. Which of the following steroid hormones is secreted in response to angiotensin II?

(A) Cortisol
(B) Aldosterone
(C) Both cortisol and aldosterone
(D) Neither cortisol nor aldosterone

17. Which of the following hormones is produced by the anterior pituitary?

(A) Oxytocin
(B) Vasopressin
(C) Both oxytocin and vasopressin
(D) Neither oxytocin nor vasopressin

18. Which of the following hormones is associated with neurophysin in secretory granules?

(A) Oxytocin
(B) Vasopressin
(C) Both oxytocin and vasopressin
(D) Neither oxytocin nor vasopressin

19. Which of the following hormones is associated with diuresis?

(A) Oxytocin
(B) Vasopressin
(C) Both oxytocin and vasopressin
(D) Neither oxytocin nor vasopressin

20. Which of the following hormones is produced from the pro-opiomelanocortin (POMC) gene?

(A) Oxytocin
(B) Vasopressin
(C) Both oxytocin and vasopressin
(D) Neither oxytocin nor vasopressin

21. A 73-year-old woman is transferred to the intensive care unit after she is found to be in septic shock. It is believed that she originally had a urinary tract infection and that the bacteria seeded her bloodstream. The critical care fellow is concerned she may not have an adequate stress response in this situation. He orders a cosyntropin test, which evaluates the body's ability to produce which of the following hormones?

(A) Oxytocin
(B) Vasopressin
(C) Cortisol
(D) Corticotropin-releasing hormone (CRH)
(E) Adrenocorticotropic hormone (ACTH)

22. A 56-year-old woman with a 60-pack year history of smoking is recently found to have a large mass in her lungs, likely a tumor. Her basic labs demonstrate a reduce serum sodium of 127 mmol/L (normal =

135–145 mmol/L) and a reduced urine osmolality. She likely has which of the following endocrine abnormalities?

(A) Cushing disease
(B) Syndrome of inappropriate anti-diuretic hormone (SIADH)
(C) Cushing syndrome
(D) Acromegaly
(E) Prolactinoma

23. A 75-year-old woman with osteoporosis complains of back pain. A magnetic resonance imaging (MRI) scan of her back confirms a compression fracture of the L3 vertebra. The attending physician begins treating the patient with morphine for pain control. Morphine is an analgesic that works similarly to which of the following endogenously produced substance?

(A) ACTH
(B) POMC
(C) Lipotropin
(D) Melanocyte-stimulating hormone (MSH)
(E) Endorphin

24. A 13-year-old boy has developed polydipsia, polyuria, polyphagia, and weight loss over the last few weeks. His parents are concerned because he woke up this morning lethargic. He was brought to the emergency room and found to have a blood glucose of 600 mg/dL. He is immediately placed on an insulin drip. Insulin works by which of the following mechanisms?

(A) Activating adenylate cyclase
(B) Binding to an intracellular receptor
(C) Activating phospholipase C
(D) Producing cyclic guanosine monophosphate (cGMP)
(E) Causing phosphorylation of tyrosine residues

25. A 43-year-old man presents to the neurologist with headache and double vision. He also complains of a milky discharge from his breast. An MRI of his head confirms the suspected diagnosis of a prolactinoma. Which of the following substances could inhibit the release of prolactin from the pituitary?

(A) Dopamine
(B) Caffeine
(C) Endorphins
(D) Renin
(E) Prostaglandin $F_{2\alpha}$

26. A 50-year-old woman complains of feeling warm all of the time. Her eyes appear as though they are bulging out of their sockets (proptosis). She sees a family physician to evaluate her condition. Her labs demonstrate a decreased level of TSH. Which of the following would you expect in this patient?

(A) Reduced blood pressure
(B) Weight gain
(C) Increased basal metabolic rate
(D) Reduced heart rate
(E) Excess sleep

27. A 43-year-old man comes to the emergency room with a headache and blurred vision. He complains that his wedding ring no longer fits him and that his favorite hat no longer fits on his head. His wife feels that his nose has become wider. He is found to have acromegaly. Which of the following metabolic effects would you expect in this patient?

(A) Decreased protein synthesis
(B) Inhibition of gluconeogenesis
(C) Inhibition of lipolysis
(D) Increased protein synthesis
(E) Gigantism

28. A 23-year-old woman is referred from an endocrinologist for weight gain, especially around the waist. She also has striae over the abdomen and a rounded appearance to her face. She is found to have Cushing disease. Which of the following would likely be found in this patient?

(A) Increased immunity
(B) Increased protein synthesis
(C) Inhibition of lipolysis
(D) Increased gluconeogenesis
(E) Decreased liver glycogen stores

29. A 56-year-old women with no known medical conditions presents to the emergency room with pain in the upper arm. She denies any trauma; however, a fracture of the humerus is found on x-ray. She is found to have an elevated PTH level. Which of the following statements best describes PTH?

(A) It lowers serum calcium.
(B) It directly promotes the absorption of calcium from the intestine.
(C) It stimulates the conversion of vitamin D to the active form.
(D) It promotes the reabsorption of phosphate from the kidney.
(E) It promotes the excretion of calcium from the kidney.

30. A 75-year-old man complains of increased urinary frequency, especially at night. He has difficulty starting to urinate (hesitancy) and often dribbles urine when he finishes. His urologist suspects benign prostatic hyperplasia and places him on a 5-α reductase inhibitor. This would decrease which of the following?

(A) Conversion of cyclic adenosine monophosphate (cAMP) to adenosine monophosphate (AMP)
(B) Release of calcium from the endoplasmic reticulum
(C) Prostaglandin synthesis
(D) Conversion of angiotensin I to angiotensin II
(E) Conversion of testosterone to dihydrotestosterone (DHT)

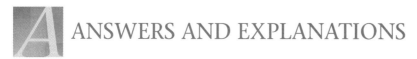

1–A. Testosterone is reduced to dihydrotestosterone (DHT), the more active hormone. Testosterone is a steroid hormone, thus it activates genes. It is a precursor of estradiol (E_2). Testosterone inhibits the synthesis of gonadotropin-releasing hormone (GnRH).

2–B. Phosphatidylinositol bisphosphate is cleaved to inositol triphosphate (IP_3) and diacylglycerol (DAG). IP_3 causes the release of Ca^{2+} from the endoplasmic reticulum, while DAG activates protein kinase C. Parathyroid hormone (PTH) stimulates the release of Ca^{2+} from bone, and 1,25-dihydroxycholecalciferol (1,25-DHC) stimulates the absorption of Ca^{2+} from the intestine.

3–B. When iodine is deficient in the diet, the thyroid does not make normal amounts of thyroid hormone. Consequently, there is less feedback inhibition of thyrotropin-releasing hormone (TRH) and thyroid-stimulating hormone (TSH) production and release. Low levels of thyroid hormone result in decreased heat production.

4–E. GnRH stimulates the release of two pituitary hormones—luteinizing hormone (LH) and follicle-stimulating hormone. Growth hormone-releasing hormone (GRH) stimulates the release of growth hormone (GH); TSH stimulates the release of triiodothyronine (T_3) and tetraiodothyronine; and prolactin-releasing hormone (PRH) stimulates the release of prolactin (PRL). Insulin-like growth factor (IGF) stimulates growth.

5–C. In contrast to what is seen with all the other pituitary hormones, the hypothalamus tonically suppresses prolactin (PRL) secretion from the pituitary. Dopamine serves as the major prolactin-inhibiting factor.

6–C. Thyroxine inhibits the release of TSH by the anterior pituitary.

7–A. LH binds to receptors on Leydig cells and stimulates the release of testosterone.

8–D. GH stimulates the release of IGF by the liver and other tissues.

9–B. PRL stimulates the synthesis of milk proteins.

10–A. LH stimulates the corpus luteum to produce progesterone.

11–E. FSH stimulates maturation of the ovarian follicle, which produces estradiol.

12–D. Steroid hormones do not act through second messengers. They enter the cell and activate genes.

13–C. Steroid hormones are synthesized from cholesterol. Cortisol and aldosterone are made in the adrenal cortex.

14–C. Steroid hormones bind to receptors, and the complexes subsequently bind to DNA, activating genes. 1,25-DHC, thyroid hormone, and retinoic acid (from vitamin A) act in the same fashion.

15–A. Glucocorticoids, such as cortisol, activate the gene for phosphoenolpyruvate carboxykinase (PEPCK).

16–B. Angiotensin II stimulates the synthesis and secretion of aldosterone.

17–D. Oxytocin and vasopressin are produced by the hypothalamus and stored in and secreted from the posterior pituitary.

18–C. Both oxytocin and vasopressin are bound to neurophysins.

19–D. Vasopressin has an antidiuretic action. Neither oxytocin nor vasopressin acts as a diuretic.

20–D. The pro-opiomelanocortin (POMC) gene product is produced by the anterior pituitary. Both oxytocin and vasopressin are produced by the posterior pituitary.

21–C. The primary stress hormone in the body is cortisol. Normally corticotropin-releasing hormone (CRH) form the hypothalamus stimulates the release of adrenocorticotropic hormone (ACTH) from the anterior pituitary. ACTH then acts on the adrenal gland to produce cortisol. Cosyntropin is a synthetic ACTH injected to stimulate the release of cortisol to evaluate an appropriate stress response. Oxytocin is involved in labor during birth and milk ejection afterwards. Vasopressin comes from the posterior pituitary and controls volume status and blood pressure.

22–B. This patient has a metabolic derangement consistent with the syndrome of inappropriate antidiuretic hormone (SIADH). This can be due to trauma to the head or, in this case, be a paraneoplastic syndrome associated with lung tumors. Cushing disease is a result of increased cortisol, which, when due to a pituitary adenoma secreting tumor, is referred to a Cushing syndrome. Acromegaly results from growth hormone excess, and a prolactinoma would cause amenorrhea and galactorrhea in a female.

23–E. Morphine and other opioids are agonists of the endogenously produced endorphins. Endorphins result from the proteolytic cleavage of pro-opiomelanocortin (POMC). The two main peptides produced from POMC include ACTH, which stimulates cortisol production, and lipotropin. Lipotropin is further processed to melanocyte-stimulating hormone (MSH) and endorphins.

24–E. Insulin binds to extracellular receptors, promoting dimerization and subsequent phosphorylation of tyrosine residues on the intracellular portion of the receptor. This triggers a cascade of signals that promote the metabolic effects of this molecule. Hormones like epinephrine bind to G protein–coupled receptors with activation of adenylate cyclase. Steroid hormones are lipid soluble and diffuse through the cell membrane, binding intracellular receptors that activate gene transcription. Parathyroid hormone mediates its effects, at least in part, by activating phospholipase C. Lastly, atrial natriuretic peptide activates guanylate cyclase, which produces cyclic guanosine monophosphate (cGMP).

25–A. Dopamine normally inhibits the release of prolactin from the anterior pituitary. When there is damage to the dopamine-producing neurons of the hypothalamus or drugs are given to inhibit dopamine, prolactin levels increase, resulting in galactorrhea. Caffeine inhibits phosphodiesterase and, therefore, the conversion of cyclic adenosine monophosphate (cAMP) to adenosine monophosphate (AMP). Endorphins are produced by proteolytic processing of POMC from the anterior pituitary. Renin is produced by the kidney and cleaves angiotensinogen to angiotensin I. Prostaglandin $F_{2\alpha}$ is important in stimulating uterine contractions during delivery.

26–C. This patient presents with signs and labs consistent with hyperthyroidism. Thyroid hormone is an important regulator of basal metabolic rate and increased levels, with subsequent decreased TSH, result in an increased metabolic rate. The other choices, including reduced blood pressure, weight gain, and excess sleep, are all seen with hypothyroidism.

27–D. Acromegaly results from a growth hormone–producing tumor of the anterior pituitary. Growth hormone (GH) is an important metabolic regulator, and its actions are often antagonistic to insulin. As such, increased GH levels results in increased protein synthesis, increased gluconeogenesis, and increased lipolysis. Gigantism results from GH excess in children, before the closing of the growth plates of bones.

28–D. Patients with Cushing disease have excess levels of cortisol. Excess of this important metabolic regulator leads to decreased protein synthesis, often resulting in easy bruisability and thinning of the skin, causing striae. Steroids inhibit the immune response and are often administered exogenously to control autoimmune diseases. Lipolysis is increased, as is gluconeogenesis. This ultimately results in increased liver glycogen stores.

29–C. This patient likely has a PTH-producing tumor of the parathyroid. PTH is an important regulator of calcium homeostasis. It stimulates the conversion of vitamin D to the active form, which, in turn, promotes the absorption of calcium from the intestine as well as reabsorption of calcium from the kidney filtrate. It functions to increase serum calcium by liberating calcium phosphate from bone, making it weaker and prone to fracture. PTH prevents accumulation of phosphate by promoting it's excretion from the kidneys.

30–E. Dihydrotestosterone (DHT) is a growth factor for prostate cells and a 5-α reductase inhibitor would decrease the conversion of testosterone to DHT, thus shrinking the prostate and reducing the patient's symptoms. Caffeine inhibits the conversion of cAMP to AMP. The signaling intermediate phosphatidylinositol bisphosphate (PIP$_2$) inhibits the release of calcium from the endoplasmic reticulum. Prostaglandin synthesis is inhibited by lipocortin. Angiotensin-converting enzyme (ACE) inhibitor, which is used in the control of blood pressure, is used to inhibit the conversion of angiotensin I to angiotensin II.

DNA Replication and Transcription

I. Nucleic Acid Structure

A. The structure of DNA

1. *Chemical components of DNA*
   a. Each polynucleotide chain of DNA contains nucleotides, which consist of a **nitrogenous base** (A, G, C, or T), **deoxyribose,** and **phosphate** (Figure 1-19).
   b. The bases are the **purines** adenine (A) and guanine (G), and the **pyrimidines** cytosine (C), and thymine (T).
   c. **Phosphodiester bonds** join the 3'-carbon of one sugar to the 5'-carbon of the next (Figure 21-1).
2. *DNA double helix*
   a. Each DNA molecule is composed of two **polynucleotide chains** joined by hydrogen bonds between the bases (Figure 21-2).
      (1) **Adenine** on one chain forms a base pair with **thymine** on the other chain.
      (2) **Guanine** base pairs with **cytosine.**
      (3) The **base sequences** of the two strands are **complementary.** Adenine on one strand is matched by thymine on the other, and guanine is matched by cytosine.
   b. The **chains are antiparallel.** One chain runs in a **5' to 3'** direction; the other chain runs **3' to 5'** (Figure 21-3).
   c. The double-stranded molecule is twisted to form a **helix** with major and minor grooves (Figure 21-4).
      (1) The **base pairs** that join the two strands are **stacked** like a spiral staircase in the interior of the molecule.
      (2) The **phosphate groups** are on the outside of the double helix. Two acidic groups of each phosphate are involved in phosphodiester bonds. The third is free and dissociates its proton at physiologic pH, giving the molecule a **negative charge** (see Figure 21-1).
      (3) The **B form of DNA,** first described by Watson and Crick, is right handed and contains **10 base pairs per turn.**
      (4) Other forms of DNA include the A form, which is similar to the B form but more compact, and the Z form, which is left handed and has its bases positioned more toward the periphery of the helix.

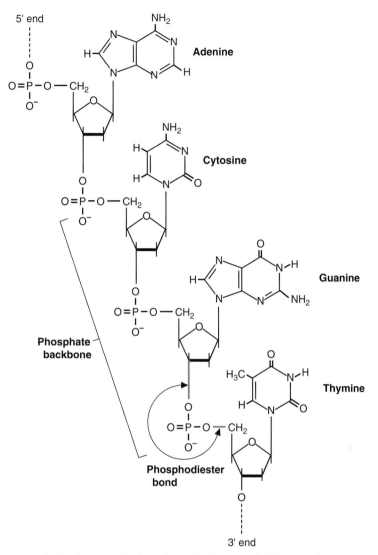

Figure 21-1   A segment of a polynucleotide strand. This strand contains thymine and deoxyribose, so it is a segment of DNA.

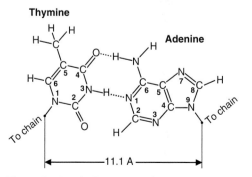

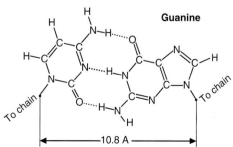

Figure 21-2   The base pairs of DNA.

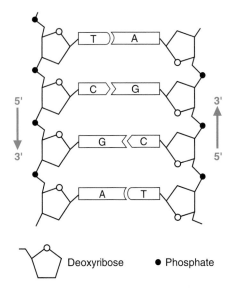

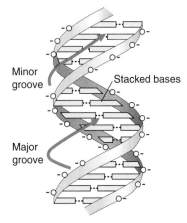

Figure 21-3 Antiparallel strands of DNA. Note that the strands run in opposite directions. A = adenosine; C = cytosine; G = guanosine; T = thymine.

3. *Denaturation, renaturation, and hybridization*
   a. **Denaturation: Alkali** or **heat** causes the **strands** of DNA to **separate** but does not break phosphodiester bonds.
   b. **Renaturation:** If strands of DNA are separated by heat and then the **temperature** is slowly **decreased** under the appropriate conditions, **base pairs reform**, and complementary strands of DNA come back together.
   c. **Hybridization:** A single strand of DNA pairs with complementary base sequences on another strand of DNA or RNA.
4. *DNA molecules are extremely large*
   a. The entire chromosome of the bacterium *Escherichia coli* is circular and contains more than 4×10^6 base pairs.
   b. The DNA molecule in the longest human chromosome is linear and is over 7.2 cm long.
5. *Packing of DNA in the nucleus*
   a. The **chromatin** of eukaryotic cells consists of DNA complexed with histones in **nucleosomes** (Figure 21-5).
      (1) **Histones** are relatively small, basic proteins with a high content of **arginine** and **lysine**. (Prokaryotes do not have histones.)

Figure 21-4 The DNA double helix.

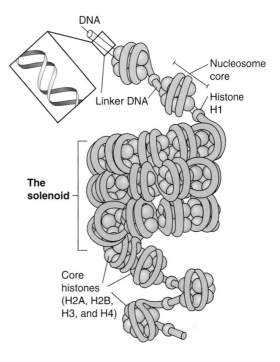

Figure 21-5 A polynucleosome. (Adapted from Olins DE, Olins AL: Nucleosomes: The structural quantum in chromosomes. *American Scientist* 66:708, 1978.)

  (2) Eight histone molecules form an octamer, around which approximately 140 base pairs of DNA are wound to form a nucleosome core.

  (3) The DNA that joins one nucleosome core to the next is complexed with histone H1.

 b. The "beads on a string" nucleosomal structure of chromatin is further compacted to form solenoid structures (helical, tubular coils).

6. *Mitochondrial DNA*

 a. The mitochondrial genome is a **double-stranded circular DNA** molecule found within the **mitochondrial matrix.**

  (1) The genetic code for the mitochondria is slightly different than that of genomic DNA.

  (2) The genome codes for 13 **protein subunits of the electron transport chain,** a large and small **ribosomal RNA (rRNA)**, and 22 **transfer RNAs (tRNAs)**.

 b. **Mitochondrial DNA is maternally inherited.**

  (1) Mitochondria from the egg contribute exclusively to the zygote.

  (2) The mitochondria autonomously reproduce, and therefore, all the mitochondria are of maternal origin.

 c. **Mitochondrial DNA has a high mutation rate** (~5–10 times greater than the nuclear genome).

> *cc 21.1* Mitochondrial DNA is used by medical anthropologists to **establish evolutionary relationships** between different species and ethnic groups.

B. **The structure of RNA**

 1. *RNA differs from DNA*

 a. The polynucleotide structure of RNA is similar to DNA except that RNA contains the sugar **ribose** rather than deoxyribose and uracil (U) rather than thymine. (A small amount of thymine is present in tRNA.)

b. RNA is generally **single stranded** (in contrast to DNA, which is double stranded).

   (1) When **strands loop back** on themselves, the bases on opposite sides can pair: adenine with uracil (A–U) and guanine with cytosine (G–C).

   (2) **RNA molecules have extensive base pairing**, which produces secondary and tertiary structures that are important for RNA function.

   (3) RNA molecules recognize DNA and other RNA molecules by base pairing.

c. Some **RNA molecules** act as **catalysts** of reactions; thus, RNA, as well as protein, can have enzymatic activity.

   (1) **Ribozymes,** usually precursors of rRNA, remove internal segments of themselves, splicing the ends together.

   (2) RNAs also act as **ribonucleases,** cleaving other RNA molecules (e.g., RNase P cleaves tRNA precursors).

   (3) **Peptidyl transferase,** an enzyme in protein synthesis, consists of RNA.

2. Messenger RNA (mRNA) contains a cap structure and a poly(A) tail.

a. The **cap** consists of methylated guanine triphosphate (GTP) attached to the hydroxyl group on the ribose at the 5′ end of the mRNA.

   (1) The N7 in the guanine is methylated.

   (2) The 2′-hydroxyl groups of the first and second ribose moieties of the mRNA also may be methylated (Figure 21-6).

---

cc **21.2** Many viruses, such as the **influenza virus,** transfer the 7-methyl G cap from host cell mRNAs to viral mRNA, which functions to increase mRNA stability and increase translation of the mRNA.

---

b. The **poly(A) tail** contains up to 200 adenine (A) nucleotides attached to the hydroxyl group at the 3′ end of the mRNA.

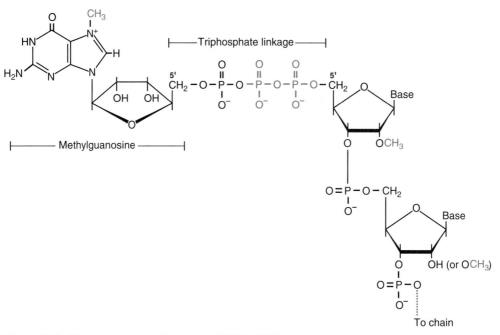

Figure 21-6   The cap structure of messenger RNA (mRNA).

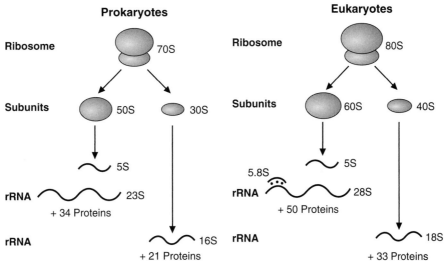

Figure 21-7   The composition of ribosomes. rRNA = ribosomal RNA; S = sedimentation coefficients.

3. **rRNA** contains many loops and extensive base pairing.
   a. rRNA molecules differ in their sedimentation coefficients (S). They associate with proteins to form **ribosomes** (Figure 21-7).
   b. **Prokaryotes** have three types of rRNA: 16S, 23S, and 5S rRNA.
   c. **Eukaryotes** have four types of cytosolic rRNA: 18S, 28S, 5S, and 5.8S rRNA. Mitochondrial ribosomes are similar to prokaryotic ribosomes.
4. **tRNA** has a cloverleaf structure and contains modified nucleotides. tRNA molecules are relatively small, containing about 80 nucleotides.
   a. In eukaryotic cells, many nucleotides in tRNA are modified. Modified nucleotides containing **pseudouridine (Ψ)**, **dihydrouridine (D)**, and **ribothymidine (T)** are present in most tRNAs (Figure 21-8).
   b. All tRNA molecules have a similar **cloverleaf structure** even though their base sequences differ (Figure 21-9).
      (1) The first loop from the 5′ end, the **D loop**, contains dihydrouridine.
      (2) The middle loop contains the **anticodon**, which base pairs with the codon in mRNA.
      (3) The third loop, the **TΨC loop**, contains both ribothymidine and pseudouridine.
      (4) The **CCA sequence** at the 3′ end carries the amino acid.

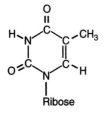

Ribothymidine (T)

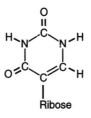

Pseudouridine (ψ)

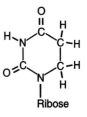

Dihydrouridine (D)

Figure 21-8   Three modified nucleosides found in most transfer RNAs (tRNAs).

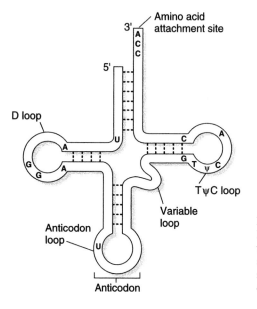

Figure 21-9 The cloverleaf structure of transfer RNA (tRNA). Bases that commonly occur in a particular position are indicated by *letters*. Base pairing in stem regions is indicated by *dashed lines* between strands. Ψ = pseudouridine, T = ribothymidine; D = dihydrouridine.

 Mutation in the **mitochondrial tRNAs** for phenylalanine, leucine, lycine, and histidine have been associated with the disorder known as **MERFF syndrome**, or **myoclonus epilepsy associated with ragged-red fibers**. These patients have myoclonic seizures of the limbs or the entire body. Impairment of the ability to coordinate movements (**ataxia**) and an abnormal accumulation of lactic acid in the blood (**lactic acidosis**) may also be present in affected individuals.

II.   Synthesis of DNA (Replication)

A.   **Mechanism of replication**

1. **Replication** is bidirectional and semiconservative (Figure 21-10).
   a. **Bidirectional** means that replication begins at a site of origin and simultaneously moves out in both directions from this point.
      (1) Prokaryotes have one site of origin on each chromosome.
      (2) Eukaryotes have multiple sites of origin on each chromosome.
   b. **Semiconservative** means that, following replication, each daughter molecule of DNA contains one intact parental strand and one newly synthesized strand joined by base pairs.
2. **Replication forks are the sites at which DNA synthesis is occurring.**
   a. The **parental strands** of DNA separate, and the helix unwinds ahead of a replication fork (Figure 21-11).
   b. **Helicases** unwind the helix, and single-strand binding proteins hold it in a single-stranded conformation.
   c. **Topoisomerases** act to prevent the extreme supercoiling of the parental helix that would result as a consequence of unwinding at a replication fork.
   d. Topoisomerases break and rejoin DNA chains.

cc 21.4 The cancer drug **etoposide (VP-16)** inhibits **topoisomerase** and is widely used in the treatment of lung, ovarian, testicular, and prostate cancer.

   e. **DNA gyrase**, a topoisomerase, is found only in prokaryotes.

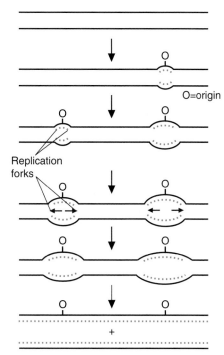

Figure 21-10 Replication of a eukaryotic chromosome. *Solid lines* are parental strands. *Dotted lines* are newly synthesized strands. Synthesis is bidirectional from each point of origin (O).

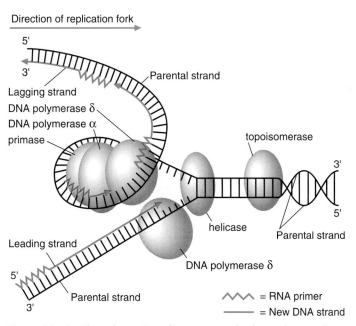

Figure 21-11 The eukaryotic replication complex located at a replication fork. The lagging strand loops around the complex. Single-strand binding proteins (not shown) are attached to the regions of single-stranded DNA.

> *cc* **21.5** **Quinolone antibiotics,** such as **ciprofloxacin,** inhibit **DNA gyrase** and are used for numerous infections including complicated **urinary tract infections** and lower respiratory tract infections.

3. **DNA polymerases catalyze the synthesis of DNA.**
   a. **Prokaryotes** have three DNA polymerases: **pol I, pol II,** and **pol III.** Pol III is the replicative enzyme, and pol I is involved in repair.
   b. **Eukaryotes** have five DNA polymerases: α, β, γ, δ, and ε.
      (1) DNA polymerase α is involved in replication of nuclear DNA.
      (2) Polymerase δ acts in conjunction with α during replication.
      (3) Polymerases β and ε are involved in repair of nuclear DNA, and γ functions in mitochondria.
   c. **DNA polymerases** can only copy a DNA template in the 3′ to 5′ direction and produce the newly synthesized strand in the 5′ to 3′ direction.
   d. **Deoxyribonucleoside triphosphates** (dATP, dGTP, dTTP, and dCTP) are the precursors for DNA synthesis.
      (1) Each precursor pairs with the corresponding base on the template strand and forms a phosphodiester bond with the hydroxyl group on the 3′-carbon of the sugar at the end of the growing chain (Figure 21-12).

> *cc* **21.6** Many of the antivirals used in the treatment of human immunodeficiency virus (HIV) are **analogs of deoxyribonucleoside triphosphates.** For instance, the drug **zidovudine (AZT, ZDV)** is an analog of thymidine, which lacks the 3′-hydroxyl for the addition of the next nucleotide, thereby inhibiting the viral DNA polymerase. **Dideoxyinosine (ddI)** and **zalcitabine (ddC)** are similar agents used to treat HIV.

      (2) Pyrophosphate is produced and cleaved to two inorganic phosphates.

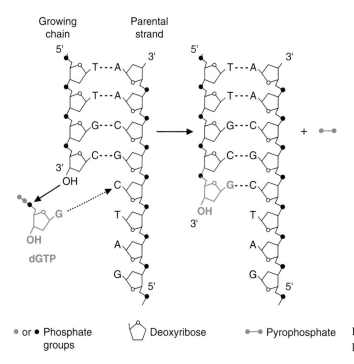

● or ● Phosphate groups   ⬠ Deoxyribose   ●—● Pyrophosphate   **Figure 21-12** The action of DNA polymerase.

4. **DNA polymerase** requires a **primer** (Figure 21-13).
   a. DNA polymerases **cannot initiate** synthesis of new strands.
   b. **RNA serves as the primer** for DNA polymerase in vivo. The RNA primer, which contains about 10 nucleotides, is formed by copying of the parental strand in a reaction catalyzed by **primase.**
   c. **DNA polymerase** adds deoxyribonucleotides to the 3'-hydroxyls of the RNA primers and subsequently to the ends of the growing DNA strands.
   d. **DNA parental (template) strands** are copied simultaneously at replication forks, although they run in opposite directions.

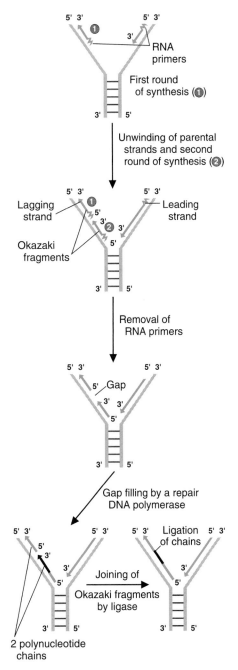

Figure 21-13 Mechanism of DNA synthesis at the replication fork. Two rounds of polymerase action are shown (❶ and ❷). The number of nucleotides added in each round is much larger than shown; in eukaryotes, about 10 ribonucleotides and 200 deoxyribonucleotides are polymerized on the lagging strand. Synthesis on the leading strand is continuous. The unshaded regions of the *arrows* indicate the nucleotides added by the repair action of a DNA polymerase.

(1) The **leading strand** is formed by continuous copying of the parental strand that runs 3' to 5' **toward** the replication fork.

(2) The **lagging strand** is formed by discontinuous copying of the parental strand that runs 3' to 5' **away from** the replication fork.

- As more of the helix is unwound, synthesis of the lagging strand begins from another primer. The short fragments formed by this process are known as **Okazaki fragments.**
- The RNA **primers are removed by nucleases** (e.g., RNase H), and then the resulting **gaps are filled** with the appropriate deoxyribonucleotides by another DNA polymerase.
- Finally, the **Okazaki fragments are joined by DNA ligase**, an enzyme that catalyzes formation of phosphodiester bonds between two polynucleotide chains.

e. In eukaryotic cells, about 200 deoxyribonucleotides are added to the lagging strand in each round of synthesis, whereas in prokaryotes, 1000 to 2000 are added.

5. The **fidelity of replication** is very high, with an overall error rate of 10^{-9} to 10^{-10}.

a. **Errors** (insertion of an inappropriate nucleotide) that occur during replication can be corrected by editing during the replication process. This proofreading function is performed by a 3' to 5' exonuclease activity associated with the polymerase complex.

b. **Post-replication repair processes** (e.g., mismatch repair) also increase the fidelity of replication.

> *cc* **21.7** Many **viruses** encode their own polymerases, which **lack the fidelity of host cell polymerases.** This makes viruses more prone to mutations that can lead to **changes in viral antigens** that allow them to **avoid the immune response.** Such changes result in the **antigenic shift** of **influenza virus,** leading to the need for route **vaccinations** in some people.

B. Mutations

1. **Changes in DNA** molecules cause mutations. After replication, these changes result in a permanent alteration of the base sequence in the daughter DNA.

2. **Changes causing mutations** include:
   a. **Uncorrected errors** made during replication
   b. **Damage** that occurs to replicating or nonreplicating DNA caused by oxidative deamination, radiation, or chemicals, resulting in cleavage of DNA strands or chemical alteration or removal of bases

3. **Types of mutations** include:
   a. **Point mutations** (substitution of one base for another)

> *cc* **21.8** α_1-**Antitrypsin deficiency** most commonly arises from a single amino acid substitution due to a **point mutation.** Patients accumulate misfolded protein in the endoplasmic reticulum of hepatocytes. Lack of this important anti-protease leads to **emphysema** and **cirrhosis.**

b. **Insertions** (addition of one or more nucleotides within a DNA sequence)

> *cc* **21.9** **Huntington disease** results from the addition of **multiple CAG repeats** within the huntington protein, leading to large stretches of glutamine **(polyglutamine repeats)** within the protein. Aggregation of this protein in neuronal tissue leads to **atrophy of the caudate** nucleus of the brain. Patients manifest with **involuntary choreiform movements,** depression, and cognitive impairment.

c. **Deletions** (removal of one or more nucleotides from a DNA sequence)

> *cc* **21.10** The most common mutation in **cystic fibrosis** is the **ΔF508 muta-tion.** Deletion of the codon for phenylalanine (F) at the 508 position of the **cystic fibrosis transmembrane conductance regulator** (CFTR) results in absence of this protein on the cell surface with resultant thickening of airway secretions. Patients suffer from **recurrent pulmonary infections** that are potentially life threatening.

C. **DNA repair** (Figure 21-14)

  1. In general, repair involves three steps:
     a. **Removal** of the segment of DNA that contains a damaged region or mismatched bases
     b. **Filling in the gap** by action of a DNA polymerase that uses the undamaged sister strand as a template
     c. **Ligation** of the newly synthesized segment to the remainder of the chain
  2. **Endonucleases, exonucleases,** a DNA **polymerase,** and a **ligase** are required for repair.

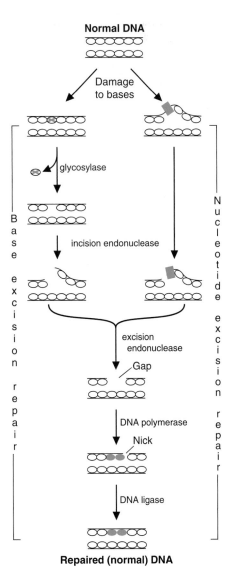

Figure 21-14 Base excision and nucleotide excision repair of DNA. Circles indicate normal bases; x and ■ indicate damaged bases. The actual number of nucleotides removed (the size of the gap) is larger than that shown.

3. **Nucleotide excision repair** involves the removal of a group of nucleotides (including the damaged nucleotide) from a DNA strand.
4. **Base excision repair** involves a specific glycosylase that removes a damaged base by hydrolyzing an *N*-glycosidic bond, producing an apurinic or apyrimidinic site, which is cleaved and, subsequently, repaired.
5. **Mismatch repair** involves the removal of the portion of the **newly synthesized strand** of recently replicated DNA that contains a pair of mismatched bases.
    a. Bacteria recognize the newly synthesized strand because, in contrast to the parental strand, it has not yet been methylated.
    b. The recognition mechanism in eukaryotes is not known.

D. **Rearrangements of genes**

1. Several processes produce new combinations of genes, thus promoting genetic diversity.
2. **Recombination** occurs between homologous DNA segments, that is, those that have very similar sequences.
3. **Transposition** involves movement of a DNA segment from one site to a non-homologous site. Transposons ("jumping genes") are mobile genetic elements that facilitate the movement of genes.

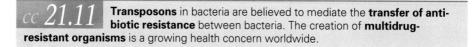

cc 21.11 **Transposons** in bacteria are believed to mediate the **transfer of antibiotic resistance** between bacteria. The creation of **multidrug-resistant organisms** is a growing health concern worldwide.

E. **Reverse transcription**

1. Synthesis of DNA from an **RNA template** is catalyzed by reverse transcriptase.
2. **Retroviruses** contain RNA as their genetic material.
    a. The retroviral RNA serves as a template for synthesis of DNA by reverse transcriptase.
    b. The DNA that is generated can be inserted into the genome (chromosomes) of the host cell and be expressed.

cc 21.12 **HIV** is **the retrovirus** that causes acquired immune deficiency syndrome (**AIDS**) in humans. **Hepatitis C,** a virus that causes **hepatitis, cirrhosis,** and hepatocellular carcinoma, is another human virus that encodes for a **reverse transcriptase.**

3. Reverse transcriptase also may play a role in normal development.

III. Synthesis of RNA (Transcription)

A. **RNA polymerase**

1. RNA polymerase can **initiate** the synthesis of new chains. A primer is not required.
2. The DNA template is copied in the 3′ to 5′ direction, and the RNA chain grows in the 5′ to 3′ direction.
3. **Ribonucleoside triphosphates** (ATP, GTP, UTP, and CTP) serve as the precursors for the RNA chain. The process is similar to that for DNA synthesis (see Figure 21-12).

B. **Synthesis of RNA in bacteria**

1. The RNA polymerase of *E. coli* contains **four subunits:** $\alpha_2\beta\beta'$, which form the core enzyme; and a fifth subunit, the sigma factor (σ), which is required for initiation of RNA synthesis.

> *cc* **21.13**   **Rifampin** is a bactericidal antibiotic that **inhibits the β-subunit of bacterial DNA-dependent RNA polymerase.** It is used in the treatment of **tuberculosis** or as prophylaxis against some forms of bacterial meningitis.

2. Genes contain a **promoter region** to which RNA polymerase binds.
    a. Promoters contain the consensus sequence **TATAAT** (called the Pribnow or TATA box) about 10 bases upstream from (before) the start point of transcription.
    b. A **consensus sequence** consists of the most commonly found sequence of bases in a given region of all DNAs tested.
    c. A **second consensus sequence (TTGACA)** is usually located upstream from the Pribnow box, about 35 nucleotides (–35) from the start point of transcription.
3. When RNA polymerase binds to a **promoter**, local unwinding of the DNA helix occurs, so that the DNA strands partially separate. The polymerase then begins transcription, copying the template strand.
    a. As the polymerase moves along the DNA, the next region of the double helix unwinds, while the single-stranded region that has already been transcribed rejoins its partner.

> *cc* **21.14**   **Actinomycin D** is an antibiotic-type compound that binds to DNA and **inhibits the elongation of the RNA transcription by RNA polymerase.** Although highly toxic, it is used in the treatment of **some pediatric cancers** like neuroblastoma, Wilms tumor, and sarcomas.

    b. Termination occurs in a region in which the transcript forms a hairpin loop that precedes four U residues.
    c. The ρ (rho) factor aids in the termination of some transcripts.
4. **mRNA** is often produced as a **polycistronic transcript** that is translated as it is being transcribed.
    a. A polycistronic mRNA produces several different proteins during translation, one from each cistron.
    b. *E. coli* mRNA has a short half-life. It is degraded in minutes.
5. **rRNA** is produced as a **large transcript** that is cleaved, producing the 16S rRNA that appears in the 30S ribosomal subunit.
    a. The 23S and 5S rRNAs appear in the 50S ribosomal subunit.
    b. The 30S and 50S ribosomal subunits combine to form the 70S ribosome.
6. **tRNA** usually is produced from **larger transcripts** that are cleaved. One of the cleavage enzymes, RNase P, contains an RNA molecule that acts as a catalyst.

C. **Synthesis of RNA in nuclei of eukaryotes**

1. *mRNA synthesis* (Figure 21-15)
    a. Eukaryotic genes that produce mRNA contain a **basal promoter** region. This region binds transcription factors, which are proteins that bind RNA polymerase II. Promoters contain a number of conserved sequences.

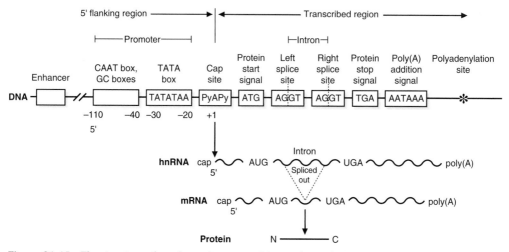

Figure 21-15 The structure of a eukaryotic gene and its products. As is customary, DNA sequences are given for the nontemplate strand. The DNA template strand, of course, is present. Its sequence is complementary and antiparallel to that of the nontemplate strand. The sequence of the RNA transcript is identical to that of the corresponding region of the nontemplate strand of the DNA, except that, in RNA, U replaces T. hnRNA = heterogeneous nuclear RNA; mRNA = messenger RNA; Py = pyrimidine.

      (1) A **TATA** (Hogness) **box,** containing the consensus sequence TATATAA, is located about 25 base pairs upstream (−25) from the transcription start site.

      (2) A **CAAT box** is frequently found about 70 base pairs upstream from the start site.

      (3) **GC-rich regions** (GC boxes) often occur between −40 and −110 base pairs upstream from the start site.

  b. **Enhancers** are DNA sequences that function in the **stimulation** of the transcription rate.

      (1) Enhancers can be located thousands of base pairs upstream or downstream from the start site.

      (2) Other sequences called **silencers** function in the **inhibition** of transcription.

  c. **RNA polymerase II** initially produces a large primary transcript called **heterogeneous nuclear RNA (hnRNA),** which contains exons and introns.

> *cc* **21.15** α-**Amanitin** is a cellular toxin that binds and inhibits **RNA polymerase II,** thereby **halting mRNA synthesis** and ultimately protein synthesis. Ingestion of *Amanita phalloides* **mushroom** (death cap), which produces the toxin, results in severe gastrointestinal symptoms, **liver toxicity,** and, potentially, death.

      (1) **Exons** are sequences within a transcript that appear in the mature **mRNA.**

      (2) **Introns** are sequences within the primary transcript that are **removed** and do not appear in the mature mRNA.

  d. **Processing of hnRNA** yields mature mRNA, which enters the cytoplasm through nuclear pores (Figure 21-16).

      (1) The **primary transcript** (hnRNA) is capped at its 5′ end as it is being transcribed.

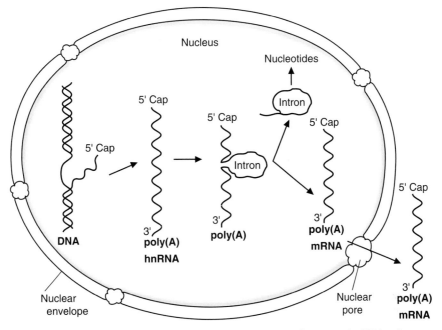

Figure 21-16 Synthesis of messenger RNA (mRNA) in eukaryotes. hnRNA = hetero-geneous nuclear RNA.

(2) A **poly(A) tail**, 20 to 200 nucleotides in length, is added to the 3′ end of the transcript.

(3) The sequence AAUAAA in hnRNA serves as a signal for cleavage of the hnRNA and addition of the poly(A) tail by poly(A) polymerase. ATP serves as the precursor.

(4) **Splicing** reactions remove introns and connect the exons.

   • The **splice point** at the **left** flank of an intron usually has the sequence AG followed by an **invariant GU**. At the **right** flank, an **invariant AG** is frequently followed by GU (see Figure 21-15).

   • Small nuclear RNAs complexed with protein (**snRNPs**) (e.g., U1 and U2) are involved in the cleavage and splicing process. A **lariat** structure is generated during the splicing reaction (see Figure 21-16).

> *cc 21.16*   The most common cause of **β-thalassemia** are defects in **mRNA splicing of the β-globin gene.** Mutations that affect the splicing create aberrant transcripts that are degraded before they are translated. If patients inherit a single mutated gene (**thalassemia minor**), the disease manifests with a **mild anemia.** However, patients with homozygous mutations (**thalassemia major**) have **severe transfusion-dependent anemia.**

(5) Some hnRNAs contain 50 or more exons that must be spliced correctly to produce functional mRNA. Other hnRNAs have no introns.

2. *rRNA synthesis and assembly of ribosomes* (Figure 21-17)

   a. A **45S precursor** is produced by RNA polymerase I from rRNA genes located in the fibrous region of the nucleolus. Many copies of the genes are present, linked together by spacer regions.

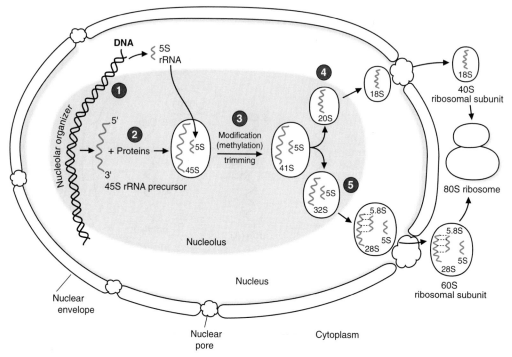

Figure 21-17   Synthesis of ribosomal RNA (rRNA) and assembly of ribosomes.

    b. The **45S** precursor is modified by methylation and undergoes a number of cleavages that ultimately produce 18S rRNA and 28S rRNA; the latter is hydrogen bonded to a 5.8S rRNA.

    c. **18S rRNA** complexes with proteins and forms the 40S ribosomal subunit.

    d. The **28S, 5.8S, and 5S rRNAs** complex with proteins and form the 60S ribosomal subunit. 5S rRNA is produced by RNA polymerase III outside of the nucleolus.

    e. The **ribosomal subunits** migrate through the nuclear pores into the cytoplasm where they complex with mRNA, forming 80S ribosomes. (Because sedimentation coefficients reflect both shape and particle weight, they are not additive.)

    f. rRNA precursors can contain introns that are removed during maturation. In some organisms, the enzymatic activity that removes rRNA introns resides in the rRNA precursor. No proteins are required. These autocatalytic RNAs are known as **ribozymes.**

  3. *tRNA synthesis* (Figure 21-18)

    a. **RNA polymerase III** is the enzyme that produces tRNA. The promoter is located within the coding region of the gene.

    b. **Primary transcripts** for tRNA are cleaved at the 5′ and 3′ ends.

    c. Some precursors contain **introns** that are removed.

    d. During processing of tRNA precursors, **nucleotides are modified.**

      (1) Post-transcriptional modification includes the conversion of uridine to pseudouridine (Ψ), ribothymidine (T), and dihydrouridine (D).

      (2) Other unusual nucleotides are also produced.

    e. Addition of the sequence **CCA** to the **3′ end** is catalyzed by nucleotidyl transferase.

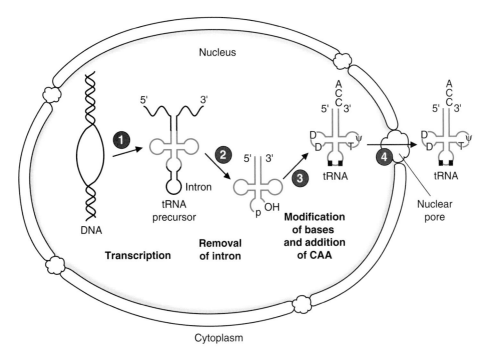

Figure 21-18   Synthesis of transfer RNA (tRNA). D, T, Ψ, and ■ are unusual nucleotides produced by post-transcriptional modifications.

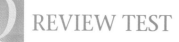

REVIEW TEST

*Directions: Each of the numbered questions or incomplete statements in this section is followed by answers or by completions of the statement. Select the **one** lettered answer or completion that is **best** in each case.*

1. In DNA, on a molar basis, which of the following statements is correct?

(A) Adenine equals thymine.
(B) Adenine equals uracil.
(C) Guanine equals adenine.
(D) Cytosine equals thymine.
(E) Cytosine equals uracil.

2. Which of the following sequences is complementary to the DNA sequence 5'-AAGTCCGA-3'?

(A) 5'-AAGUCCGA-3'
(B) 3'-TTCAGGCT-5'
(C) 5'-TTCAGGCT-3'
(D) 3'-TCGGACTT-5'

3. Okazaki fragments are formed on the _____ strands and in the _____ direction.

(A) Leading; 3'–5'
(B) Lagging; 3'–5'
(C) Leading; 5'–3'
(D) Lagging; 5'–3'

4. Transcription is directly involved in which of the following steps in the flow of genetic information?

(A) DNA to RNA
(B) RNA to DNA
(C) DNA to DNA
(D) RNA to protein

5. The messenger RNA (mRNA) produced in transcription is most similar to which of the following?

(A) The noncoding strand
(B) The coding strand
(C) The template strand
(D) The 3' to 5' strand of the parental DNA

6. The initial RNA produced during the translation of DNA to RNA, which contains both the coding exons and the noncoding introns, is known as which of the following?

(A) Amino-acetyl transfer RNA (tRNA)
(B) mRNA

(C) Ribosomal RNA (rRNA)
(D) Heterogeneous nuclear RNA

7. The action of DNA polymerases requires which of the following?

(A) A 5'-hydroxyl group
(B) Deoxyuridine triphosphate (dUTP)
(C) NAD+ as a cofactor
(D) A 3'-hydroxyl group
(E) Cytosine triphosphate (CTP)

8. Which of the following phrases describes nucleosomes?

(A) Single ribosomes attached to mRNA
(B) Complexes of DNA and newly transcribed RNA
(C) Subunits of chromatin
(D) Structures that contain DNA in the core with histones wrapped around the surface
(E) Complexes of protein and the 45S rRNA precursors found in the nucleolus

9. A common mutagenic event is the deamination of cytosine in DNA to form uracil. If the damaged strand is replicated, a CG base pair in DNA will be converted to which of the following pairs?

(A) TA base pair
(B) GC base pair
(C) GG base pair
(D) UG base pair

10. Eukaryotic genes that produce mRNA are best described as by which of the following phrases?

(A) Contain a TATA box downstream from the start site of transcription
(B) Can contain a CAAT box in the 5' flanking region
(C) Are transcribed by RNA polymerase III
(D) Contain long stretches of thymine nucleotides that produce the poly(A) tail of mRNA
(E) Do not contain introns

11. A 23-year-old man presents to his family physician with a painless swelling of his testicles. An ultrasound is suspicious for a neoplasm, and a biopsy confirms the presence of cancer. He is referred to an oncologist, who begins treatment with the topoisomerase inhibitor etoposide. The normal function of this enzyme is to do which of the following?

(A) Repair nuclear DNA in the event of DNA damage
(B) Unwind the DNA helix during replication
(C) Break and rejoin the DNA helix during replication
(D) Prevent the single strands of DNA from re-annealing during replication
(E) Lay down RNA primers for DNA polymerase

12. A 33-year-old, homosexual man is recently diagnosed with human immunodeficiency virus (HIV). His CD4+ T-cell count is dramatically decreased, and he has a high HIV viral load. He is referred to an infectious disease clinic where they begin him on a nucleoside analog. These drugs inhibit DNA synthesis because they lack which of the following properties required for normal DNA polymerization?

(A) A 5′ phosphate
(B) A 3′-hydroxyl
(C) A 7-methyl G cap
(D) A poly(A) tail
(E) A consensus sequence

13. A 53-year-old man is referred to a neurologist because he is beginning to develop spastic-like movements in his lower limbs. A magnetic resonance imaging (MRI) scan of the head is performed that shows loss of mass in the caudate nucleus. A presumptive diagnosis of Huntington disease is made, and genetic tests are ordered. Which of the following types of mutations is exemplified by this disease?

(A) Genetic insertion
(B) Genetic deletion
(C) Point mutation
(D) Transposition
(E) Mismatch repair

14. A 37-year-old, female immigrant from Thailand develops fevers, night sweats, weight loss, and a blood-tinged cough. While in the emergency room, an infectious disease doctor is consulted and immediately prescribes a multidrug regimen that includes rifampin. Rifampin inhibits RNA transcription because it inhibits which enzyme?

(A) DNA-dependent DNA polymerase
(B) DNA-dependent RNA polymerase
(C) RNA-dependent DNA polymerase
(D) RNA-dependent RNA polymerase
(E) Reverse transcriptase

15. Two couples present to the emergency room with severe nausea, vomiting, and diarrhea. One of the patients admits that she served a salad at the dinner party to which she had added a few mushrooms she picked on a hike earlier. With such information, it is likely that their symptoms are a result of inhibition of what molecular event?

(A) Inhibition of RNA polymerase II
(B) Inhibition of RNA polymerase I
(C) Inhibition of RNA splicing
(D) Inhibition of RNA polyadenylation
(E) Inhibition of RNA polymerase III

16. A 23-year-old diabetic woman reports having fevers and pain on urination. Physical examination reveals costovertebral tenderness, and her urinary analysis shows the presence of bacteria in her urine. Her physician suspects a complicated urinary tract infection and begins ciprofloxacin, a quinolone antibiotic that inhibits which of the following enzymes?

(A) Eukaryotic topoisomerase
(B) Helicase
(C) Ribozymes
(D) Gyrase
(E) Poly(A) polymerase

17. A 4-year-old child is referred by the pediatrician to a pediatric neurologist after presenting with myoclonic seizures and lactic acidosis. The neurologist orders a muscle biopsy, and the pathology returns with the appearance of "ragged red fibers." The parents are informed that the child has MERFF syndrome, a mitochondrial DNA (mtDNA) disorder. Which of the following statements best explains mtDNA?

(A) It is inherited equally from both parents.
(B) It is replicated with increased fidelity with respect to nuclear DNA.
(C) It shares the same genetic code as nuclear DNA.
(D) It is a double-stranded circular DNA.
(E) It encodes all the proteins necessary for the electron transport chain.

18. A 34-year-old man of Italian descent is seen for a yearly physical. He has no complaints and is in good health. However, he does relay a family history of anemia, and a complete blood count demonstrates a mild anemia; the physician suspects thalassemia minor in the patient. Thalassemia is most often due to a defect in RNA splicing, which is best explained by which of the following statements?

(A) Poly(A) RNA is the initial transcript produced, which is subsequently spliced to mRNA.
(B) The coding region of the gene is found on introns.
(C) The coding sequences of the gene are found on exons.
(D) All human genes require splicing of introns.
(E) The left flank of the intron contains the nucleotides AG followed by an invariant GU.

19. A 4-year-old child, on a well-child check-up, is found to have a large flank mass. A computed tomography (CT) scan demonstrates a large mass arising from the kidney, and a subsequent biopsy reveals a diagnosis of Wilms tumor. A pediatric oncologist starts chemotherapy containing the transcription inhibitor actinomycin D. Which of the following statements is correct regarding transcription?

(A) Eukaryotes often produce poly-cistronic mRNA.
(B) RNA polymerase requires a primer.
(C) The RNA chain grows in the 3' to 5' direction.
(D) Rho factor is critical for initiation of RNA synthesis.
(E) The TATA box contains a consensus sequence for the binding of RNA polymerase.

20. A second-year medical student looking to match into a competitive residency and joins a laboratory studying gene regulation in a mouse model of hepatocellular carcinoma. He isolates nucleic acids from the cells after exposure to a known carcinogen and has the sequences analyzed. He is surprised to find that some of the nucleotides are pseudouridine and ribothymidine. Which type of nucleic acid has the student likely isolated?

(A) tRNA
(B) rRNA
(C) hnRNA
(D) mRNA
(E) snRNP

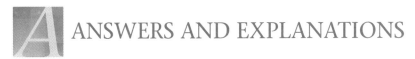

1–A. On a molar basis, DNA contains equal amounts of adenine and thymine and of guanine and cytosine. Uracil is not found in DNA.

2–B. Complementary sequences base pair with each other (A with T, C with G). The strands run in opposite directions. 5'-AAGTCCGA-3' base pairs with 3'-TTCAGGCT-5' (or with the RNA sequence 3'-UUCAGGCU-5').

3–D. Okazaki fragments are formed because there are interruptions on the lagging strands and replication is always in the 5'-3' direction.

4–A. Transcription is the synthesis of RNA, using a DNA template. DNA synthesis using a DNA template is replication, whereas producing protein from the mRNA template is translation.

5–A. The messenger RNA (mRNA) produced in transcription is an identical copy of the noncoding strand (aside from the RNA using uracil in place of thymidine) since the coding strand is the template.

6–D. The initial RNA produced by transcription of the DNA template, containing the unspliced introns, is known as heterogeneous nuclear RNA (hnRNA). Following splicing out of the introns and other modifications, such as the addition of a polyadenylated 3' sequence, the RNA is then mRNA.

7–D. DNA polymerase requires dATP, dTTP, dGTP, and dCTP as precursors that add to the 3'-hydroxyl group at the 3' end of the growing chain.

8–C. Nucleosomes are subunits of chromatin (the complex of DNA and proteins in the nucleus). They consist of a core composed of two molecules of each of the four histones (H2A, H2B, H3, and H4) with 140 base pairs of DNA wrapped around the surface. Histone H1 binds to the linker DNA that joins one nucleosome core to the next.

9–A. When the DNA is replicated, U in the template strand will pair with A in the daughter strand. Subsequent rounds of replication will cause the original CG base pair to become a TA base pair.

10–B. Eukaryotic genes contain a TATA box and often contain a CAAT box in the 5' flanking region, upstream from the start site for transcription. RNA polymerase II transcribes these genes, producing hnRNA, which is modified and processed to form mRNA. A cap is added at the 5' end and poly(A) is added to the 3' end post-transcriptionally; they are not encoded in the DNA. These genes contain introns, which are removed during processing of hnRNA.

11–C. Topoisomerase creates double-stranded breaks ahead of the replication fork to relieve the supercoiling induced by the action of helicase, which unwinds the DNA helix during replication. DNA polymerase I is important in repairing DNA damage. Single-strand binding proteins prevent the separated strands from re-annealing. Primase is required to lay down primers for DNA replication by DNA polymerase.

12–B. DNA polymerase requires a 3'-hydroxyl on the deoxyribonucleotide, to which the 5' phosphate of the subsequent nucleotide is attached. Nucleoside analogs inhibit polymerization because they lack the 3' OH for chain elongation. A 7-methyl G cap and a poly(A) tail are added to eukaryotic mRNA to stabilize the transcript. A consensus sequence is a DNA sequence that is found at the promoter and functions to bind RNA polymerase for the transcription of genes.

13–A. Huntington disease is a neurodegenerative disorder that results from the genetic insertion of CAG trinucleotide repeats within the Huntington gene. Cystic fibrosis is an example of a genetic disease caused by genetic deletion. Point mutations may cause disease when they occur in coding or noncoding regions, such as the point mutation in the α-antitrypsin coding sequence or the mutations in introns found in β-thalassemia. Transposition is a phenomenon in lower organisms and results in "jumping genes." Many heritable cancer syndromes are due to defects in mismatch repair.

14–B. Rifampin is an important agent in a multidrug regimen for tuberculosis. It works by inhibiting the β subunit of bacterial DNA-dependent RNA polymerase (RNA polymerase). A DNA-dependent DNA polymerase, such as Pol I, directs DNA replications, whereas Pol III is involved with DNA repair. An RNA-dependent DNA polymerase is known as reverse transcriptase. Only RNA viruses code for RNA-dependent RNA polymerases.

15–A. α-Amanitin, from the *Amanita phalloides* mushroom, inhibits RNA polymerase II, the enzyme required for RNA synthesis. RNA polymerase I is responsible for the synthesis of ribosomal RNA, and RNA polymerase II produces tRNA. Small ribonucleoproteins (SNPs) are important in RNA splicing. RNA poly A polymerase normally adds stretches of adenine residues to the 3′ end of mRNA.

16–D. Quinolone antibiotics inhibit DNA gyrase, a prokaryotic topoisomerase, and are important drugs in the treatment of urinary tract infections. Eukaryotic topoisomerase inhibitors include etoposide, which is used in the treatment of some cancers. There are no current drugs regimens that target helicase, which is the enzyme that unwinds DNA during replication, or poly(A) polymerase. Although ribozymes, which are autocatalytic RNAs, are interesting drug targets, no such therapy currently exists.

17–D. Mitochondrial DNA is a small double-stranded circular DNA within the mitochondria. It is inherited exclusively from the mother because the ovum contributes the cytoplasm to the zygote. The replication machinery is less evolved than nuclear DNA and replicates with mutations rates of 5–10× greater. The genetic code of mitochondria is slightly different than that of the nuclear genome. Finally, it encodes only 13 of the numerous subunits of the electron transport chain.

18–C. The coding region of any gene is located in an exon. Some, but not all, human genes contain introns, which are spliced out. The splice point at the left flank of an intron usually has the sequence AG followed by an invariant GU. At the right flank, an invariant AG is frequently followed by GU.

19–E. RNA polymerase binds to specific sequences on DNA, the TATA box in eukaryotic cells (Hogness box) and prokaryotes (Pribnow box). Usually only prokaryotic cells produce polycistronic mRNA. RNA polymerase, unlike DNA polymerase, does not require a primer. The RNA chain grows in the 5′ to 3′ direction, off the DNA copied 3′ to 5′. The rho factor (ρ) is critical in termination, whereas the sigma factor (σ) aids in bacterial transcriptional initiation.

20–A. tRNAs are often post-transcriptionally modified bases, including the conversion of uridine to pseudouridine and ribothymidine. rRNAs often contain proteins as well as RNA components, as do snRNPs (small nuclear RNAs complexed with protein) involved in splicing. hnRNA is processed, including the removal of introns, to produce mRNA.

chapter 222

RNA Translation and Protein Synthesis

I. Protein Synthesis (Translation of Messenger RNA [mRNA])

A. **The genetic code** (Table 22-1)

1. The **genetic code** is the collection of codons that specify all the amino acids found in proteins.
2. A **codon is a sequence of three bases** (triplet) in messenger RNA (mRNA) (5′ to 3′) that specifies (corresponds to) a particular amino acid. During translation, the successive codons in an mRNA determine the sequence in which amino acids add to the growing polypeptide chain.
3. The **genetic code is degenerate** (redundant). Each of the 20 common amino acids has at least one codon; many amino acids have numerous codons.
4. The genetic code is **nonoverlapping** (i.e., each nucleotide is used only once).
   a. It begins with a start codon (**AUG**) near the 5′ end of the mRNA.
   b. It ends with a termination (stop) codon (**UGA, UAG, or UAA**) near the 3′ end.
5. The code is **commaless** (i.e., there are no breaks or markers to distinguish one codon from the next).
6. The code is **nearly universal.** The same codon specifies the same amino acid in almost all species studied; however, some differences have been found in the codons used in mitochondria.
7. The **start codon** (AUG) determines the **reading frame.** Subsequent nucleotides are read in sets of three, sequentially following this codon.

B. **Effect of mutations on proteins**

1. Mutations in DNA are transcribed into mRNA and thus can cause changes in the encoded protein.
2. The various types of mutations that occur in DNA have different effects on the encoded protein.
3. **Point mutations** occur when one base in DNA is replaced by another, altering the codon in mRNA.
   a. **Silent mutations** do not affect the amino acid sequence of a protein (e.g., CGA to CGG causes no change, since both codons specify arginine).
   b. **Missense mutations** result in one amino acid being replaced by another (e.g., CGA to CCA causes arginine to be replaced by proline).

TABLE 22-1	*The Genetic Code*				
First Base	**Second Base**				**Third Base**
(5′)	*U*	*C*	*A*	*G*	**(3′)**
U	Phe	Ser	Tyr	Cys	U
	Phe	Ser	Tyr	Cys	C
	Leu	Ser	Term	Term	A
	Leu	Ser	Term	Trp	G
C	Leu	Pro	His	Arg	U
	Leu	Pro	His	Arg	C
	Leu	Pro	Gln	Arg	A
	Leu	Pro	Gln	Arg	G
A	Ile	Thr	Asn	Ser	U
	Ile	Thr	Asn	Ser	C
	Ile	Thr	Lys	Arg	A
	Met	Thr	Lys	Arg	G
G	Val	Ala	Asp	Gly	U
	Val	Ala	Asp	Gly	C
	Val	Ala	Glu	Gly	A
	Val	Ala	Glu	Gly	G

cc 22.1 **Hereditary hemochromatosis** (HH) is one of the most common of genetic diseases. It is associated with two well-known **missense mutations** in the **HFE gene,** namely the **C282Y** mutation, a substitution of tyrosine for cysteine at amino acid 282; and the **H63D** mutation, with a substitution of aspartic acid for histidine at position 63. These **mutations are used to screen** "at-risk populations" for this **disorder of iron metabolism,** which results in **cirrhosis, diabetes, skin pigmentation,** and **heart failure.**

   c. **Nonsense mutations** result in premature termination of the growing polypeptide chain (e.g., CGA to UGA causes arginine to be replaced by a stop codon).

  4. Insertions occur when a base or a number of bases are added to DNA. They can result in a protein with more amino acids than normal.

  5. Deletions occur when a base or a number of bases are removed from DNA. They can result in a protein with fewer amino acids than normal.

  6. Frameshift mutations occur when the number of bases added or deleted is not a multiple of three. The reading frame is shifted so that completely different sets of codons are read beyond the point where the mutation starts.

cc 22.2 **Duchenne muscular dystrophy** (DMD) is an **X-linked** disorder due to a **frameshift mutation** in the muscle protein **dystrophin.** A frameshift occurs, resulting in premature translation and no **functional protein.** Patients have **proximal muscle weakness** and muscle fibrosis, with death occurring as a result of **cardiac or respiratory failure.**

C. Formation of aminoacyl-transfer RNAs (tRNAs) (Figure 22-1)

  1. Amino acids are activated and attached to their corresponding **tRNAs** by highly specific enzymes known as aminoacyl-tRNA synthetases.

  2. Each aminoacyl-tRNA synthetase recognizes a particular amino acid and the tRNAs specific for that amino acid.

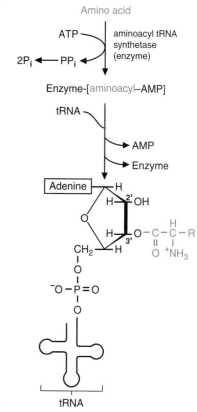

Figure 22-1   Formation of aminoacyl-transfer RNA (tRNA).

cc *22.3*   **Anti–Jo-1 antibodies** are autoantibodies to the histidyl-tRNA **synthetase.** These antibodies, as well as antibodies to other tRNA synthetases, are found in patients with **polymyositis,** a condition characterized by **arthralgias,** arthritis, and **proximal muscle weakening.**

3. An **amino acid first** reacts with adenosine triphosphate (ATP), forming an enzyme complex (aminoacyl-adenosine monophosphate [AMP]) and pyrophosphate, which is cleaved to 2 inorganic phosphates (P_i).
4. The **aminoacyl-AMP** then **forms an ester** with the 2'- or 3'-hydroxyl of a tRNA specific for that amino acid, producing an aminoacyl-tRNA and AMP.
5. Once an amino acid is attached to a tRNA, insertion of the amino acid into a growing polypeptide chain depends on the codon–anticodon interaction (Figure 22-2).

D.   Initiation of translation (Figure 22-3)

1. In eukaryotes, methionyl-tRNA$_i$^Met binds to the small **ribosomal subunit.**
   a. The **5' cap** of the mRNA binds to the small subunit, and the first AUG codon base pairs with the anticodon on the methionyl-tRNA$_i$^Met.
   b. The methionine that initiates protein synthesis is subsequently removed from the N-terminus of the polypeptide.

cc *22.4*   **Streptomycin,** an antibiotic, inhibits the initiation of protein synthesis as it **binds to the 30S subunit** and distorts the structure of the assembling initiation complex.

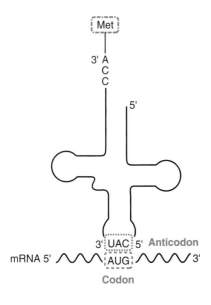

Figure 22-2   Antiparallel binding of aminoacyl-transfer RNA (tRNA) to messenger RNA (mRNA).

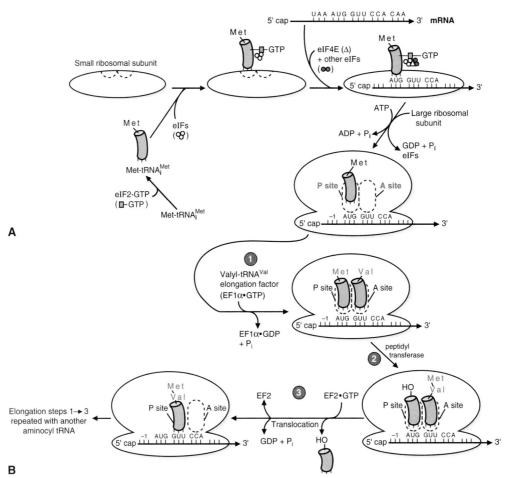

Figure 22-3   The initiation (**A**) and elongation (**B**) reactions of protein synthesis. eIFs are initiation factors in eukaryotes (IFs in prokaryotes). EF-1 and EF-2 are eukaryotic elongation factors corresponding with EF-Tu and EF-G in prokaryotes. A site = aminoacyl site; P site = peptidyl site.

c. **In bacteria,** the methionine that initiates protein synthesis is **formylated** and is carried by tRNA$_f^{Met}$.

> *CC 22.5* **Tetracyclines** are a class of antibiotics that bind to the **30S ribosomal subunit,** thereby blocking the access of the aminoacyl-tRNA to the mRNA-ribosomal complex.

> *CC 22.6* **Aminoglycosides,** such a gentamicin, are a class of antibiotics that bind to the 30S **ribosomal** subunit, thus interfering with the assembly of the functional ribosomal apparatus.

d. **Prokaryotes do not contain a 5′ cap** on their mRNA. An mRNA sequence upstream from the translation start site (the Shine-Dalgarno sequence) binds to the 3′ end of 16S ribosomal RNA (rRNA).

2. The **large ribosomal subunit binds,** completing the initiation complex.
   a. The methionyl-tRNA$_i^{Met}$ is bound at the **P (peptidyl) site** of the complex.
   b. The **A (acceptor or aminoacyl) site** of the complex is unoccupied.

> *CC 22.7* Both **erythromycin** and **clindamycin** are antibiotics that inhibit protein synthesis as they **bind the 50S ribosomal subunit** of bacteria. This results in inhibition of translocation of the growing peptide.

3. **Initiation factors (IFs), ATP, and guanosine triphosphate (GTP)** are required for formation of the initiation complex.
   a. The **initiation factors** are designated IF-1, IF-2, and IF-3 in prokaryotes. In eukaryotes, they are designated eIF-1, eIF-2, and so on. Seven or more may be present.
   b. Release of the initiation factors involves hydrolysis of GTP to guanosine diphosphate (GDP) and inorganic phosphate (P$_i$).

E. **Elongation of polypeptide chains** (see Figure 22-3B)

1. The addition of each amino acid to the growing polypeptide chain involves binding of an aminoacyl-tRNA at the A site, formation of a peptide bond, and translocation of the peptidyl-tRNA to the P site.

2. *Binding of aminoacyl-tRNA to the A site* (see Step 1, Figure 22-3B)
   a. The **mRNA codon** at the A site determines which aminoacyl-tRNA will bind.

> *CC 22.8* The antibiotic **puromycin** is an analog of **aminoacyl-tRNA.** It inhibits both prokaryotic as well as eukaryotic **translation** as it acts as a chain terminator in protein synthesis.

   (1) The codon and the anticodon bind by base pairing that is antiparallel (see Figure 22-2).
   (2) Internal methionine residues in the polypeptide chain are added in response to AUG codons. They are carried by tRNA$_m^{Met}$, a second tRNA specific for methionine.

b. An **elongation factor** (EF) (EF-Tu in prokaryotes and EF-1 in eukaryotes) and hydrolysis of GTP are required for binding.

3. *Formation of a peptide bond* (see Step 2, Figure 22-3B)

   a. A peptide bond forms between the amino group of the aminoacyl-tRNA at the **A site** and the carbonyl of the aminoacyl group attached to the tRNA at the **P site**. Formation of the peptide bond is catalyzed by **peptidyl transferase**, which is rRNA.

   > *CC* **22.9** **Chloramphenicol,** an antibiotic rarely used due to the potential to develop decreased white blood cells, **inhibits peptidyltransferase,** thus halting protein synthesis.

   b. The tRNA at the P site now does not contain an amino acid. It is "uncharged."
   c. The growing polypeptide chain is attached to the tRNA in the A site.

4. *Translocation of peptidyl-tRNA* (see Step 3, Figure 22-3B)

   a. The peptidyl-tRNA (along with the attached mRNA) moves from the A site to the P site, and the uncharged tRNA is released from the ribosome. An **elongation factor** (EF-2 in eukaryotes or EF-G in prokaryotes) and the hydrolysis of **GTP** are required for translocation.

   > *CC* **22.10** **Diphtheria toxin** is produced from phage genes incorporated into the bacterium *Corynebacterium diphtheriae.* The toxin causes diphtheria, a lethal disease of the respiratory tract. The A fragment of the toxin catalyzes the adenosine diphosphate **(ADP)-ribosylation** of **EF-2,** thus inhibiting translocation in eukaryotes.

   b. The next codon in the mRNA is now in the A site.
   c. The elongation and translocation steps are repeated until a termination codon moves into the A site.

F. **Termination of translation**

   1. When a termination codon (UGA, UAG, or UAA) occupies the A site, release factors cause the newly synthesized polypeptide to be released from the ribosome.
   2. The ribosomal subunits dissociate from the mRNA.

G. **Polysomes** (Figure 22-4)

   1. More than one ribosome can be attached to a single mRNA at any given time. The complex of mRNA with multiple ribosomes is known as a **polysome.**
   2. Each ribosome carries a nascent polypeptide chain that grows longer as the ribosome approaches the 3′ end of the mRNA.

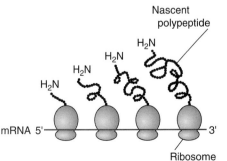

Figure 22-4 A polysome. mRNA = messenger RNA.

H. **Post-translational processing**

- After synthesis is completed, **proteins can be modified** by phosphorylation, glycosylation, ADP-ribosylation, hydroxylation, and addition of other groups.

I. **Synthesis and release of secretory proteins**

1. **Secretory proteins,** destined for release from the cell, are synthesized on ribosomes attached to the **rough endoplasmic reticulum (RER)** in eukaryotic cells.
2. A **hydrophobic signal sequence** at the N-terminus of a secretory protein causes the nascent protein to pass into the lumen of the RER. The signal sequence is cleaved from the N-terminus, and the protein may be glycosylated within the RER.
3. The protein travels in vesicles to the **Golgi,** where it may be glycosylated further and is packaged in secretory vesicles.
4. **Secretory vesicles** containing the protein travel from the Golgi to the cell membrane. The protein is released from the cell by **exocytosis.**

II.   Regulation of Protein Synthesis

A. **Regulation of protein synthesis in prokaryotes**

1. *Relationship of protein synthesis to nutrient supply*
    a. **Prokaryotes** respond to changes in their supply of nutrients in a way that allows them to obtain or conserve energy most efficiently.
       (1) Prokaryotes, such as *Escherichia coli,* require a source of **carbon,** which is usually a sugar that is oxidized for energy.
       (2) A source of **nitrogen** is also required for the synthesis of amino acids from which structural proteins and enzymes are produced.
    b. *E. coli* uses **glucose** preferentially whenever it is available. The enzymes in the pathways for glucose utilization are made **constitutively** (i.e., they are constantly being produced).
    c. **If glucose is not present** in the medium but another sugar is available, *E. coli* produces the enzymes and other proteins that allow the cell to derive energy from that sugar. The process by which synthesis of the enzymes is regulated is called **induction.**
    d. **If an amino acid is present in the medium,** *E. coli* does not need to synthesize that amino acid and conserves energy by ceasing to produce the enzymes required for its synthesis. The process by which synthesis of these enzymes is regulated is called **repression.**
2. *Operons*
    a. An operon is a **set of genes** that are **adjacent** to one another in the genome and are coordinately controlled; that is, the genes are either all turned on or all turned off (Figure 22-5).
    b. The **structural genes** of an operon **code** for a series of different proteins.
       (1) A single **polycistronic mRNA** is transcribed from an operon. This single mRNA codes for all the proteins of the operon.
       (2) A series of **start** and **stop codons** on the polycistronic mRNA allows a number of different proteins to be produced at the translational level from the single mRNA.
    c. Transcription begins near a **promoter region,** which is located upstream from the group of structural genes.

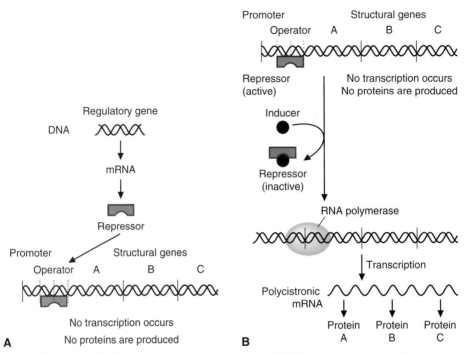

Figure 22-5 An inducible operon (e.g., the *lac* operon). **(A)** If the inducer is absent, the repressor is active and binds to the operator, preventing RNA polymerase from binding. Thus, transcription does not occur. **(B)** If the inducer is present, it binds to and inactivates the repressor, which then does not bind to the operator. Therefore, RNA polymerase can bind and transcribe the structural genes.

> **d.** Associated with the promoter is a short sequence, the **operator**, which determines whether or not the genes are expressed.
> **e.** **Binding of a repressor protein** to the operator region prevents binding of RNA polymerase to the promoter and **inhibits transcription** of the structural genes of the operon.
> **f.** Repressor proteins are encoded by regulatory genes, which may be located anywhere in the genome.
>
> **3.** *Induction (see Figure 22-5B)*
>
>> **a.** Induction is the process whereby an **inducer** (a small molecule) stimulates transcription of an operon.
>> **b.** The inducer is frequently a sugar (or a metabolite of the sugar), and the proteins produced from the inducible operon allow the sugar to be metabolized.
>>> **(1)** The inducer binds to the **repressor**, inactivating it.
>>> **(2)** The inactive repressor does not bind to the operator.
>>> **(3)** **RNA polymerase**, therefore, can **bind** to the promoter and **transcribe** the operon.
>>> **(4)** The structural **proteins** encoded by the operon are **produced**.
>> **c.** The **lactose (*lac*) operon** is **inducible**.
>>> **(1)** A metabolite of lactose, **allolactose**, is the inducer.
>>> **(2)** Proteins produced by the genes of the *lac* operon allow the cell to oxidize lactose as a source of energy. Gene Z produces a **β-galactosidase;** gene Y, a lactose permease; and gene A, a transacetylase.
>>> **(3)** The *lac* operon is induced only in the **absence of glucose**. It exhibits **catabolite repression** (see II A 6).

4. *Repression*
   a. Repression is the process whereby a **corepressor** (a small molecule) **inhibits transcription** of an operon.
   b. The **corepressor** is usually an amino acid, and the proteins produced from the repressible operon are involved in the synthesis of the amino acid.
      (1) The corepressor binds to the repressor, activating it.
      (2) The active repressor binds to the operator.
      (3) **RNA polymerase**, therefore, cannot bind to the promoter, and the operon is not transcribed.
      (4) The cell stops producing the structural proteins encoded by the operon.
   c. The **tryptophan (*trp*) operon** is **repressible.**
      (1) **Tryptophan** is the corepressor.
      (2) The proteins encoded by the *trp* operon are involved in the synthesis of tryptophan.
      (3) The *trp* operon is repressed in the presence of tryptophan, since cells do not need to make the amino acid if it is present in the growth medium.

5. *Positive control*
   a. Some operons are turned on by mechanisms that **activate transcription.**
   b. When the repressor of the arabinose (*ara*) operon binds arabinose, it changes conformation and becomes an activator that stimulates binding of RNA polymerase to the promoter. The operon is then transcribed, and the proteins required for oxidation of arabinose are produced.

6. *Catabolite repression* (Figure 22-6)
   a. Cells preferentially use **glucose** when it is available.
   b. Some operons (e.g., *lac* and *ara*) are not expressed when glucose is present in the medium. These operons require **cyclic adenosine monophosphate (cAMP)** for their expression.
      (1) Glucose causes cAMP levels in the cells to decrease.
      (2) When glucose decreases, cAMP levels rise.
      (3) **cAMP** binds to the catabolite-activator protein (**CAP**).
      (4) The **cAMP-protein complex** binds to a site near the **promoter** of the operon and facilitates binding of RNA polymerase to the promoter.
   c. The *lac* operon exhibits **catabolite repression.**
      (1) In the **presence of lactose** and the **absence of glucose**, the *lac* repressor is inactivated, and the high levels of cAMP facilitate binding of RNA polymerase to the promoter.
      (2) The **operon is transcribed**, and the proteins that allow the cells to utilize lactose are produced.

7. *Attenuation*
   a. In bacterial cells, **transcription and translation occur simultaneously.**
   b. Attenuation occurs by a mechanism by which **rapid translation** of the nascent transcript causes **termination of transcription.**
   c. As the transcript is being produced, if ribosomes attach and **rapidly translate** the transcript, a secondary structure is generated in the mRNA that is a **termination signal** for RNA polymerase.
   d. If **translation is slow**, this termination structure does not form, and **transcription continues.**
      (1) Multiple codons for the amino acid are located near the translation start site of the mRNA.
      (2) When cells contain low levels of the amino acid (which is produced by the enzymes encoded by the operon), less aminoacyl-tRNA is available to bind to these codons, and translation slows.

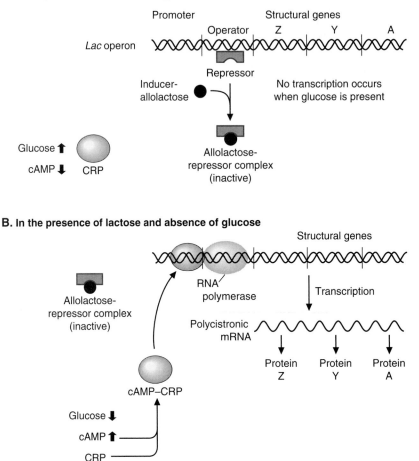

A. In the presence of lactose and glucose

B. In the presence of lactose and absence of glucose

Figure 22-6 Catabolite repression. The operon is transcribed only when glucose is low. Cyclic adenosine monophosphate (cAMP) is elevated, and the inducer binds to the repressor, inactivating it. Under these conditions, the cAMP–CRP complex forms and binds to the DNA, facilitating the initiation of transcription by RNA polymerase. The *lac* operon exhibits catabolite repression.

    e. The *trp* operon is regulated by attenuation.
  8. Factors, such as sigma, affect RNA polymerase activity. These factors bind to the core RNA polymerase and increase its ability to bind to specific promoters.

B. Differences between eukaryotes and prokaryotes

  1. Eukaryotic cells undergo differentiation, and the organisms go through various developmental stages.
  2. Eukaryotes contain nuclei. Therefore, transcription is separated from translation. In prokaryotes, transcription and translation occur simultaneously.
  3. DNA is complexed with histones in eukaryotes, but not in prokaryotes.
  4. The **mammalian genome** contains about **1000 times more DNA** than *E. coli* (10^9 versus 10^6 base pairs).
  5. Most **mammalian** cells are **diploid.**
  6. The **major part of the genome** of mammalian cells **does not code for proteins.**

7. **Some eukaryotic genes**, like most bacterial genes, **are unique** (i.e., they exist in one or a small number of copies per genome).
8. **Other eukaryotic genes**, unlike bacterial genes, **have many copies** in the genome (e.g., genes for tRNA, rRNA, histones).
9. Relatively **short, repetitive DNA sequences** are dispersed throughout the eukaryotic genome. They do not code for proteins (e.g., Alu sequences).
10. **Eukaryotic genes contain introns.** Bacterial genes do not.
11. **Bacterial genes** are organized in **operons** (sets that are under the control of a single promoter). **Each eukaryotic gene has its own promoter.**

C. **Regulation of protein synthesis in eukaryotes**

1. Regulation can result from changes in genes or from mechanisms that affect transcription, processing, and transport of mRNA, mRNA translation, or mRNA stability.
2. *Changes in genes*
   a. **Genes can be lost** (or partially lost) from cells, so that functional proteins can no longer be produced (e.g., during differentiation of red blood cells).
   b. **Genes can be amplified.**

   > cc *22.11* Gene amplification is common in tumor cells. For instance, in one of the most common childhood solid tumors, **neuroblastoma,** patients have up to **300 copies** of the growth-promoting **N-*myc* gene.**

   c. **Segments of DNA can move** from one location to another on the genome, associating with each other in various ways so that different proteins are produced.

   > cc *22.12* Both **T and B lymphocytes undergo DNA rearrangements,** with loss of intervening DNA (Figure 22-7). Such rearrangements create a **single transcriptional unit** for the formation of a diverse repertoire of **antibodies and T-cell receptors** for a competent immune system.

   d. **Modification** of the **bases in DNA** affects the **transcriptional activity** of a gene.
      (1) Cytosine can be methylated at its 5 position.
      (2) The greater the extent of methylation, the less readily a gene is transcribed.

   > cc *22.13* **Globin genes** are more **extensively methylated** in nonerythroid cells than in erythroid cells, in which they are expressed.

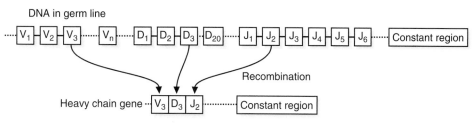

Figure 22-7 Rearrangement of DNA. Specific V, D, and J segments from among a large number of potential sequences in the DNA of precursor cells combine to form the heavy-chain gene from which lymphocytes produce immunoglobulins (antibodies).

3. *Regulation of the level of transcription*

a. Histones, which are small, basic proteins associated with the DNA of eukaryotes, act as nonspecific repressors.

b. The **expression** of specific genes is stimulated by **positive** mechanisms.

c. Inducers (e.g., steroid hormones) enter cells, bind to protein receptors, interact with chromatin in the nucleus, and **activate specific genes.**

> *cc* **22.14** **Synthetic retinoids** are potent inducers of numerous genes involved in **embryogenesis.** Exposure to the retinoid **isotretinoin,** for the treatment of acne **during pregnancy,** has been associated with a range of **birth defects** due to inappropriate patterns of **retinoid-induced gene expression.**

d. Some genes have **more than one promoter.** Thus, the promoter that is used can differ under different physiologic conditions or in different cell types.

4. *Regulation during processing and transport of mRNA*

a. Regulatory mechanisms that occur during capping, polyadenylation, and splicing can alter the amino acid sequence or the quantity of the protein produced from the mRNA. Editing of mRNA also occurs, and the rate of degradation of mRNA is also regulated.

b. Alternative splice sites can be used to produce different mRNAs.

> *cc* **22.15** The use of different splice sites results in the production of **calcitonin in the C cells of the thyroid** or alternatively, in the brain, the neuropeptide **calcitonin gene-related peptide** (CGRP) (Figure 22-8).

c. Alternative polyadenylation sites can be used to generate different mRNAs.

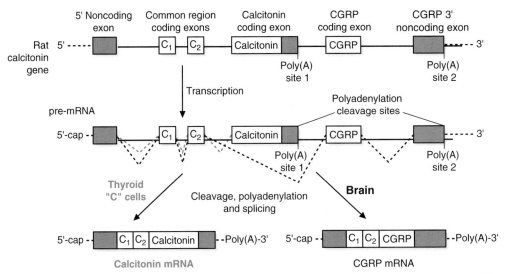

Figure 22-8 Alternative splicing of the calcitonin gene. In thyroid cells, heterogeneous nuclear RNA (hnRNA) transcribed from the calcitonin gene is processed to form the messenger RNA (mRNA) that produces calcitonin. In the brain, the same transcript of this gene is spliced differently. The first polyadenylation site is cleaved out, and a second polyadenylation site is used. The protein product is the calcitonin gene-related protein (CGRP).

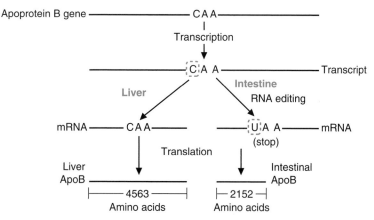

Figure 22-9   RNA editing. In liver, the apoprotein B (Apo B) gene produces a protein (Apo B100) that contains more than 4000 amino acids. It is the major apoprotein of very low–density lipoprotein (VLDL). In intestinal cells, the same gene produces a protein that contains only 48% of this number of amino acids. This protein (Apo B48) is the major apoprotein of chylomicrons. "Editing" of mRNA (conversion of a C to a U) generates a stop codon in the intestinal mRNA.

 Immunoglobin M (IgM) genes contain **two distinct polyadenylation sites.** One poly A site is at the 3′ end of the hydrophobic transmembrane region, found in IgM that is anchored to the cell surface. The second poly A site is at the 5′ end of the transmembrane region. Alternative splicing at this second poly A site results in a soluble **secreted IgM molecule.**

 d. **mRNAs can be degraded** by nucleases after their synthesis in the nucleus and before their translation in the cytoplasm. Some mRNA are degraded more rapidly than others.

 e. **RNA editing** involves the alteration ("editing") of bases in mRNA after transcription (Figure 22-9).

5. **Protein synthesis** can be **regulated at the translational level,** during the initiation or elongation reactions.

cc 22.17 **Heme stimulates the synthesis of globin** by preventing the phosphorylation and consequent **inactivation of eIF-2,** a factor involved in initiation of protein synthesis.

cc 22.18 **Interferon-α,** an antiviral cytokine, has several important functions to prevent the spread of viral infection. It stimulates the **synthesis of 2′,5′-oligo(A),** which activates a nuclease that **degrades mRNA.** Additionally, it stimulates the **phosphorylation of eIF-2,** causing **inhibition of initiation.**

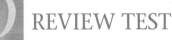

*Directions: Each of the numbered questions or incomplete statements in this section is followed by answers or by completions of the statement. Select the **one** lettered answer or completion that is **best** in each case.*

1. Which of the following is not a characteristic of the genetic code?

(A) It is a triplet code.
(B) It is nonoverlapping and without punctuation.
(C) It is degenerate in that one codon may code for more that one amino acid.
(D) It is nearly universal.

2. Which of the following statements is not correct concerning aminoacyl-transfer RNA (tRNA) synthetases?

(A) They recognize and hydrolyze incorrect aminoacyl-tRNAs that may have been produced.
(B) The bond between the tRNA and amino acids is an amide bond.
(C) There several aminoacyl-tRNA synthetases for every amino acid.
(D) Charging an aminoacyl-tRNA synthetase with an amino acid is an energetically favorable reaction.

3. Which of the following structures is formed by many ribosomes simultaneously associated with a single messenger RNA (mRNA), along which there are numerous nascent polypeptide chains in various states of translational completion?

(A) Polycistronic mRNA
(B) Nucleosome
(C) Polysome
(D) The 3′–5′ strand of the parental DNA

4. Which one of the following changes in mRNA (caused by a point mutation) would result in translation of a protein identical to the normal protein?

(A) UCA → UAA
(B) UCA → CCA
(C) UCA → UCU
(D) UCA → ACA
(E) UCA → GCA

5. Which of the following statements best describes methionine?

(A) It is the amino acid used for initiation of the synthesis of all proteins.
(B) It is generally found at the N-terminus of proteins isolated from cells.
(C) It requires a codon other than AUG to be added to growing polypeptide chains.
(D) It is formylated when it is bound to tRNA in eukaryotic cells.

6. Which of the following statements about bacteria is correct?

(A) They contain 80S ribosomes.
(B) They initiate protein synthesis with methionyl-tRNA.
(C) They are insensitive to chloramphenicol.
(D) They synthesize proteins on mRNA that is in the process of being transcribed.

7. Which of the following is required for initiation of protein synthesis in the cytosol of eukaryotic cells?

(A) A 40S ribosomal subunit
(B) Initiation factor (IF)-2
(C) Methionyl-tRNA$_f^{Met}$
(D) Uracil triphosphate (UTP)
(E) Elongation factor (EF)-2

8. In bacterial operons that are inducible, which of the following occurs?

(A) The inducer binds to the repressor and activates it.
(B) The inducer stimulates binding of RNA polymerase to the promoter.
(C) A regulatory gene produces an inactive repressor.
(D) Structural genes that are adjacent on the DNA are coordinately expressed in response to the inducer.
(E) Each of the structural genes produces a separate mRNA.

376

9. When cyclic adenosine monophosphate (cAMP) levels are relatively high in *Escherichia coli,* which of the following occurs?

(A) Lactose is not required for transcription of the *lac* operon.
(B) Glucose levels in the medium are low.
(C) The repressor is bound to the *lac* operon if lactose is present.
(D) The enzymes for the metabolism of lactose are not induced.

10. Which of the following statements about regulation of protein synthesis in eukaryotes is correct?

(A) A gene that is methylated is transcribed more readily than one that is not methylated.
(B) Genes cannot undergo rearrangements that allow cells to produce new proteins.
(C) Red blood cells do not produce hemoglobin mRNA because they lack the appropriate gene.
(D) Recognition of alternative polyadenylation sites allows cells to produce proteins that have different N-terminal regions.
(E) Steroid hormones activate genes that are specifically repressed by histones.

11. The sequence for a portion of a gene responsible for a lysosomal storage disease (Tay-Sachs) has been determined. The normal gene sequence and the mutant gene sequence are given below. (There is a dot above every fifth base and a number above every tenth base.)

        •   10   •   20   •

Normal CGTATATCCTATGGCCCTGACCCAG

Mutant CGTATATC̲T̲A̲T̲C̲CTATGGCCCTGAC

The amino acid sequence in this region of the normal protein is Arg-Ile-Ser-Tyr-Gly-Pro-Asp. Which of the following statements best explains this portion of the gene sequence?

(A) The messenger RNA produced from this region of the mutant gene codes for the amino acid sequence given above.
(B) The codon used for arginine in this sequence is AGA.
(C) The mutant protein will be shorter than the normal protein.
(D) The mutant gene contains a deletion that causes a frameshift mutation.
(E) The mutant gene has a point mutation.

12. A 53-year-old man sees his family physician with concerns that his skin is "bronzing." He is found to have diabetes as well as an elevated ferritin (a sign of iron overload). The physician suspects hemochromatosis and finds the patient carries a mutation where tyrosine is substituted for cysteine at position 282 (C282Y) of the HFE gene. The patient is diagnosed with hemochromatosis, which is a disease that results from which type of mutation?

(A) Silent
(B) Missense
(C) Nonsense
(D) Frameshift
(E) Deletion

13. A 43-year-old woman is referred to a rheumatologist for progressive weakness, including difficulty getting out of her chair and climbing the stairs. A full rheumatologic workup reveals the patient likely has polymyositis with anti-Jo-1 antibodies. The physician explains to her that she has autoantibodies directed against histidinyl-tRNA synthetase. Which of the following best describes this protein?

(A) The formation of aminoacyl-tRNA synthetase does not require any energy.
(B) Initiation of transcription requires the interaction of aminoacyl-tRNA synthetase with the 30S subunit of the ribosome.
(C) Each aminoacyl-tRNA synthetase recognizes a particular amino acid and a particular tRNA for that amino acid.
(D) It is inhibited by puromycin, an analog of aminoacyl-tRNA synthetase.
(E) It attaches amino acids to the 5′ end of tRNA.

14. A 54-year-old man develops a nonproductive cough and a low-grade fever. He visits his family physician who suspects mycoplasma pneumonia. The physician decides to treat the patient empirically with erythromycin. Which of the following describes the mechanism of erythromycin?

(A) Binds to the 5′ cap of RNA
(B) Inhibits the 30S ribosomal subunit
(C) Binds to the Shine-Dalgarno sequence
(D) Inhibits the initiation factor IF-1
(E) Inhibits the 50S ribosomal subunit

15. A 5-year-old child from rural West Virginia is seen by his family physician for a week-long cough that sounds like a "whoop." The doctor learns that the child's vaccinations are not up to date, and he is yet to receive all his pertussis vaccinations. One way in which pertussis toxin causes cell death is through the inhibition of EF-2. Which of the following statements best explains EF-2?

(A) Translocation of peptidyl-tRNA depends on a functional EF-2.
(B) It is required for initiation of protein synthesis.
(C) It is also inhibited by chloramphenicol.
(D) The protein functions as a peptidyl transferase.
(E) The protein that performs a similar function in prokaryotes is eIF-1.

16. A third-year medical student joins a laboratory that studies gene regulation. The lab uses bacteria to study gene expression and metabolic regulation after exposure to toxic compounds. The hope is that what is learned in this prokaryotic system can explain the way eukaryotic cells respond to such insults. Which of the following statements explains both prokaryotic and eukaryotic genes?

(A) They both have diploid genomes.
(B) They both organize their DNA with histones.
(C) They both have short repetitive DNA sequences throughout their genome.
(D) They both organize their genes into operons.
(E) They both use the same genetic code.

17. A 23-year-old man is seen in the gastroenterologist's office for a referral for a family history of α-antitrypsin deficiency. The physician arranges for the interventional radiologist to perform a liver biopsy, which demonstrates the accumulation of nonsecreted protein in the cell. Which of the following statements is true of proteins like α-antitrypsin that are normally to be secreted from the cell?

(A) They are synthesized on ribosomes attached to the smooth endoplasmic reticulum.
(B) They contain a hydrophilic signal sequence.
(C) The signal sequence is found on the C-terminus of the protein.
(D) Glycosylation takes place only in the endoplasmic reticulum.
(E) Proteins travel from the endoplasmic reticulum to the Golgi and are ultimately secreted by exocytosis.

18. Bacterial cells growing in a medium containing glucose and all 20 amino acids are transferred to a medium in which the only sugar is lactose and NH_4^+ is the only source of nitrogen. Concerning cells growing in the second medium, compared with those growing in the first medium, which of the following statements is most correct?

(A) cAMP levels will be lower.
(B) Catabolite-activator protein (CAP) protein (cAMP-binding protein) will be bound to the *lac* promoter.
(C) The *lac* repressor will be bound to the *lac* operator.
(D) RNA polymerase will not bind to the *trp* promoter.
(E) Attenuation of transcription of the *trp* operon will increase.

19. Gene transcription rates and mRNA levels were determined for an enzyme that is induced by glucocorticoids. Compared with untreated levels, glucocorticoid treatment caused a 10-fold increase in the gene transcription rate and a 20-fold increase in both mRNA levels and enzyme activity. These data indicate that a primary effect of glucocorticoid treatment is to decrease which of the following?

(A) The activity of RNA polymerase II
(B) The rate of mRNA translation
(C) The ability of nucleases to act on mRNA
(D) The rate of binding of ribosomes to mRNA
(E) The activity of RNA polymerase III

20. A scientist is studying post-transcriptional processing in human stem cells. He clones an unknown segment of DNA to express the gene in culture. However, when he sequences the protein, he finds that one of the amino acids does not match the amino acid that would be predicted from the genetic code. After exhaustive confir-mation, he suspects that RNA editing has taken place. Which of the following is an example of RNA editing in humans?

(A) Production of calcitonin and calcitonin-related peptide from the same gene
(B) Production of cell surface immuno-globulin M (IgM) and secreted IgM from the same gene
(C) Increased expression of N-*myc* in neu-roblastoma cells
(D) The production of apoprotein (Apo) B48 from the transcript for Apo B100
(E) The disappearance of globulin genes in response to heme

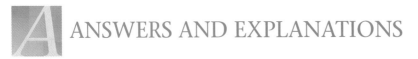

ANSWERS AND EXPLANATIONS

1–C. Although one amino acid may be generated by more than one codon (degenerate), only one amino acid is translated by a codon (unambiguous).

2–A. The recognition of the incorrect match between transfer RNA (tRNA) and amino acid is one checkpoint to assure the accuracy in protein synthesis.

3–A. The messenger RNA (mRNA) produced in transcription is an identical copy of the noncoding strand (aside from the RNA using uracil in place of thymidine) since the coding strand is the template.

4–C. UCA is a codon for serine. If the C were replaced by A → UAA, it is converted to a termination codon; UCA → CCA converts it to a proline codon; UCA → ACA converts it to a threonine; and, lastly, the U → G to an alanine codon. Translation to UCU would produce no change in the protein, since UCU is also a codon for serine.

5–A. Methionine, the amino acid that initiates the synthesis of proteins, is subsequently cleaved from the protein. The only codon for methionine is AUG, which serves as the codon for methionine residues within a protein as well as the initiating residue. The methionyl-transfer RNA (tRNA) for initiation is formylated in bacterial cells and in mitochondria.

6–D. Bacteria contain 70S ribosomes that are sensitive to chloramphenicol. They initiate protein synthesis with methionine that is formylated. Because bacteria do not have nuclei, ribosomes bind to mRNA as it is being synthesized, so that translation begins before transcription is completed.

7–A. Methionyl-tRNA (not formylated Met-tRNA), initiation factor eIF-2, and guanosine triphosphate (GTP) bind to the 40S ribosomal subunit. The cap of mRNA binds, and the ribosomal subunit moves along the mRNA until the first AUG codon pairs with the anti-codon on the tRNA. The 60S subunit is added, and protein synthesis is initiated. EF-2 is used during the elongation process in eukaryotes, and IF-2 is a prokaryotic initiation factor.

8–D. In induction, a regulatory gene produces an active repressor, which is inactivated by binding to the inducer. The inducer prevents binding of the repressor to the operator, rather than stimulating binding of RNA polymerase. The structural genes are coordinately expressed. Transcription yields a single, polycistronic mRNA, which is translated to produce a number of different proteins.

9–B. Cyclic adenosine monophosphate (cAMP) is involved in catabolite repression. Bacterial cells preferentially use glucose. When glucose is low, cAMP rises. cAMP forms a complex with the catabolite-activator protein (CAP), and the complex binds near the *lac* promoter region, facilitating the binding of RNA polymerase. Lactose must be present to inactivate the repressor, so that the operon can be expressed.

10–C. A gene that is methylated is less readily transcribed than one that is not methylated. In cells that become antibody-producing lymphocytes, segments of genes are rearranged to form the V, D, and J regions of the gene that will produce an antibody in the mature cell. Red blood cells have lost their nuclei, so they do not produce mRNA. Polyadenylation sites are at the C-terminus of a protein. Histones are nonspecific repressors of gene expression.

11–C. The mutant gene has a four-base insertion (TATC) starting at position 9. Consequently, a frameshift occurs, and the mutant gene encodes a protein with a different amino acid sequence beyond this point. The insertion causes the sequence TGA at position 22 to come into frame. This corresponds with UGA, a termination codon in the mRNA. Therefore, the mutant protein will be shorter than the normal protein. Although AGA is a codon for arginine (Arg), another codon for Arg is used in this sequence.

12–B. A missense mutation results from a nucleotide change, which results in a codon for a different amino acid, as is the case of the C282Y mutation in hereditary hemochromatosis. A silent mutation does not result in an amino acid change, by definition, due to the degenerate nature of the genetic code. A frameshift mutation, as in muscular dystrophy, can result in premature termination of protein synthesis with a dysfunctional protein. Deletion mutations, as in cystic fibrosis, result in the loss of one or more amino acids.

13–C. Each aminoacyl-tRNA synthetase recognizes a single amino acid and the particular tRNA for that amino acid. The formation of the aminoacyl-tRNA requires the hydrolysis of adenosine triphosphate (ATP) as the amino acid is added to the 5′ end of the tRNA. The initiation of transcription requires the interaction of the small ribosomal subunit and a methionyl-tRNA.

14–C. Erythromycin, as well as chloramphenicol, inhibits the 50S ribosomal subunit of bacteria. Aminoglycosides, like gentamicin, tetracycline, and streptomycin, inhibit the 30S ribosomal subunit. The ribosomes bind to the 5′ cap of the RNA in eukaryotes and at a consensus sequence known as the Shine-Dalgarno sequence at the 5′ end of prokaryotic mRNA. Initiation factor (IF)-1, IF-2, and IF-3 are bacterial initiation factors required for the formation of the initiation complex, although they are not the targets of any antibiotic.

15–A. The translocation of peptidyl-tRNA along the mRNA requires the elongation factor EF-2 as well as the hydrolysis of GTP. A similar factor, EF-Tu, performs the same function in prokaryotes. Initiation of protein synthesis requires several initiation factors, designated eIF-1, eIF-2, etc., in eukaryotes. Peptidyl transferase is an rRNA involved in formation of the peptide bond between the amino acid groups within the A and P sites of the ribosome. Chloramphenicol inhibits the peptidyl transferase.

16–E. The genetic code is nearly universal, although there are some differences in mitochondria. Only eukaryotes have a diploid genome, which is organized into chromatin with the aid of highly positively charged histones. Only eukaryotes have numerous short repetitive DNA sequences throughout their genome, like Alu sequences. Lastly, prokaryotes, but not eukaryotes, organize transcriptional units as operons.

17–E. Proteins destined to be secreted travel from the endoplasmic reticulum to the Golgi on their way to be excreted by the cell. Ribosomes attach to the rough endoplasmic reticulum with the aid of a hydrophobic signal sequence at the N-terminus of the protein. Glycosylation takes place in both the endoplasmic reticulum, as well as the Golgi.

18–B. In the absence of glucose and the presence of lactose, the *lac* repressor will be inactive, cAMP levels will rise, and CAP protein will bind to the *lac* promoter, stimulating transcription of the operon. Tryptophan levels in the cell will be low; thus, the repressor for the *trp* operon will be inactive, and the operon will be transcribed by RNA polymerase. Attenuation of transcription of this operon will decrease.

19–C. If the rate of degradation of the mRNA is not altered by glucocorticoids, the increase in mRNA levels should reflect the increase in transcription rate. Because the increase in mRNA level is greater than the increase in transcription rate, the glucocorticoids must also be increasing mRNA stability (i.e., decreasing the rate of degradation by nucleases). The activity of RNA polymerase II is increased (transcription is increased), and the rate of translation (the binding of ribosomes to mRNA) is increased (the enzyme activity is increased).

20–D. RNA editing results in the production of apoprotein (Apo) B48 from the same transcript as that for Apo B-100. A CAA codon is edited to a UAA codon, resulting in premature stop and the production of the shorter B48 molecule from the same transcript as the longer B100 transcript. The production of calcitonin and calcitonin-related peptide is a consequence of alternative splicing. The production of cell surface immunoglobulin M (IgM) and secreted IgM from the same gene occurs as the result of alternative polyadenylation sites. The disappearance of globulin mRNAs in the presence of heme results from heme's ability to prevent phosphorylation of eIF-2, halting the initiation of protein translation. The increased expression of N-*myc* in neuroblastoma tumors occurs as a result of DNA amplification and does not occur as a result of post-transcriptional regulation.

The Biochemistry of Cancer

I. Cell Cycle

A. Cells destined to **divide** into two identical daughter cells normally progress through a sequence of duplicating the cell contents (**interphase**), nuclear division (**mitosis**), and cytoplasmic division (**cytokinesis**).

B. G_0 is the **quiescent state** in which cells, which are not in the process of cellular division, are maintained.

> 1. At this point, the cells contain the **diploid number of genetic material (2n)**, where n represents the number of homologous chromosomes, which number **23 in humans.**
> 2. These cells **express proteins** required for cellular housekeeping as well as proteins required to perform the specialized function of that cell type.

C. Interphase

> 1. **Interphase is the period between cell divisions**, which is further divided into the following distinct periods: gap 1, synthesis, and gap 2 (Figure 23-1).
> 2. G_1 **(gap 1):** Point of entry for cells to divide. A time of intense messenger RNA **(mRNA) transcription** for the production of proteins required to produce a full complement for the **resultant two daughter cells,** as well as producing all the proteins required for the **duplication of the genome.**
> 3. **S (synthesis):** Results in the **semiconservative replication** of cellular DNA with the production of two copies of the cellular DNA (**4n**).
> 4. G_2 **(gap 2):** The cell prepares for cell division with further protein and organelle synthesis. Also, the integrity of the **replicated DNA is assessed** prior to proceeding to mitosis.

D. Mitosis (see Figure 23-1)

> 1. The process of nuclear division further broken into the following microscopically discernable stages: prophase, metaphase, anaphase, and telophase.
> 2. *Prophase* is the initial stage of the process of mitosis encompassing the following changes:
>> a. **Chromosomes** can be identified with the condensation of the newly replicated chromatin. This is promoted by the phosphorylation of histone H1.

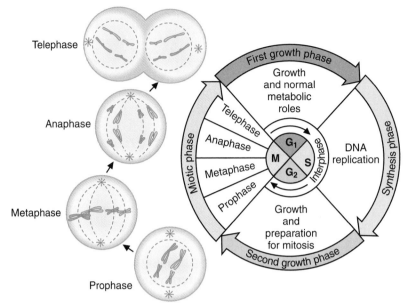

Figure 23-1 Diagram displaying the phases of the cell cycle along with the cellular changes associated with each stage of mitosis.

   b. The organization network of structural proteins, known as the **centrioles**, begins moving to opposite poles of the cell.
   c. Breakdown of proteins known as **lamins**, results in dissolution of the nuclear membrane, as the genetic material will be segregated to opposite sides of the cell during the division process.
 3. *Metaphase* is the most distinctively visualized stage (see Figure 23-1).
   a. Duplicated genetic material, **sister chromatids**, line up along the **equatorial plane** of the cell.
   b. Cytoskeletal elements **radiating from the polar centrioles** connect to the junction between the two sister chromatids, the **kinetochores.**
 4. *Anaphase* is the "action" stage of the process.
   a. Separation of the two sister chromatids occurs by movement toward the polar centrioles on the network of cytoskeletal elements.

> *cc 23.1* The chemotherapy agent paclitaxel **(Taxol)** prevents the **cytoskeletal** remodeling required to complete the migration of the replicate chromatids to the cell poles for the formation of replicated daughter cells. It is an important agent in the treatment of many cancers, including breast cancer.

   b. This process is simultaneous for all chromosomes, ensuring the **segregation of equal genetic material** (2n) to the daughter cells.
 5. *Telophase*
   a. **Decondensation of chromosomes** occurs, with the return of less highly organized chromatin.
   b. A new nuclear membrane is formed encapsulating the newly divided daughter genomes.
   c. **Cytokinesis**, the final step in telophase as well as cell division, requires **the pinching off of the plasma membrane** and the formation of two separate membrane-bound daughter cells.

II. Control of the Cell Cycle

A. The progression of the cell cycle

1. This progression is orchestrated through an elaborate series of check points.
2. They are mediated by interactions between proteins such as cyclins, cyclin-dependent kinases (CDKs), and cyclin-dependent kinase inhibitors (CDK-Is).

B. The entry into the cell cycle

1. *The $G_0 \to G_1$ transition* (Figure 23-2)
   a. Cells in the G_0 phase may remain so **indefinitely** as in the case of **neuronal or cardiac muscle cells** or, under certain circumstances, may enter into the cell cycle (as is often the case with epithelial **cells of the gastrointestinal tract**).
   b. The transition of cells from $G_0 \to G_1$ is contingent on the presence of one or more **growth factors,** which are produced when cells of a certain type are required.
2. *The $G_1 \to S$ transition* (see Figure 23-2)
   a. The boundary between the G_1 and S phase is often referred to as the **restriction point.** Once cells traverse this boundary, the cell is committed to completion of the S phase.
   b. **Cyclin D** levels begin to rise late in G_1 and bind to constitutively expressed **CDK4 and CDK6.**
   c. CDK4 and CDK6 **phosphorylate cyclin D,** which, together as cyclin D–CDK4 or cyclin D–CDK6 complexes, **phosphorylate** the nuclear **retinoblastoma (Rb) protein.**
   d. **Rb** protein is normally bound to and **inhibits transcription factor E2F,** which is **released when Rb is phosphorylated** by the cyclin–CDK complexes.
   e. E2F then is free of its Rb-mediated repression, resulting in the **activation of genes** required for **cell cycle progression.**
   f. The progression of the cell cycle can be inhibited by a family of the **CDK inhibitors, p21, p27, and p57.**
3. *The $G_2 \to M$ transition* (see Figure 23-2)
   a. With the continued growth of the G_2 phase, a group of cyclins, predominantly **cyclin A and cyclin B,** begin to accumulate.

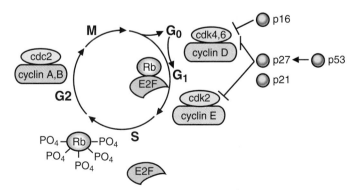

Figure 23-2 Diagram displaying the multiple proteins involved in the transitions between various points in the cell cycle.

    b. Cyclin A associates with **CDK1** and **CDK2,** which form activated complexes required for progression through the cell cycle.

    c. Targets of the G_2 phase CDKs include **topoisomerase,** which, when phosphorylated, results in **condensation of chromosomes** and phosphorylation of **lamins** with the fragmentation of the nuclear membrane.

C. Progression through the various phases of mitosis requires the phosphorylation of numerous proteins, primarily by the cyclin B–CDK1 complex.

III. Oncogenes

A. When expressed **normally in growth and development,** oncogenes are referred to as **proto-oncogenes.**

    1. The aberrant expression of oncogenes results in entry of the cell into the cell cycle with **abnormal cell growth,** suggesting a **gain of function.**

    2. There are several classes of such genes, which perturb cell growth through a variety of mechanisms.

B. Growth factors

    1. Aberrant production of these proteins or response to the signals they elicit (in cells normally in the G_0 phase) **can result in aberrant transition from $G_0 \rightarrow G_1$, with subsequent uncontrolled growth.**

    2. *Growth factors*

      a. Overexpression of a member of these **polypeptide growth hormones** stimulates the proliferation of restricted cell types, leading to their aberrant growth.

      b. Fibroblast growth factors (FGFs) is a family of proteins that is normally expressed during the proliferation of cells required for **normal wound healing,** but overexpression can lead to tumor formation.

      c. Platelet-derived growth factor (PDGF) is a polypeptide that is normally important for **extracellular matrix production,** but overexpression may result in proliferation as a result of **autocrine stimulation.**

    3. *Growth factor receptors*

      a. The normal binding of growth factors to their receptors results in signal transduction in response to receptor dimerization.

      b. Several growth factor receptors have been identified that are capable of **activation, even in the absence of specific ligand.** Many of these receptors have intracellular domains that function as **tyrosine kinases.**

      c. Epidermal growth factor (EGF) **receptors** (EGFR): There are at least three members of the family of tyrosine kinase receptors, *erb* **b-1,** *erb* **b-2,** and *erb* **b-3,** which, when mutated, lead to errant signaling and growth in the absence of the cognate ligand.

cc **23.2** Overexpression of the growth factor receptor *erb* **b-1,** also known as **HER2/neu,** is associated with the development of breast cancers. Patients who **overexpress HER2** (human epidermal growth factor receptor 2) in their breast tumors can be treated with a monoclonal antibody to HER2, trastuzumab **(Herceptin),** which blocks signaling through this oncogenic pathway.

> *cc* 23.3 **Gefitinib (Iressa)** is an orally active small-molecule **inhibitor of the EGFR tyrosine kinase** currently used in the treatment of non–small-cell **carcinoma of the lung** and is being actively explored in the treatment of other cancers.

    d. Rearranged during Transfection (RET): Although this tyrosine kinase receptor does not directly bind growth factors, it is important in the transduction of a signal upon binding of glial cell line–derived neurotrophic factor (GDNF), with mutations resulting in autonomous growth-promoting signals in the absence of ligand binding.

> *cc* 23.4 **Mutations in RET** are commonly associated with **multiple endocrine neoplasia (MEN) syndromes,** including **MEN1,** which is characterized by pancreatic, pituitary, and parathyroid tumors, and **MEN2,** which is characterized by adrenal, thyroid, and parathyroid tumors.

C. Signal Transducing Proteins

    1. The next level at which defects in cell growth and development can occur is at the level of **downstream signal transduction** proteins. Two such examples are given: the ras gene and nonreceptor tyrosine kinase proteins.

    2. The **ras gene** (Figure 23-3)

        a. A guanine triphosphate (GTP)–**binding protein** anchored to the **inner cell membrane** via a covalently attached **farnesyl moiety.**

            (1) In the **inactive state,** Ras binds guanosine diphosphate (GDP).

            (2) In stimulation of the cell by growth factor–ligand interactions, Ras **exchanges GTP for GDP,** leading to activation of downstream signaling events.

        b. The Ras protein has **intrinsic GTPase activity,** terminating the signal transduction events when **GTP is hydrolyzed back to GDP,** returning Ras to its **inactive** state.

> *cc* 23.5 **Ras** is the **most commonly mutated oncogene in cancer,** with 10–20% of tumors harboring mutations in ras. Ras mutations are found in a large number of tumors of the colon, pancreas, and thyroid.

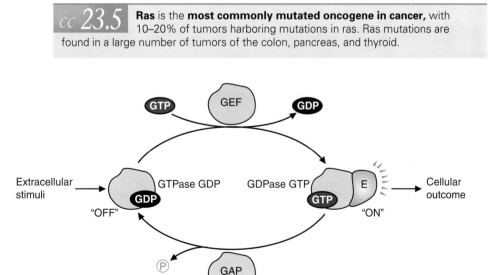

Figure 23-3   Molecular control of ras activation. Note the presence of the GTPase-activating protein (GAP), of which neurofibromatosis (NF)-1 is an example.

3. Another important grouping of signaling molecule is the **nonreceptor tyrosine kinase proteins.**
   a. These proteins include molecules such as the proto-oncogenes **abl** and **src.**
   b. These proteins function as **intermediaries** in signal transduction pathways resulting in the promoters of cellular growth.

D. **Nuclear transcription proteins**

1. These transcription proteins, such as the proto-oncogene **myc**, integrate divergent growth-promoting pathways and ultimately lead to the production of proteins that allow the cell to advance through the cell cycle.
2. Nuclear transcription factors contain amino acid sequences dictating three-dimensional motifs such as **helix-loop-helix, leucine zipper,** and **zinc finger domains,** which allow them **to bind to DNA.**

> *cc* **23.6** The nuclear transcription protein **WT-1,** coded for on chromosome **11p13,** is mutated in **Wilms tumors.** Wilms tumors are the most common **tumors of the kidney** in children.

3. Such genes are **rapidly induced** when quiescent cells receive signals to divide and are rapidly translocated to the nucleus to mediate **gene transcription.**

E. **Cell cycle regulators**

1. Alterations in the normal function of cyclins, CDKs, and inhibitors often results in unchecked cell growth.
2. **Cyclin D:** Increased expression of this regulator of the $G_1 \rightarrow S$ **transition** is commonly found in tumors.
3. **CDK4:** This regulator is among the most commonly altered genes in this class of genes.
4. **CDK inhibitors:** Alterations in the CDK-Is **p16, p21,** and **p27** are all found in various cancers.

IV. Tumor-Suppressor Genes

A. **Tumor-suppressor genes are cellular proteins,** which when lost, result in uncontrolled cell growth.

B. **Cell surface molecules**

1. **There are numerous cell surface molecules that antagonize normal cell growth and development.**
2. **Transforming growth factor (TGF)-β receptor** mediates its inhibitory effects by stimulating the production of CDK-Is.
3. The protein product of the deleted in colon carcinoma (DCC) gene regulates cell growth through the integration of signals from the cellular environment.

C. **Molecules that regulate signal transduction**

1. These molecules possess an antagonistic role to the actions of intracellular proto-oncogenes.

2. **Neurofibromatosis (NF)-1** gene product and **GTPase-activating protein** (GAP) activates **the GTPase function of Ras,** converting GTP to GDP and **suppressing** the growth-promoting function of **ras** (see Figure 23-3).

> *cc* **23.7** **von Recklinghausen disease,** which is also known as **neurofibromatosis-1,** results from **mutations of NF-1.** This **autosomal recessive** disorder results in the development of **café-au-lait spots,** as well as multiple tumors of the peripheral nerve sheath (**schwannomas**) and tumors of the 7th cranial nerve (**acoustic neuromas**).

3. **Adenomatous polyposis coli (APC)** gene product promotes the **degradation of β-catenin,** which otherwise normally translocates to the nucleus to induce cellular proliferation.

> *cc* **23.8** **Familial adenomatous polyposis (FAP)** syndromes result from mutations of the APC gene located on **chromosome 5.** Such patients have a **100% chance** of developing **colon cancer.**

D. **Molecules that regulate nuclear transcription**

1. Several tumor-suppressor genes residing in the nucleus encode proteins that play an important role in the integration of growth-promoting and growth-inhibiting signals.
2. The **retinoblastoma (Rb)** gene, as discussed, is an important negative regulator of cell growth.

> *cc* **23.9** Patients with **retinoblastoma (Rb) mutation** are prone to the development of **tumors of the retina** early in life and **osteosarcomas** of the bone later in life.

3. **p53** has an important gate-keeper role in cellular proliferation.
   a. p53 is **induced when DNA is damaged** by irradiation, ultraviolet (UV) light, or chemical mutagenesis.
   b. p53 then exerts its growth-inhibitory function in one of two ways to assure adequate **repair of the damaged DNA before proceeding through the cell cycle.**
      (1) p53 induces the transcription of the **CDK-I p21,** which **inhibits** the CDK/cyclin-mediated **phosphorylation of Rb** required for the cell to transition to the S phase.
      (2) If DNA damage inflicted upon the cell cannot be successfully repaired, **p53 mediates the transcription of genes implicated in the process of programmed cell death, or apoptosis** (see cc 23.10 and cc 23.11).

> *cc* **23.10** Mutations in the tumor-suppressor gene, **p53,** are the **most common molecular alterations in cancer,** with over 50% of human tumors harboring mutations in p53.

> *cc* **23.11** **Germline mutations in p53** result in **Li-Fraumeni syndrome.** Patients in families with a history of Li-Fraumeni syndrome inherit one mutant copy of p53 in their cells, thereby requiring only one sporadic mutation in their other allele to develop cancer. These patients develop sarcomas, breast cancers, tumors of the central nervous system, and leukemias at an increased frequency and decreased age compared with normal individuals.

V. Apoptosis

A. Apoptosis is defined as the programmed destruction of the cell.

1. It is characterized by a decrease in cell volume, mitochondrial destabilization, chromatin condensation with nuclear fragmentation, and cellular dispersion into fragmented apoptotic bodies without the release of cellular material.
2. Apoptosis is the **endpoint of a cascade** of converging events that **results in cell death.**
   a. **Growth factor withdrawal** occurs with the activation of the proto-oncogene myc in conditions of sparse nutrients in the cellular milieu.
   b. Signals are provided by the **pro-apoptotic cytokines,** tumor necrosis factor **(TNF),** and **Fas ligand,** whose receptors stimulate the activation of pro-apoptotic enzymes, **caspases.**

> *cc* **23.12** Agents such as **infliximab (Remicade)** and **etanercept (Enbrel)** are biologic agents that are used in the treatment of **autoimmune diseases.** These drugs trigger TNF receptors on autoreactive immune cells, inducing these cells to undergo apoptosis.

   c. Activation of the **pro-apoptotic gene Bax** by the tumor-suppressor gene p53 occurs if DNA mutations detected during the G_1/S checkpoint cannot be repaired with adequate fidelity.

B. Terminal events in the process of apoptosis

1. The release of the electron transport chain protein **cytochrome c** located on the outer mitochondrial membrane is a **critical regulator** in the process of apoptosis.
   a. Cytochrome c is normally prevented from translocating out of the mitochondria by the **anti-apoptotic gene, bcl-2** (Figure 23-4).
   b. The exiting of cytochrome c occurs via the mitochondrial channel protein **Bax.**
   c. The **relative abundance of *bcl*-2 and Bax** determines the ultimate fate of the cell.
   d. If **Bax predominates,** cytochrome c is liberated through the channel and associates with the cytoplasmic molecule, pro-apoptotic protease activating factor (**Apaf-1**).

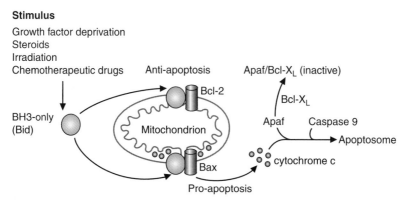

Figure 23-4 Pathways in the process of apoptosis. Apaf, pro-apoptotic protease activating factor.

e. Apaf-1 then activates a **cascade of proteolytic events** via the activation of **caspases.**

2. **Caspases** contain both "C" (**cysteine**) and "aspase" (**aspartic acid**) **protease activity,** and once activated, they begin the apoptotic cascade.

a. Caspases normally exist in the cytoplasm as inactive **zymogens** until stimulated through any of the major pathways triggering apoptosis.

b. Caspases degrade intracellular proteins and **activate DNases**, with resultant DNA fragmentation, or **DNA laddering**, which is characteristic of apoptosis.

C. The normal programmed cell death pathway, when perturbed, can also result in the **accumulation of cells and uncontrolled cell growth.**

VI. Mechanism of Oncogenesis

A. Numerous mechanisms exist to create the genetic changes that result in uncontrolled cell growth.

B. Point mutations

1. Point mutations are changes in the individual nucleotides in the gene encoding either proto-oncogenes or tumor-suppressor genes that can result in cancer.

2. **Ras: Mutations in codon 12** of the ras proto-oncogene results in the **loss of GTPase activity.** This results in continuous activation and the conversion to an oncogene.

3. **p53:** A wide spectrum of point mutations have been reported, and most **compromise the ability to survey the integrity of the replicate genome** during the cell cycle, with gradual increase in **additional mutations** in other critical regulators of cell growth.

C. Chromosomal translocations

1. Such translocations occur during chromosomal replication, with whole segments of different chromosomes becoming aberrantly attached and fused, resulting in two distinct mechanisms of aberrant growth factor production.

2. *Insertional inactivation*

a. Insertional activation results when normally tightly **regulated growth-promoting genes** come under the control of the regulatory elements of **constitutively expressed** genes due to the close proximity resulting from the **repositioning of chromosomal elements** not normally in juxtaposition.

b. Insertional activation is illustrated by the **t(8;14)** translocation with the expression of the **myc** oncogene (normally **on chromosome 8**), under the control of the immunoglobulin **(Ig) gene** promoter (normally on **chromosome 14**).

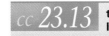 **t(8;14)** is associated with the development of high-grade **Burkitt lymphoma,** a type of B-cell malignancy.

c. Similarly, the **t(14;18)** translocation results in the control of the anti-apoptotic gene, **bcl-2,** (normally on **chromosome 18**) by the regulators of the **Ig gene** (**chromosome 14**).

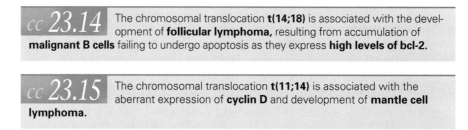

cc 23.14 The chromosomal translocation **t(14;18)** is associated with the development of **follicular lymphoma,** resulting from accumulation of **malignant B cells** failing to undergo apoptosis as they express **high levels of bcl-2.**

cc 23.15 The chromosomal translocation **t(11;14)** is associated with the aberrant expression of **cyclin D** and development of **mantle cell lymphoma.**

3. *Chimeric protein formation*
   a. This results when the reading frame of a protein becomes fused, in-frame, with that of another protein by virtue of a genetic rearrangement between chromosomes.
   b. **bcr-abl** fusion protein results for the translocation between **chromosomes 9 and 22**, with the formation of the **Philadelphia chromosome.**

   cc 23.16 **Chronic myelogenous leukemia** (CML), a hematopoietic malignancy of nearly mature cells of the myeloid lineage (i.e., neutrophils) results from the **t(9;22) translocation.**

   (1) The resultant protein, **p210**, is derived from the fusion of the proto-oncogene **c-abl** (from **chromosome 9**) and the **bcr** gene (from **chromosome 22**).
   (2) p210 **abl** is a potent tyrosine kinase with **50-fold greater activity of the normal gene**, resulting in dramatic cell cycle progression.

   cc 23.17 **Imatinib (Gleevec)** is a recently developed **tyrosine kinase inhibitor** that inhibits the active site of the **p210** gene and is used in the treatment of **CML.** It has also been found to inhibit the receptor tyrosine kinase c-Kit, which is overexpressed in some gastrointestinal stromal tumors. It is one of the first drugs developed solely based on rational drug design.

   c. Other such translocations are known to occur between multiple transcription factors, resulting in inappropriate protein production and subsequent cell growth.

   cc 23.18 The translocation **t(15;17)** results in a mutant form of **the retinoic acid receptor** that blocks white blood cell differentiation, leading to an accumulation of immature cells and the development of a form of **acute myelogenous leukemia (AML).**

4. *Gene amplification*
   a. Defined as overexpression of proto-oncogenes, gene amplification can result from aberrant duplication of their DNA sequences, often resulting in several hundred copies of the proto-oncogene and in abnormal growth.
   b. These duplicated regions can be seen on the chromosome as **homogeneous staining regions (HSRs).**

   cc 23.19 **Breast cancers** are routinely screened for the presence of an **amplified HER2/neu oncogene.** HER2/neu expression has been associated with a **poor prognosis.** However, patients with HER2/neu overexpression are candidates for **Herceptin therapy.**

c. In the event that the HSRs cause genetic instability, these amplified regions form **double minute (dm) chromosomes.**

> *cc 23.20* **N-*myc,*** which is normally found on **chromosome 2,** is often **grossly amplified** in one of the most common pediatric solid tumors, **neuro-blastoma.** Up to 300 copies of the N-*myc* gene have been found both as HSRs and dms. **N-*myc* amplifications carry a poor prognosis in neuroblastoma.**

VII. Molecular Carcinogenesis

A. As cells proceed through the multiple rounds of division during the growth and maintenance of the organism, mistakes in the replication of the genome are inevitable. As the cell is subjected to insults, such as chemicals, radiant energy, or viruses, the normal DNA repair mechanisms may become overwhelmed, leading to the chemical changes that result in mutations.

B. Chemical carcinogenesis

1. Both natural and synthetic compounds are capable of damaging cells either directly, after being acted upon by the cell, or in synergy with other chemicals (Table 23-1).

TABLE 23-1	*Association of Environmental and Industrial Exposures with Various Cancers*	
	Substance	Cancer
cc 23.21	Aniline dyes	Bladder cancer
cc 23.22	Asbestos	Mesotheliomas
cc 23.23	Radon	Lung cancer
cc 23.24	Arsenic	Skin cancer
cc 23.25	Chromium and nickel	Lung cancer
cc 23.26	Vinyl chloride	Angiosarcoma of the liver
cc 23.27	Diethylstilbestrol (DES)	Vaginal cancer
cc 23.28	Nitrosamines (food preservatives)	Stomach cancer

2. *Initiators*
   a. These compounds cause direct damage to cellular macromolecules, but their effects are not sufficient, in and of themselves, for tumor formation.
   b. Direct acting compounds are usually **highly reactive electrophiles,** such as **alkylating agents,** that **form adducts** with various cellular components (DNA, RNA, proteins, or lipids).

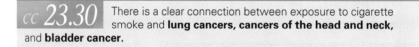

| *CC 23.29* | **Aflatoxin B$_1$** is associated with the development of the most common cancer worldwide, **liver cancer.** This substance is produced by molds that grow on desperately needed grains that are consumed by developing nations. |

   c. Indirect acting compounds (procarcinogens)
      (1) This larger group requires enzymatic activation to produce an **ultimate carcinogen.**
      (2) This enzymatic conversion is often the product of the **P450 monooxygenase system.**
      (3) Such enzyme systems are capable of transforming **polyaromatic hydrocarbons,** such as **benzopyrene,** into a reactive species that binds to GC base pairs in DNA, creating **distortions in the helical structure** of DNA.

| *CC 23.30* | There is a clear connection between exposure to cigarette smoke and **lung cancers, cancers of the head and neck,** and **bladder cancer.** |

3. *Promoters*
   a. These compounds are noncarcinogenic but facilitate the abnormal growth of cells that have been exposed to initiators.
   b. These compounds facilitate tumor formation by **stimulating proliferation of the cell mutated by the initiator.**

C. Radiation carcinogenesis

   1. DNA and other macromolecules are capable of being damaged by different wavelengths of electromagnetic radiation including both ultraviolet (UV) and ionizing radiation.
   2. UV radiation from the sun is responsible for causing mutations in DNA by the formation of **dimers between two adjacent pyrimidines (thymine dimers),** which must be removed for normal replication to proceed.
   3. Ionizing radiation: High-energy radiation (**x-rays and γ rays**) causes direct damage **to DNA** and **creates highly reactive hydroxyl and hydrogen radicals** that further interact with various cellular macromolecules.

D. Viral carcinogenesis

   1. Viruses, both DNA and RNA, have evolved numerous strategies for promoting the aberrant growth of their host cell types.
   2. *DNA viruses*
      a. Human papilloma virus (HPV): Members of this family are capable of causing **abnormal cell cycle progression** as the HPV **viral E6 protein binds** to and facilitates the degradation of **cellular p53,** whereas another viral protein **E7 perturbs** the normal function of the protein **Rb.**

cc **23.31** HPVs, particularly the more aggressive subtypes **HPV 16 and HPV 18,** are closely associated with the development of **cervical cancers.** The development of the **Papanicolaou (Pap) smear** to detect abnormal cervical cells has expedited the screening for cervical cancer, dramatically improving the early detection and treatment of this previous leading gynecologic malignancy.

b. **Epstein-Barr virus (EBV)** causes abnormal accumulation of cells through the production of the protein **LMP-1,** which promotes the expression of **bcl-2,** leading to protection from the normal **apoptotic pathways** that trigger cell death.

cc **23.32** EBV is associated with several malignant conditions including Burkitt lymphoma, Hodgkin lymphoma, and nasopharyngeal carcinoma (especially in Southeast Asia).

c. **Hepatitis B virus (HBV):** Although this virus does not encode any known oncoproteins, its association with human liver cancer has been clearly demonstrated as most likely multifactorial.

cc **23.33** HBV is the leading cause of **hepatocellular carcinoma** worldwide. It is believed that the repeated viral damage to liver cells followed by regeneration leads to increased accumulation of mutations, which culminates in the development of liver cancer. As mentioned before, **aflatoxin B_1** also promotes hepatocellular pathology and, along with HBV, works as **co-carcinogen,** synergistically increasing the development of liver cancer.

3. *RNA viruses*
   a. RNA **retroviruses** have clearly demonstrated a link to carcinogenesis through two distinct mechanisms.
   b. **Insertional activation** occurs when viral regulatory elements come **in juxtaposition with cellular proto-oncogenes** upon **retroviral integration,** resulting in aberrant expression of host cell genes and leading to uncontrolled growth.

cc **23.34** **Human T-cell lymphotrophic virus (HTLV)-1** is an oncogenic RNA virus. HTLV-1 plays a causative role in the development of a rare set of human T-cell **leukemias and lymphomas.**

   c. **Viral oncogenes:** Some animal retroviruses contain **viral homologues (v-oncs)** of normal **cellular proto-oncogenes (c-oncs),** which, when expressed in high levels, lead to cellular transformation.

VIII. DNA Repair and Carcinogenesis

A. The cell has evolved several mechanisms for the **repair of DNA** damaged by the multitudes of insults encountered in the environment. Multiple proteins exist to correct such errors in two major DNA repair pathways (Table 23-2).

B. Nucleotide excision repair

1. This repair mechanism is responsible for **surveying the topology of the DNA double helix** and **removing such local distortions.**

TABLE 23-2	Hereditary DNA Repair Defect Syndromes		
	Genetic Syndrome	**Defective Repair System**	**Associated Malignancies**
cc 23.35	Ataxia telangiectasia	DNA damage as a result of **ionizing radiation**	T-cell leukemias and lymphomas
cc 23.36	Bloom syndrome	DNA damage as a result of **UV exposure**	Skin cancers
cc 23.37	Fanconi anemia	DNA cross-linking repair with sensitivity to **nitrogen mustards**	Nonlymphoid hemato-poietic malignancies
cc 23.38	Li-Fraumeni syndrome	Germline mutations in **p53**	Multiple cancers, especially neoplasms of breast, soft tissue, and central nervous system
cc 23.39	Hereditary non-polyposis colon carcinoma (HNPCC)	Defect in **DNA mismatch repair**	Colon cancer as well as other gastrointestinal malignancies
cc 23.40	Xeroderma pigmentosum	DNA damage due to **UV-induced thymidine dimers**	Skin and ocular cancers

UV = ultraviolet.

2. This occurs through endonuclease cleavage of the damaged bases and restoration of the original segment through the concerted actions of a DNA polymerase **using the intact strand as a template,** to correct the complementary strand.

C. **Mismatch repair**

1. Sometimes during replication, DNA polymerases insert nucleotides that defy the normal **Watson-Crick base pairing** (i.e., a G may pair with a T instead of the normal A to T pairing.)
2. Such "misspellings" need to be recognized and corrected before perpetuation of the error to the next round of division.

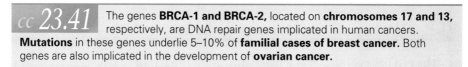

cc 23.41   The genes **BRCA-1 and BRCA-2,** located on **chromosomes 17 and 13,** respectively, are DNA repair genes implicated in human cancers. **Mutations** in these genes underlie 5–10% of **familial cases of breast cancer.** Both genes are also implicated in the development of **ovarian cancer.**

IX. Molecular Progression of Cancer

A. Many genetic alterations are required for the approximately **10^9 tumor cells required to form 1 gram of tissue mass,** which corresponds to the smallest clinically detectable mass.

1. Every human cancer reveals the **activation of several oncogenes and the loss of two or more tumor-suppressor genes.**
2. This is evidenced in the molecular model of colon carcinogenesis known as the adenoma-carcinoma sequence (Figure 23-5).

B. Tumor growth

1. Numerous variables contribute to the growth of transformed cells.
2. *Growth factors*
   a. Many tumors require the presence of various **hormones or other growth factors** to fuel the growth of the tumor mass.
   b. The lack of such factors retards the developing mass.

> cc *23.42* **Breast cancers** are often responsive to estrogens. Therefore, once breast cancers have been shown to express **estrogen receptors,** the estrogen antagonist **tamoxifen** is often used as anti-hormonal therapy in such patients.

3. *Angiogenesis*
   a. Tumor cell growth requires the presence of nutrients and oxygen and due to normal diffusion limits, tumors can only grow to a thickness of **approximately 2 mm without a nutrient supply.**
   b. As such, **hypoxic conditions** elicit the production of **angiogenic molecules,** such as **vascular endothelial growth factor (VEGF),** which promotes vascularization of the growing tumor mass.

> cc *23.43* **Avastin** is a monoclonal antibody that **inhibits VEGFs,** thus inhibiting new blood vessel formation. Avastin is used in the treatment of **colon cancer**

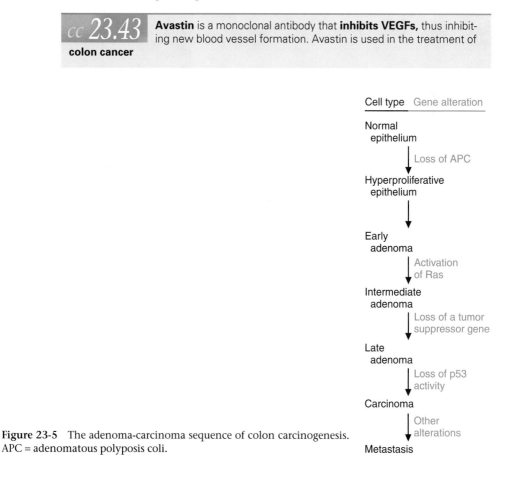

Figure 23-5 The adenoma-carcinoma sequence of colon carcinogenesis. APC = adenomatous polyposis coli.

C. Invasion

1. In order to disseminate throughout the body, the cancer must gain access to the circulation. This requires **breaking through the basement membrane**, the thick extracellular matrix that separates tissue layers.
2. Such steps are facilitated by the rendering of various proteases, such as **matrix metalloproteases (MMPs)**, **cathepsin D** (a cysteine protease), and **urokinase-type plasminogen activator** (a serine protease).

D. Metastasis. Once in the circulation, tumor cells alter the expression of adhesion molecules, allowing them to deposit as **"seeds"** to distant sites, which serve as the **"soil"** for continued growth of the transformed cells.

X. Molecular Markers in Cancer Biology

A. There are **numerous proteins** that are **overexpressed in cancer cells**. Some are actually capable of being detected in the serum of patients with specific cancers. Many of these proteins are simple markers and have no special significance with respect to the pathology of the disease.

B. It is important to note that many of these proteins lack either the specificity or sensitivity to use as screening tests. Their true utility is in monitoring the progression of the disease once confirmed or in monitoring therapy or recurrence (Table 23-3).

TABLE 23-3	*Molecular Markers in Cancer Biology*	
	Marker	Cancer
cc 23.44	Carcinoembryonic antigen (CEA)	Colon cancer
cc 23.45	Human chorionic gonadotropin (hCG)	Trophoblastic tumors; testicular tumors
cc 23.46	Calcitonin	Medullary carcinoma of the thyroid
cc 23.47	Catecholamines	Tumors of the adrenal cortex
cc 23.48	Prostate-specific antigen (PSA)	Prostate cancer
cc 23.49	Cancer antigen (CA)-125	Ovarian cancer
cc 23.50	CA 19-9	Pancreatic cancer
cc 23.51	α-Fetoprotein (AFP)	Liver cancer; testicular tumors

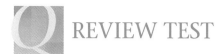

*Directions: Each of the numbered questions or incomplete statements in this section is followed by answers or by completions of the statement. Select the **one** lettered answer or completion that is **best** in each case.*

1. During which stage of mitosis are duplicated chromosomes found aligned along the equatorial plane of the cell?

(A) Prophase
(B) Metaphase
(C) Anaphase
(D) Telophase
(E) Interphase

2. During which phase of the cell cycle is cellular integrity assessed prior to mitosis?

(A) G_0
(B) G_1
(C) S
(D) G_2
(E) Interphase

3. Which of the following structures is the location of attachment for newly replicated sister chromatids to the cellular cytoskeleton?

(A) Centrioles
(B) Equatorial plane
(C) Diploid
(D) Kinetochore
(E) Telomere

4. Which family of proteases executes the final steps in the process of programmed cell death?

(A) Cyclins
(B) Caspases
(C) Telomerases
(D) Phosphorylases
(E) Kinases

5. Exit of which of the following molecules from the mitochondria precipitates the events of apoptosis?

(A) Pro-apoptotic protease activating factor (Apaf-1)
(B) Bax
(C) DNase
(D) Cytochrome c

(E) Vascular endothelial growth factor (VEGF)

6. Which of the following is the most commonly mutated oncogene in cancer?

(A) p53
(B) abl
(C) ras
(D) myc
(E) BRCA

7. Mutations in which of the following proteins accounts for the most common genetic alterations in the development of cancer?

(A) Ras
(B) RET (rearranged during transfection)
(C) bcl-2
(D) p53
(E) Wilms tumor (WT-1)

8. Which apoptosis-promoting protein functions antagonistically to the anti-apoptotic effects of bcl-2?

(A) Transforming growth factor (TGF)-β
(B) Bax
(C) Tumor necrosis factor (TNF)
(D) p210
(E) abl

9. Enzymes of which type are responsible of converting procarcinogens into ultimate carcinogens?

(A) P450 mono-oxygenases
(B) Caspases
(C) c-oncs
(D) Matrix metalloproteases
(E) Lamins

10. Which of the following molecules, produced by tumor cells in response to hypoxia, stimulates the formation of new blood vessels?

(A) Fas
(B) LMP-1

(C) VEGF
(D) TGF-β
(E) p210

11. A 56-year-old woman is recently diagnosed with breast cancer. She undergoes a lumpectomy and a lymph node dissection, which shows that there are tumor cells that have migrated to the lymph nodes. Her oncologist recommends chemotherapy including the agent paclitaxel (Taxol), which inhibits microtubules. During which phase of the cell cycle would this drug be most active?

(A) Cytokinesis
(B) Metaphase
(C) Anaphase
(D) Telophase
(E) Interphase

12. A 47-year-old man, with no known family history of cancer, develops changes in his bowel habits, including pencil caliber stools with occasional blood in the stools. A colonoscopy and biopsy confirms the diagnosis of adenocarcinoma of the colon. Furthermore, the tumor is found to have mutation in the ras protein. Which of the following correctly describes this protein?

(A) A nonreceptor tyrosine kinase
(B) A nuclear transcription protein
(C) A polypeptide growth factor
(D) A receptor tyrosine kinase
(E) A guanosine triphosphate (GTP)–binding protein

13. A 7-year-old child presents to the pediatrician for the development of numerous pigmented lesion on his body (café-au-late spots). He also complains of difficulty hearing and ringing in his ears, for which a magnetic resonance imaging (MRI) scan confirms the presence in the cerebellopontine angle (acoustic neuroma). He is diagnosed with neurofibromatosis-1. The defective protein in this patient normally has which of the following functions?

(A) Activates the GTPase function of ras
(B) Integrates signals from the extracellular environment

(C) Mediates proliferation of cells during normal wound healing
(D) Acts as a transcription factor
(E) Is the primary regulator for the G_1 to S transition of the cell cycle

14. A 23-year-old woman develops a tumor of the soft tissue of her arm (sarcoma) and is being evaluated by an oncologist. On history, he learns that her older brother had leukemia when he was 12 years old. Furthermore, the patient's grandmother died of a brain tumor, and her aunt has breast cancer. With this clustering of tumors, the oncologist suspects Li-Fraumeni syndrome and orders molecular studies on the patient's tumor for which of the following genes?

(A) TNF
(B) p53
(C) WT-1
(D) Retinoblastoma (Rb)
(E) RET

15. A 53-year-old man presents to the physician because he is fatigued and "not feeling himself." The doctor orders a routine set of tests, which demonstrates a white blood cell count of 85,000/mL (normal, 3,000–10,000/mL). Molecular studies suggest that he has chronic myelogenous leukemia. Which of the following translocations is associated with this disorder?

(A) t(8;14)
(B) t(14;18)
(C) t(11;14)
(D) t(9;22)
(E) t(15;17)

16. A 35-year-old woman is found to have breast cancer. A core biopsy is sent for molecular studies to guide treatment. The pathology reports that the tumor is HER2/neu positive. Which of the following correctly describes HER2?

(A) A tumor-suppressor gene
(B) An anti-apoptotic gene
(C) A growth factor receptor
(D) A steroid hormone
(E) A cell cycle regulator

17. A 45-year-old man develops painless lymph node swelling. He sees a surgeon, who biopsies one of the lymph nodes. The pathology report returns indicating the presence of t(14;18), which is diagnostic for follicular lymphoma. The gene aberrantly expressed in this cancer, bcl-2, normally has which of the following functions?

(A) Prevents the exit of cytochrome c from the mitochondria
(B) Provides a channel for the exit of cytochrome c from the mitochondria
(C) Activates a cascade of events by activating caspases
(D) Cleaves intracellular proteins
(E) Functions as a DNAse

18. A 22-year-old woman, who has had much unprotected intercourse since the age of 12, visits a gynecologist for her first Pap smear. The results return positive for atypical cells, indicative of human papilloma virus (HPV) infection. Which of the following correctly describes HBV's effects on cell growth?

(A) Viral E7 degrades cellular p53
(B) Causes insertional inactivation of critical genes
(C) Viral E6 perturbs the normal function of cellular Rb
(D) Viral LMP-1 prevents the expression of cellular bcl-2
(E) Viral E6 degrades cellular p53

19. While on an aid mission to central Africa with Doctors Without Borders, a physician encounters a 23-year-old man with what appears to be metastatic liver cancer. The grain storage facility outside his village was found to be contaminated with aflatoxin B_1. In addition, which of the following might act as a co-carcinogen in the development of this patient's cancer?

(A) Human T-cell lymphotrophic virus (HTLV-1)
(B) Hepatitis B virus (HBV)
(C) Asbestos
(D) Vinyl chloride
(E) Aniline dyes

20. A 23-year-old woman is seen for a lump in her breast that she palpated on self-breast exam. You further learn that her mother and her aunt both had breast and ovarian cancer. Given this presentation, you suspect the patient may have a mutation in which of the following genes involved in DNA repair?

(A) BRCA-1
(B) Hereditary nonpolyposis colon carcinoma (HNPCC)
(C) Ataxia telangiectasia
(D) p53
(E) Rb

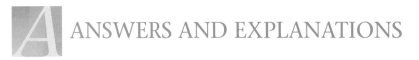

1–B. Duplicated chromosomes can be found at the center of the cell, the metaphase plate, attached to the spindle apparatus by the kinetochore.

2–D. The integrity of the DNA replicated during the S (synthesis) phase of the cell cycle is assessed during gap 2 (G_2). It is at this point that proteins such as p53 act to halt the cell, while DNA damage is corrected before mitosis is allowed to proceed.

3–D. Kinetochores are the structures that connect the two newly replicated sister chromatids. During metaphase, as the chromosomes line up along the equatorial plane, these kinetochores serve as the site of attachment for the cellular cytoskeleton. As mitosis progresses, the sister chromatids are pulled to opposite centrioles in the cell, resulting in even distribution of the cellular DNA.

4–B. Caspases are pro-enzymes that, once activated by the protein pro-apoptotic protease activating factor (Apaf-1), function as cysteine and aspartic acid proteases that digest intracellular proteins in response to pro-apoptotic signals.

5–D. The exit of cytochrome c from the mitochondria is an irreversible step in the apoptotic pathway. Normally, bcl-2 prevents the exit of cytochrome c from the inner mitochondria, thereby preventing apoptosis.

6–C. Ras is the most commonly mutated oncogene in cancer, whereas p53 mutations, a tumor-suppressor gene, are the most common genetic alterations found in cancer. It is important to realize that clinically apparent tumors have multiple genetic abnormalities including mutations in multiple oncogenes and tumor-suppressor genes.

7–D. Mutations on p53 are the most common genetic alterations in cancer. Known as the "guardian of the genome," p53 normally prevents the cell from replicating in light of DNA damage. Mutations in p53 are seen in over 50% of human cancers.

8–B. The pro-apoptotic protein Bax is a membrane ion-channel protein that allows the release of cytochrome c from the mitochondria, thereby irreversibly committing the cell to undergo apoptosis. The relative concentrations of bcl-2 and Bax are thought to determine the balance of pro- and anti-apoptotic signals.

9–A. Enzymes of the P450 mono-oxygenase family are responsible for metabolizing many endogenous as well as exogenous chemicals and drugs. Unfortunately, they are able to convert procarcinogens like benzopyrenes, which are found in cigarette smoke, into ultimate carcinogens. These oxidized compounds can then disrupt normal DNA, resulting in mutations.

10–C. Vascular endothelial growth factor (VEGF) is produced by normal tissue as well as tumor cells under hypoxic stress. Establishment of a vascular supply is critical for tumors to grow beyond a few cell layers.

11–C. The ability of paclitaxel (Taxol) to inhibit microtubule formation results in the cell being unable to complete anaphase appropriately. The replicated chromatids are unable to move to opposite ends of the cell for daughter cell formation. Metaphase occurs when the sister chromatids align on the equatorial plane. Telophase and cytokinesis are not completed if anaphase does not occur. Very few chemotherapy agents work during interphase.

12–E. Ras is a guanosine triphosphate (GTP)–binding protein, which is turned on when it is bound to GTP and shut off when it hydrolyzes GTP to guanosine diphosphate (GDP). Mutations that destroy this hydrolytic activity are among the most common in cancer, resulting in continuous growth-promoting signals. Abl and src are two nonreceptor tyrosine kinases, whereas the epidermal growth factor receptor is a receptor tyrosine kinase. Myc is an example of a nuclear transcription factor. Fibroblast growth factor is a typical example of a polypeptide growth factor implicated in cancer.

13–A. Neurofibromatosis-1 (NF-1) is a GTPase-activating protein (GAP), whose normal function is to promote the hydrolysis of GTP by ras, thereby shutting down ras signaling. Deleted in colon carcinoma (DCC) is an example of a gene that integrates signals from the extracellular environment. Fibroblast growth factor (FGF) has an important function in wound healing, and its aberrant expression is sometimes found in tumors. WT-1, the protein mutated in Wilms tumor, is a nuclear transcription factor. Cyclin D, which is mutated in some tumors, is the primary regulator of the G_1 to S transition of the cell cycle

14–B. Li-Fraumeni syndrome is a familial DNA repair syndrome caused by mutation in the tumor-suppressor gene p53. p53 is the most common genetic alteration in cancer, and patients with familial mutation have an increased predisposition to soft tissue neoplasms, leukemias, central nervous system tumors, and breast cancer. Tumor necrosis factor (TNF) is a pro-apoptotic molecule. WT-1 is muted in Wilms tumor, the most common malignancy of the kidney in children. Patients with hereditary retinoblastoma (Rb) mutations develop retinoblastoma and/or osteosarcomas. RET is mutated in patients with some thyroid tumor and those with multiple endocrine neoplasias (MEN).

15–D. Chronic myelogenous leukemia is associated with t(9;22), the Philadelphia chromosome, with the production of the aberrant bcr-abl protein. There are several other important chromosomal translocations associated with blood and lymph cancers, including t(8;14) found in Burkitt lymphoma, t(14;18) found in follicular lymphoma, t(11;14) found in mantle cell lymphoma, and finally, t(15;17) found in the M3 variant of acute myelogenous leukemia.

16–C. HER2/neu (human epidermal growth factor receptor 2) is a growth factor receptor that is sometimes overexpressed in breast cancer. Considered to be a marker of poor prognosis, patients who overexpress this protein can be treated with trastuzumab (Herceptin), which is a monoclonal antibody that blocks growth-promoting signals. p53 is a tumor-suppressor gene, whereas bcl-2 is an anti-apoptotic gene. Estrogen is a steroid hormone that is a growth factor for breast tumors that overexpress the receptor. Cyclin D is a cell cycle regulator that is aberrantly expressed in mantle cell lymphoma and other tumors.

17–A. Bcl-2 is an anti-apoptotic gene that prevents the exit of cytochrome c from the mitochondria. Overexpression of the gene, as in follicular lymphoma, results in accumulation of cells failing to undergo normal apoptosis. Other important players in apoptosis include Bax, which is a channel for the exit of cytochrome c from the mitochondria, and Apaf-1, which activates the various caspases. Activated caspases then cleave intracellular proteins, whereas DNAses cleave DNA.

18–E. Human papilloma virus (HPV) infection is a causative agent of cervical cancer and is acquired as a sexually transmitted disease. Its oncogenic potential is related to the viral E6 protein, which disrupts cellular growth by degrading cellular p53. The viral E7 perturbs the normal function of Rb. Retroviruses can cause cancer because they can cause insertional inactivation of key growth-controlling genes. The Ebstein-Barr virus (EBV) LMP-1 protein results in cancer through its ability to prevent the expression of bcl-2.

19–B. Hepatocellular carcinoma is the most common cancer in the world. Worldwide, hepatitis B virus (HBV) is a major contributor to the development of this cancer. It acts as a co-carcinogen with aflatoxin B_1. Human T-cell lymphotrophic virus (HTLV-1), a retrovirus related to human immunodeficiency virus (HIV), is associated with a form of leukemia/lymphoma. Asbestos, used as an insulator, is closely associated with a tumor of the pleural linings of the lung, a mesothelioma. Vinyl chloride is associated with a rare form of liver cancer, angiosarcoma. Finally, aniline dyes, used in the clothing industry, have been associated with bladder cancer.

20–A. BRCA-1 is a gene implicated in breast and ovarian cancer. Approximately 5% of breast cancers are due to mutations in this gene, and a strong family history of both breast and ovarian cancer is highly suspicion, especially in such a young patient. Hereditary nonpolyposis colon carcinoma (HNPCC) is associated with familial colon cancer. Patients with ataxia telangiectasia mutations have an increase in leukemias and lymphomas. p53 is a DNA repair gene; however, Rb is not.

Techniques in Biochemistry and Molecular Biology

I. Biotechnology Involving Recombinant DNA

A. **Strategies for obtaining copies of genes or fragments of DNA**

1. Short sequences of DNA (**oligonucleotides**) can be synthesized in vitro and used as **primers** for DNA synthesis or as **probes** for detection of DNA or RNA sequences.
2. Restriction endonucleases **cleave DNA into fragments.**
   a. Restriction endonucleases recognize short sequences in DNA and cleave both strands within this region (Figure 24-1).
   b. Most of the DNA sequences recognized by these enzymes are **palindromes** (i.e., both strands of DNA have the same base sequence in the 5′ to 3′ direction).
      (1) The enzyme *Eco*RI cleaves a region between an A and a G on each strand, generating two products.
      (2) The single-stranded regions of the products allow them to reanneal or to recombine with other DNA that has been cleaved by the same restriction endonuclease.
   c. A **DNA fragment**, which contains a **specific gene**, can be isolated from the cellular genome with restriction enzymes. Genes isolated from eukaryotic cells usually contain **introns,** whereas those from bacteria do not.
   d. The messenger RNA (**mRNA**) for a gene can be isolated, and a DNA copy (**cDNA**) can be produced by reverse transcriptase. cDNA does not contain introns.

B. **Techniques for identifying DNA sequences**

1. *Use of probes to detect specific DNA or RNA sequences*
   a. A **probe** is a single strand of DNA that can **hybridize (base pair)** with a complementary sequence on another single-stranded polynucleotide composed of DNA or RNA.
   b. The probe must contain a **label,** so that it can detect complementary DNA or RNA. The label may be radioactive (so it can be detected by autoradiography) or a chemical that can be identified, for example, by fluorescence.
2. *Gel electrophoresis of DNA*
   a. Gel electrophoresis **separates** DNA **chains** of varying length. Polyacrylamide gels can be used to separate short DNA chains that differ in length by only one nucleotide. Agarose gels separate chains of larger size.

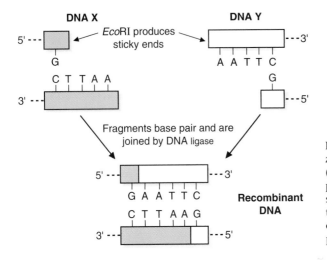

Figure 24-1 Action of restriction enzymes. *Eco*RI cleaves a palindrome (5'-GAATTC-3'). Two fragments are produced that contain complementary single-stranded regions (sticky ends). If two different DNAs (e.g., X and Y) are cleaved by *Eco*RI, the sticky ends can pair to form a recombinant DNA.

    b. Because DNA contains negatively charged phosphate groups, it will **migrate in an electric field toward the positive electrode.**

    c. Shorter chains migrate more rapidly through the pores of the gel, so **separation depends on length.**

    d. DNA **bands** in the gel can be **visualized** by various techniques, including staining with dyes (e.g., ethidium bromide) and autoradiography (if the gel contains a radioactive compound, which reacts with a photographic film). **Labeled probes** detect **specific DNA sequences.**

    e. **Blots** of gels can be made using nitrocellulose paper (Figure 24-2).

        (1) **Southern blots** are produced when a radioactive **DNA** probe hybridizes with **DNA** on a nitrocellulose blot of a gel.

> *cc 24.1* Southern blotting, named after Dr. Edward Southern, is a technique that can be used to detect mutations in DNA. It combines the use of DNA probes and restriction endonucleases.

        (2) **Northern blots** are produced when a radioactive **DNA** probe hybridizes with **RNA** on a nitrocellulose blot of a gel.

        (3) A **Western blot** is a related technique in which **proteins** are separated by gel electrophoresis and probed with **antibodies** that bind a specific protein.

  3. *DNA sequencing by the Sanger dideoxynucleotide method* (Figure 24-3)

    a. **Dideoxynucleotides** are added to solutions in which DNA polymerase is catalyzing polymerization of a DNA chain.

    b. Because a dideoxynucleotide does not contain a 3'-hydroxyl group, **polymerization of the chain is terminated** wherever a dideoxynucleotide is incorporated into the growing chain.

    c. Because the dideoxynucleotide competes with the normal nucleotide for incorporation into the growing chain, **DNA chains of varying lengths are produced.** The shortest chains are nearest the 5' end of the DNA chain (which grows 5' to 3').

    d. The sequence of the growing chain can be read (5' to 3') from the bottom to the top of the gel on which the DNA chains are separated.

  4. **DNA microarrays** or DNA chips produce a "genetic portrait" by screen for 1000s of genes simultaneously. cDNAs or oligonucleotides for different genes are spot-

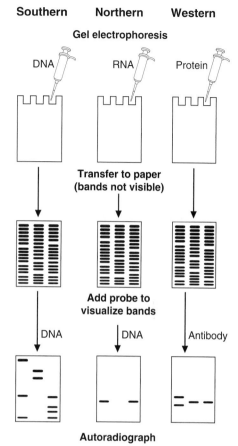

Figure 24-2   Southern, Northern, and Western blots. In Southern blots, DNA is electrophoresed, denatured with alkali, transferred to nitrocellulose paper ("blotted"), and hybridized with a DNA probe. In Northern blots, RNA is electrophoresed and hybridized with a DNA probe. (In this case, alkali is not used because RNA is already single stranded, and alkali would hydrolyze the RNA.) Western blots involve electrophoresis of proteins that are visualized by binding to antibodies. The nucleic acids and proteins can only be seen on the gel after the gel is treated with a labeled probe (i.e., labeled DNA or antibodies).

ted or arrayed individually in high density on a glass slide or on nitrocellulose paper (as blots described earlier). Probes (below) are hybridized to the microarray, and the amount of binding is quantified.
   a. Genotyping of **genomic DNA** can commence to detect mutations or polymorphisms.
   b. Gene expression uses **mRNA from two different sources** for a comparative analysis (e.g., normal vs. cancerous tissue). mRNA is converted to cDNA, and each population of cDNAs is labeled with a different fluorescent dye, mixed together, and hybridized to examine relative abundance of genes.

> *CC* **24.2**   **DNA microarrays** are used to predict response to cancer treatment. Analysis of **chronic lymphocytic leukemia (CLL)** identifies genes associated with pathogenesis, finding therapeutic targets and sensitivity or resistance to fludarabine or rituximab, which are two current treatments.

C.   **Techniques for amplifying DNA sequences**
   1.   *Polymerase chain reaction (PCR)*
      a. PCR is an **in vitro technique** used for rapidly producing large amounts of DNA (Figure 24-4).
      b. It is suitable for clinical or forensic testing because only a very small sample of DNA is required as the starting material.

A. Terminates with ddATP

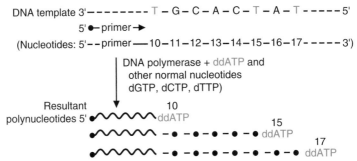

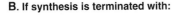

B. If synthesis is terminated with:

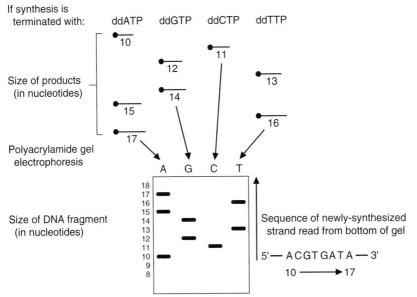

Figure 24-3 DNA sequencing by the dideoxynucleotide "Sanger" method. **(A)** A DNA template is hybridized with a primer. **(B)** DNA polymerase is added plus dATP, dGTP, dCTP, and dTTP. Either the primer or the nucleotides must have a radioactive label, so bands can be visualized on the gel by autoradiography. Samples are placed in each of four tubes, and one of the four dideoxyribonucleotides (ddNTPs) is added to each tube to cause random termination of DNA synthesis. Strands of different sizes are produced in each tube, electrophoresed, and visualized. The sequence of the newly synthesized strand is read from the bottom to the top of the gel.

> *cc* **24.3** **PCR** is used most often to detect **very low abundance nucleic acid transcripts. Human immunodeficiency virus (HIV),** with its long latency of infection, is difficult to test early after infection but can be detected with PCR. The technique is also used for detecting a three–base pair deletion, the most common mutation in **cystic fibrosis.**

2. *Cloning of DNA* (Figure 24-5)
   a. DNA from one organism ("foreign" DNA, obtained as described earlier) can be inserted into a DNA vector and used to transform cells from another organ-

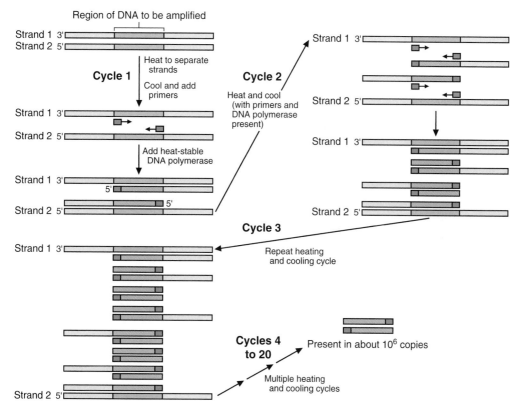

Figure 24-4 Polymerase chain reaction (PCR). The original DNA sample (strands 1 and 2) is denatured by heat. Primers (short, dark, green rectangles) are added that bind to each DNA strand when the solution is cooled. A heat-stable DNA polymerase (Taq) is added, and polymerization is allowed to proceed. The green areas represent the regions that are replicated by extension of the primers. Heating and cooling cycles are repeated until the DNA is amplified many times.

ism, usually a bacterium, that grows rapidly, replicating the foreign DNA as well as its own.

b. Large quantities of the foreign DNA can be isolated, or under the appropriate conditions, the DNA can be expressed, and its protein product can be obtained in large quantities.

D. Use of recombinant DNA techniques to detect polymorphisms

1. Humans differ in their genetic composition. **Polymorphisms** (variations in DNA sequences) occur frequently in the genome both in coding and in noncoding regions. Point mutations cause the simplest type of polymorphisms, but insertions and deletions of varying lengths also occur.

> *cc 24.4* Individual variations in DNA sequences among people occur at a frequency of approximately 1 per 1500 nucleotides. **Polymorphisms** are clinically harmless, whereas **mutations** can be detrimental and are associated with a clinical disorder.

2. *Restriction fragment length polymorphism (RFLP)*

a. Occasionally, a **mutation** occurs **in a restriction enzyme cleavage site** that is within or tightly linked to a gene.

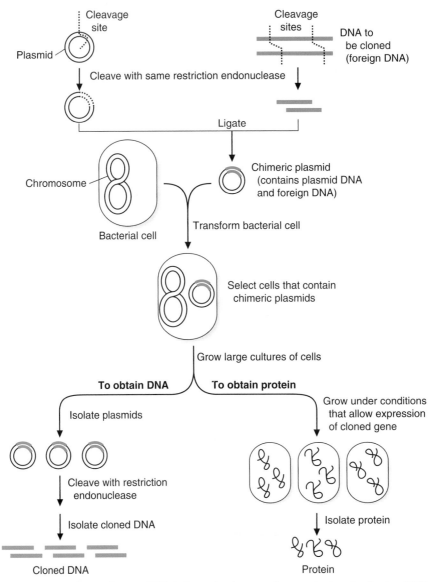

Figure 24-5 Cloning foreign DNA in bacteria. A vector for transferring the foreign DNA into the bacterium, such as a plasmid, is cleaved with the same restriction endonuclease as the foreign DNA. The plasmid and foreign DNA, both cleaved by the same restriction enzyme, are mixed together and treated with DNA ligase. Some interactions produce chimeric plasmids, containing the foreign DNA integrated into the plasmid DNA. The plasmids are introduced into bacterial host cells (transformation). Clones that contain the chimeric plasmid are selected and cultured. To obtain large quantities of the foreign DNA, the plasmids are isolated from cells and treated with the restriction enzyme to release the foreign DNA, which is then isolated. To obtain large quantities of the protein product of the foreign DNA, the cells are grown to promote synthesis of the protein, and the protein is isolated from the cells. The DNA used to express foreign proteins in bacterial cells must not contain introns because bacteria cannot remove them. Bacterial promoters must be inserted into the DNA so that the gene can be expressed.

(1) The enzyme can cleave the normal DNA at this site, but not the mutant.
(2) Thus, two smaller restriction fragments will be obtained from this region of the normal DNA, compared with only one larger fragment from the mutant.

> *cc 24.5* The classic **RFLP in prenatal disease screening** involves **sickle cell anemia.** A single nucleotide change (A → T) at codon 6 of β-globin results in a **Glu → Val** amino acid substitution, abolishing an *Mst*II restriction site. A β-globin gene probe detects different *Mst*II restriction fragments. RFLP analysis detects both the affected and unaffected alleles.

b. Sometimes, **a mutation creates a restriction site** that is not present in or near the normal gene. In this case, two smaller restriction fragments will be obtained from the mutant, and only one larger fragment will be obtained from the normal gene (Figure 24-6).

> *cc 24.6* RFLPs are considered alleles since they are heritable in a Mendelian manner. **Huntington's disease (HD)** is a progressive neurodegenerative disease with onset when patients reach their 40s. Before the human genome was sequenced, RFLP analyses identified an HD marker with appearance of 2 *Hind*III restriction sites.

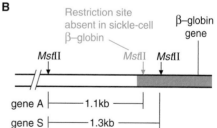

Figure 24-6 Restriction fragment length polymorphism (RFLP) is caused by loss of a restriction site. If a mutation occurs in a cleavage site for a restriction enzyme, the pattern of restriction fragments differs from normal. (A) The mutation that causes sickle cell anemia results in the loss of an *Mst*II site in the β-globin gene. (B) Samples of DNA from individuals are treated with restriction endonucleases and then subjected to electrophoresis on gels. (C) With the Southern blot technique, the restriction fragments on the gel are hybridized with a radioactive cDNA probe for the β-globin gene. The sickle cell allele produces a fragment of 1.3 kilobases (kb) when treated with *Mst*II. A normal allele produces a fragment of 1.1 kb (plus a fragment of 0.2 kb that is not seen on the gel). For a person with sickle cell disease, both alleles produce 1.3-kb restriction fragments. In a normal person, both alleles produce 1.1-kb fragments. For a carrier, both the 1.3- and 1.1-kb fragments are observed.

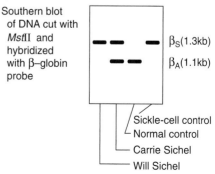

c. Normal human DNA has many regions that contain a highly **variable number of tandem repeats (VNTR).** The number of repeats differs from one individual to another (and from one allele to another).

   (1) Restriction enzymes that cleave on the left and right flanks of a VNTR produce **DNA fragments of variable length.** The length depends on the number of repeats that the DNA contains (Figure 24-7).

   (2) Fragments produced by various restriction enzymes from a number of different loci can be used to identify individuals with the accuracy of a fingerprint. Therefore, this technique is called **"DNA fingerprinting."**

---

cc 24.7   **DNA fingerprinting** is used in the legal world to determine parentage, genealogy, or other genetic relationships, or to implicate suspects in law enforcement investigations involving violent crimes. Although not a unique identifier, the combination of markers can easily exclude false suspects and narrow positive suspects to a probability of a few million-to-one.

---

3. *Single nucleotide polymorphisms (SNPs)*

  a. SNPs are single bases in DNA differing in at least 1% of the population, occurring approximately once per gene, mostly in introns (noncoding).

  b. Over 99% do not change the amino acid sequence.

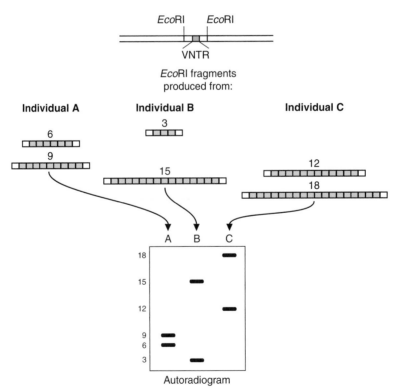

Figure 24-7 Restriction fragments produced from a gene with a variable number of tandem repeats (VNTR). DNA from three individuals, each with two alleles for this gene and a different number of repeats in each allele, was cleaved, electrophoresed, and treated with a probe for this gene. The length of the fragments depends on the number of repeats that they contain.

> *cc* **24.8** An SNP in the **APOE (apolipoprotein E)** gene is associated with an earlier onset of Alzheimer disease. Another SNP within the **chemokine-receptor gene CCR5** leads to resistance to HIV and acquired immunodeficiency syndrome (AIDS).

4. *Detection of mutations by allele-specific oligonucleotide probes*
   a. An **oligonucleotide probe** is synthesized **complementary** to a region of DNA that contains a **mutation.** A different probe is made for the normal DNA (Figure 24-8).
   b. If the *mutant* probe binds to a sample of DNA, the sample contains DNA from a *mutant* allele.
      (1) If the *normal* probe binds, the sample contains DNA from a *normal* allele.
      (2) If *both probes* bind, the sample contains DNA from both a mutant and a normal allele (i.e., the person providing the DNA sample is a carrier of the mutation).
5. *Testing for mutations by PCR*
   a. An oligonucleotide complementary to a mutant region is used as a **primer for PCR.**
   b. If the primer binds to a DNA sample (i.e., if the sample contains the mutation), amplification of the DNA occurs (i.e., the primer is extended).
   c. If the primer does not bind, extension does not occur (i.e., the DNA is normal).

> *cc* **24.9** The ability of the **PCR** to amplify the contents of a few cells has allowed detection, analysis, and early intervention by **prenatal diagnoses of parents' blood.** This method is used by couples whose family history or ethnic background may indicate that a disorder could be potentially present in a developing fetus. **Fetal diagnosis** is conducted by sampling amniotic fluid or chorionic villus cells. The DNA-based techniques described earlier are used for panels of tests have been developed to check many diseases.

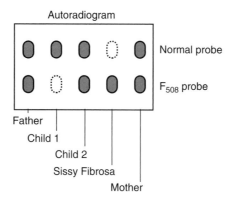

Figure 24-8 The use of oligonucleotide probes to test for cystic fibrosis (CF). Oligonucleotide probes complementary to the region where a 3-base deletion is located in the CF gene were synthesized. One probe binds only to the mutant (ΔF_{508}), and the other probe binds only to the normal region. DNA was isolated from individuals and amplified by polymerase chain reaction. Two spots were placed on nitrocellulose paper for each person. One spot was treated with the probe for the mutant region of the gene, and the other spot was treated with the probe for the normal region. Dark spots indicate binding of a probe. Only the normal probe binds to the DNA from a normal person, and only the mutant probe binds to the DNA from a person with CF. Both probes bind to DNA from a carrier. In carriers, one allele is normal and the other has the CF mutation.

E. **Alterations in the genetic composition of animals**

1. If a **gene** from another organism is **inserted into a blastocyst** (very early embryo) contributing to the germ line (eggs or sperm), a **transgenic animal** can be produced with extra genetic material in every cell. The nucleus of the fertilized egg is then transplanted into the uterus of a foster female for development.

> *cc* **24.10** A glycoprotein, Apo(a), when added to low-density lipoprotein (LDL) increases atherosclerosis risk associated with myocardial infarction, stroke, and restenosis. When fed an atherogenic diet, **Apo(a) transgenic mice developed lesions 15 times faster** than nontransgenic littermates. Mice with high levels of Apo(a) are a good model of atherosclerosis development in humans.

2. A special case of transgenesis, which is termed "**knockout,**" allows for inactivation of a given gene in all cells, which in turn creates strains of animals that lack the protein product of the gene.

> *cc* **24.11** Knockout mice are models for human diseases. A **defective leptin or leptin receptor** gene leads animals towards prodigious weight gain. Defects in metabolic pathways are explored to discover **causes of obesity** and to test drugs as possible treatments.

F. **Mapping of the human genome**

1. A massive effort was mounted to **sequence the entire** 3 billion base pairs of the **human genome,** culminating in 2001 with the publication of a "draft sequence." The results are expected to provide a better understanding of normal function and to elucidate the specific defects that result in inherited disease.

> *cc* **24.12** There are only about **30,000 genes in the human genome,** which is less than the number in rice. Current drugs in the pharmacopeia only target approximately 3% of the known genes.

G. **Gene therapy** (Figure 24-9)

1. Transgenesis with humans could eliminate disease genes, but technical and ethical issues prevail regarding using human eggs.
2. Some diseases have responded to efforts to introduce normal functioning genes into individuals with defective genes by introduction of the normal gene (**gene replacement**) in a viral vector to infect patient cells into production of the required protein.

> *cc* **24.13** Treatment of patients has commenced targeting the autoimmune disease **severe combined immunodeficiency disease (SCID).** A therapeutic correction of the defective gene by retroviral delivery into hematopoietic cells has corrected X-linked SCID by an interleukin receptor subunit and adenosine deaminase (ADA) in ADA-SCID. Problems result that require the use of other vectors for delivery.

H. **Stem cells**

1. These pluripotent cells can develop into many different cell types.
2. **Embryonic** stem cells are undifferentiated cells from an embryo with potential to become a variety of specialized cell types, whereas **adult** stem cells can differentiate to specialized cell types of the tissue from which it originated.

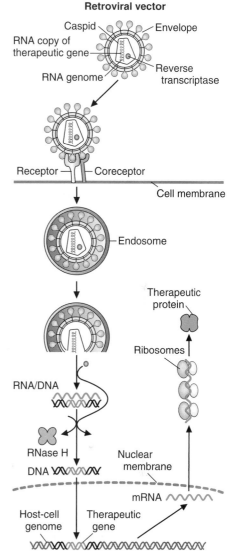

Figure 24-9 Use of retroviruses for gene therapy. The retrovirus caries an RNA copy of the therapeutic gene into the cell. The endosome that caries the virus dissolves, and the RNA and viral reverse transcriptase are released. This enzyme copies the RNA, making a double-strand DNA that integrates into the host cell genome. Transcription and translation of this therapeutic gene produces the therapeutic protein. mRNA = messenger RNA.

---

cc 24.14 The potential for human stem cells is in generating tissue for **regenerative cell-based therapy.** The need for transplantable tissue outstrips the supply. Stem cells may be able to differentiate to treat Parkinson disease, Alzheimer disease, spinal cord injury, diabetes, and heart disease.

I. **Organismal cloning** (Figure 24-10)

   1. Organismal cloning produces **genetically identical offspring** to the animal being cloned.
   2. This process removes the nucleus of an egg, replacing it with a diploid nucleus from the organism to be cloned. The egg is induced to divide and is placed in the uterus of a foster mother where gestation occurs.

---

cc 24.15 Organismal cloning has been demonstrated in animals and is an ethically and politically controversial topic for humans, with false claims abounding. **Dolly the sheep** is a clone.

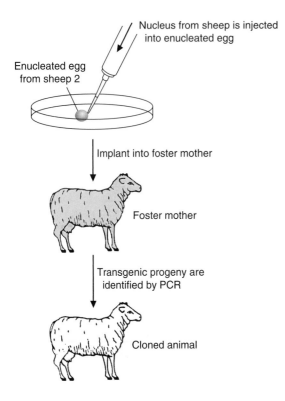

Nucleus from sheep is injected into enucleated egg

Enucleated egg from sheep 2

Implant into foster mother

Foster mother

Transgenic progeny are identified by PCR

Cloned animal

Figure 24-10 Organismal cloning of a mammal. PCR = polymerase chain reaction.

II. Technology Involving Proteins

A. **Strategies for separating proteins**

1. The **physical characteristics** that define a protein as a sum of all the properties of the **individual amino acids** are used for purifying proteins. This process of separation is done by various methods of **chromatography** (Table 24-1).

2. Another way of separating proteins with different amino acid composition is by **application of an electric field** termed **electrophoresis** that exploits charge and size of proteins. **Restriction endonucleases** cleave DNA into fragments (Table 24-2). Restriction endonucleases recognize short sequences in DNA and cleave both strands within this region (see Figure 24-1).

> **CC 24.16** The term **molecular medicine** arose upon elucidation of the amino acid substitution at **codon 6** of **Glu for HbA to Val for HbS** (sickle). Electrophoresis of hemoglobin proteins is an effective diagnostic tool since variant hemoglobins like sickle cell often have different charges.

> **CC 24.17** **Plasma protein electrophoresis** is an older diagnostic technique currently in use. Examining the size and migration of peaks, **acute and chronic inflammation responses** can be sought as well as **gammopathies and nephrotic syndrome.**

B. **Techniques for detecting single proteins (diagnostics)**

1. **Enzyme-linked immunosorbent assays** (ELISA) are based upon antibody–antibody interactions.

TABLE 24-1	*Chromatographic Techniques for Separating Biomolecules*	
Name	**Separates By**	**Brief Description**
Gel filtration	Size/Mass	Apply protein mixture to porous beads Big molecules are excluded first, small are retarded in column
Ion exchange	Charge	Apply protein mixture to charged beads Negatively charged proteins stick to positively charged proteins Negatively charged proteins come through Conversely, positive proteins stick to negative beads
Affinity	Specific ligand	Specific ligands are bound to beads to extract protein from mixture (e.g., antibody to capture antigen, peptide to capture receptor, DNA to catch transcription factor)
Liquid chromatography	Hydrophobicity or charge under pressure	Enhanced column chromatography Separate by size or hydrophobicity under high pressure Peptides, small proteins, and pieces of DNA (can differentiate 1 base pair difference)

a. Antigens are pre-coated onto plastic plates. An anti-human immunoglobulin (Ig) G is coupled to an enzyme as a second antibody, binding to human antibodies.
b. A substrate (that changes color when cleaved by an enzyme) is attached to the second antibody for detection.

TABLE 24-2	*Electrophoresis Techniques for Separating Biomolecules*	
Name	**Separates:**	**Brief Description**
DNA	Mass of DNA on agarose	A porous gel with an electric charge separates DNA by mass since there are uniform negatively charged phosphate groups
Native	Shape (radius)/protein mass; DNA by mass	For DNA, can resolve 1 base pair For proteins on shape of protein and mass, so unfolded proteins can be separated from folded ones
SDS-PAGE	Mass of proteins	Sodium dodecyl sulfate-polyacrylamide gel electrophoresis Denature proteins, add SDS detergent to unfold protein, and place uniform negative charge Electric field separates by mass
Two-dimensional (2D)	Isoelectric point (pI) and mass of proteins	First, separate proteins by pI so they stop migrating where there is **NO** net charge, and then apply to SDS-PAGE as above Resolves 1000s of proteins for proteomics

> *cc 24.18* **ELISA** is the most commonly used **test to screen for HIV infection.** It detects antibodies to HIV from blood, urine, or buccal washes. ELISA is not sensitive (false-negative) during the initial 3 to 4 weeks of infection or late in the disease when HIV-specific antibody production is low. A positive ELISA occurs approximately 22 to 26 days after acute infection. False-positive results are also possible in multiparous women, people recently vaccinated for hepatitis or influenza, or people with hematologic malignancies, multiple myeloma, alcoholic hepatitis, or primary biliary cirrhosis.

2. **Western immunoblotting** (see Figure 24.2) separates proteins by sodium dodecyl sulfate-polyacrylamide gel electrophoresis (SDS-PAGE) (see Table 24-2) and transfers them to a membrane. Often the membrane is cut into strips for testing patient samples for antibodies directed against the "blotted" protein (antigen).
   a. If there are any antibodies present that are directed against one or more of the blotted antigens, those antibodies will bind to the protein(s), whereas other antibodies will be washed away.
   b. To detect bound antibodies, anti-IgG is coupled to a reporter and, after excess second antibody is washed free, a substrate is added with the conjugate, resulting in a visible band where the primary antibody bound to the protein.

> *cc 24.19* **Western immunoblotting** confirms **HIV infection and is more specific than ELISA.** Antibodies are visualized against each viral protein. HIV-infected cells are lysed, electrophoresed, and blotted onto a membrane. The membrane is cut into strips and incubated with the serum samples from each patient. If positive, it is confirmed by the presence of the HIV viral proteins p24 OR p31 AND gp120 OR gp160.

C. **Strategies for determining protein structure**

1. **X-Ray crystallography** provides a three-dimensional structure by "seeing" how atoms arrange in a protein.
   a. Highly purified protein is crystallized and exposed to x-rays.
   b. The diffraction patterns are recorded and analyzed with computers to generate an electron density to fit the amino acid sequence. Energy minimization assures the chemical bonds are correct.

> *cc 24.20* Determining the structure of proteins by x-ray crystallography aids in drug design to interfere with pathologic function. The tyrosine kinase product of bcr-abl is implicated in **chronic myelogenous leukemia** (CML). **Abl kinase inhibitors** such as imatinib **(Gleevec)** were synthesized. The structural elucidation of rhinovirus and its cellular receptor were determined, and an antiviral agent **pleconaril** was developed to attenuate rhinoviral symptoms and shorten the duration of infection.

2. **Nuclear magnetic resonance (NMR)** is complementary to crystallography.
   a. The nuclei of some atoms (^{1}H, ^{13}C, ^{15}N) resonate at specific radio frequencies, so when atoms are close (<0.5 nm), their distances to secondary structure can be calculated. Although limited to smaller proteins (<45 kDa), crystals are not required.
   b. NMR is performed in solution and can measure the dynamic movements of a protein.

cc *24.21* The same principles of proteins in an NMR form the basis for **magnetic resonance imaging (MRI),** a nonionizing radiation source of imaging. Contrast reagents made of paramagnetic nuclei tagged to compounds examine the redistribution of water in tissue and in interstitial spaces.

3. **Mass spectrometry** measures mass:charge ratios of protein very accurately and with miniscule amounts of sample to determine the total mass (molecular weight) and the amino acid sequence of a protein.
   a. This has replaced chemical sequencing by Edman degradation, although most protein sequence information comes from translation of gene sequences.
   b. Mass data is used to search sequence databases to identify proteins in a sample.

cc *24.22* Mass spectrometry is used by **anti-doping agencies in sports** to detect the illicit use of **erythropoietin (Epo),** a hormone made by the kidney that stimulates bone marrow to make red blood cells. Epo is used by athletes to increase oxygen going to muscles, and the small difference in human and recombinant hormone is one carbohydrate residue.

D. Proteomics

1. Proteomics refers to the **PROTE**in complement of the gen**OME**, the gene *products*. Unlike the genome, the proteome changes depending on the physiologic state.
2. First, protein separation occurs by enrichment and two-dimensional gel electrophoresis (see Table 24-2). Once the proteins are separated, identification of the proteins and their modifications is accomplished by mass spectrometry (see II C 3).
3. Diversity and complexity of humans are not due to the genome, but instead, to the proteome and protein modifications, since we only have ~30,000 genes.

cc *24.23* Proteomics is initially used in finding specific **diagnostic and prognostic markers for cancers** by protein profiling. Protein expression patterns are compared between cancerous and adjoining noncancerous tissue.

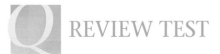

Directions: *Each of the numbered questions or incomplete statements in this section is followed by answers or by completions of the statement. Select the **one** lettered answer or completion that is **best** in each case.*

1. What biophysical technique is currently used for sequencing proteins more efficiently and faster than chemical sequencing by Edman degradation?

(A) Electrophoresis
(B) Mass spectrometry
(C) High-performance liquid chromatography (HPLC)
(D) X-ray crystallography
(E) Polymerase chain reaction (PCR)

2. A protein with several basic Lys and Arg residues has an isoelectric point (pI) of 4.3. The protein is applied to the middle of a polyacrylamide gel (see arrows in Figure below) and is subjected to electrophoresis under native conditions. The porous matrix through which the protein migrates contains a pH gradient. If the protein is subjected to the electric field (as shown) for several hours, which of the following diagrams depicts the position on the gel where the protein stops migrating?

(A) 1
(B) 2
(C) 3
(D) 4
(E) 5

3. Southern blot experiments are best described by which of the following?

(A) Can be used to map the 3′ end of RNA
(B) Can be used to identify DNA binding proteins
(C) Are used to identify the level of one specific RNA in the cell
(D) Require specific antibodies for detection
(E) Rely on the reversible denaturation of DNA

4. Northern blot analyses are useful for which of the following?

(A) Determination of nonsense mutations in a gene
(B) Determination of the relative rate of transcription of a gene
(C) Determination of a restriction map polymorphism
(D) Identification of relative level of a specific messenger RNA (mRNA)
(E) Identification of an RNA binding protein

5. What property is the most critical for the success of the PCR?

(A) DNA polymerase Klenow fragment
(B) DNA polymerase I
(C) DNA polymerase III
(D) An RNA primer
(E) Denaturation/renaturation of the DNA

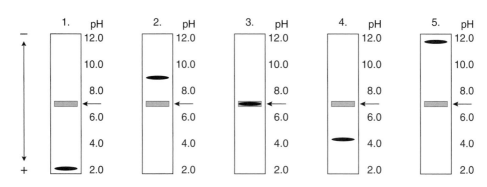

420

6. A single amino acid substitution of a protein alters its elution profile on ion exchange chromatography. Which of the following is another technique that is likely to be useful in detecting the normal and mutant forms of the enzyme?

(A) Sodium dodecyl sulfate-polyacrylamide gel electrophoresis (SDS-PAGE)
(B) Mass spectrometry
(C) Size exclusion chromatography
(D) Density gradient centrifugation
(E) PCR

7. Three single-polypeptide globular proteins have the following masses and pIs:

	Mass	pI
A	75,000	7.5
B	105,000	7.0
C	140,000	8.0

The relative rates of migration on SDS-PAGE at pH 7.5 are described by which of the following?

(A) $C > B > A$
(B) $A > B > C$
(C) $B > A > C$
(D) $C > A > B$
(E) $B > C$, with no movement of A at its pI

8. A gene you have cloned has 5′ overhangs on each end of the sequence. This will most readily be joined to a cleaved vector if the vector has which of the following?

(A) Compatible 3′ overhangs on both ends
(B) Compatible 5′ overhangs on both ends
(C) Two blunt ends
(D) Compatible 3′ overhangs on one end and a compatible 5′ end on the other end to ensure that, relative to the vector, the gene is inserted directionally in the correct orientation.
(E) Compatible 5′ overhangs on one end and a compatible 3′ end on the other end to ensure that, relative to the vector, the gene is inserted directionally in the correct orientation.

9. Moonlighting for a summer as a member of MSI (Medical Student Investigators), you have recovered a few cells with extractable DNA for forensic analysis of a crime scene. Knowing you must use PCR analysis, you decide to use 30 cycles to amplify the DNA. Using the correct primers and an excess of deoxynucleotides, you will have increased the amount of DNA by approximately which of the following?

(A) 10^{30} fold
(B) 30^2 fold
(C) 2^{10} fold (~1000 fold)
(D) 2^{30} fold (~1,000,000,000 fold)
(E) It is indeterminable since you did not measure how much DNA you started out with

10. Normal hemoglobin (HbA) and sickle cell hemoglobin (HbS) have different electrophoretic mobilities because these two proteins have different what?

(A) Amounts of bound O_2
(B) Amounts of bound 2,3-diphospho-glycerate
(C) Charges
(D) Sizes
(E) Hydrophobicity

11. A patient has a disease that is causing hyperexcretion of a protein in the urine. Which of the following representations of data from particular methods would be the fastest, easiest, and least expensive way to determine the molecular weight of the native protein in the urine?

(A) Ion exchange chromatography
(B) Size exclusion chromatography
(C) X-ray crystallography
(D) Nuclear magnetic resonance (NMR)
(E) SDS-PAGE

12. KLF6 is a key prostate cancer tumor-suppressor gene. A single nucleotide polymorphism in the coding region associated with increased risk was recently discovered. Heterozygous individuals have both the normal (Leu) and mutant (Arg). Although the single nucleotide polymorphism (SNP) was identified on the nucleotide level, you wish to separate and characterize 10 μg of each of the proteins. What approach would you use?

(A) Mass spectrometry
(B) X-ray crystallography
(C) NMR
(D) Ion exchange chromatography
(E) Affinity purification on a KLF6 polyclonal antibody column

13. A 42-year-old man presents to the emergency room and receives a neurologic consult for a slowly progressing chorea with some rigidity and an episode with seizure. There have been past episodes, and a deceased mother had choreic neurologic episodes and dementia. You suspect the patient might have Huntington's disease. You have a laboratory equipped to perform restriction fragment length polymorphism (RFLP) analyses. Which of the following adjunct techniques would you use?

(A) Western blot
(B) Northern blot
(C) Southern blot
(D) X-ray crystallography
(E) Mass spectrometry

14. A patient you have been treating for Gaucher disease, a lysosomal storage disease, comes into your office wanting to test her eager and compliant relatives who may be carriers of the disorder. The most predominant β-glucosidase defect, N370S, is present. Wanting to do this in the most expeditious and least costly manner because these are uninsured people, you would use which of the following techniques?

(A) SNP assessment
(B) DNA sequencing
(C) Allele-specific oligonucleotide probe hybridization
(D) RLFP analysis
(E) DNA fingerprinting

15. There are two primary clinical methods for separating the isozymes of creatine phosphokinase (CPK) used in the implication of various acute disorders such as myocardial infarctions and muscle injury. One

uses affinity chromatography with a specific antibody. The other uses separation of the isozymes of CPK and relies on differences in which of the following?

(A) The genes by agarose electrophoresis
(B) Net charge
(C) Affinity for creatine
(D) Affinity for adenosine triphosphate (ATP)
(E) Binding of SDS

16. Which technique is best to separate oxygenated normal HbA from oxygenated sickle cell hemoglobin (HbS) (assuming no protein aggregation) from a patient coming into a clinic?

(A) Native gel electrophoresis
(B) SDS-PAGE
(C) Gel filtration
(D) Affinity chromatography with a C-terminal antibody
(E) Ultracentrifugation

17. A patient coming into an outpatient clinic for metabolic blood work has a portion of his blood subjected to ion exchange chromatography on a carboxymethyl cellulose column. The patient's serum profile indicates less protein is binding than normal. This may indicate which of the following?

(A) Serum proteins are deficient in sialic acid residues.
(B) Serum proteins are deficient in side chains of glycosaminoglycans.
(C) Serum proteins are more negatively charged.
(D) Proteins are deficient in a substituent identical to diethylaminoethyl cellulose.
(E) The patient has a silent mutation in a hemoglobin variant.

18. A PCR assay needs to be developed to determine the human immunodeficiency virus (HIV) status of a newborn in the pediatric intensive care unit (PICU) born to a mother who is HIV positive. The primers for the assay should be which of the following?

(A) Should be antiparallel complements of two parts of a noninfected human genome

(B) Should be synthesized so, after annealing with potential infective DNA, the 5′ of primer 1 would "face" the 3′ of primer 2.

(C) Should be synthesized so, after annealing with potential infective DNA, the 5′ of both primers "face" each other.

(D) Should be synthesized with dideoxynucleotides to allow sequencing of the mutation.

(E) Should be synthesized with identical sequences to those in the HIV genome and must bind to DNA in a complementary, antiparallel manner.

19. A patient is referred to you by her obstetrician for genetic counseling for an apparent chromosomal microdeletion. To be able to test the heritability of this disorder by RFLP analyses, what is required?

(A) SDS gel electrophoresis to detect the gene product of normal and diseased individuals

(B) Mutations flanking restriction sites so the entire gene can be sequenced

(C) A unique oligonucleotide that can be amplified by successive rounds of heating, cooling, and annealing

(D) An altered restriction site closely linked to the mutation causing the disease

(E) Antibodies used with ribonucleotide probes for detection of the altered trait

20. You are counseling a patient who may have HIV. The laboratory may have to perform two different tests. The first test will be an enzyme-linked immunosorbent assay (ELISA) as a screen, and if two positive test results occur, a confirmatory Western blot will be performed. What do the ELISA and Western blots measure?

(A) ELISA measures antigen to HIV only, the Western blot measures antibody to HIV only

(B) ELISA measures antibody to HIV only, the Western blot measures antigen to HIV only

(C) ELISA measures antigen to HIV only, the Western blot measures antigen to HIV only

(D) ELISA measures antibody to HIV only, the Western blot measures antibody to HIV only

(E) ELISA measures antibodies directed against human leukocyte antigen (HLA) molecules to HIV, the Western blot measures free, circulating virus in the patient

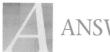 ANSWERS AND EXPLANATIONS

1–B. Mass spectrometry precisely measures the mass:charge ratio of proteins, from which the mass and sequence of a protein can be determined. Electrophoresis is used for DNA sequencing, and polymerase chain reaction (PCR) is used for amplifying nucleic acids only. High-performance liquid chromatography (HPLC) can separate proteins not sequence them, and x-ray crystallography can sequence over months and not minutes like mass spectrometry.

2–D. There are several Lys and Arg residues, but more tAsp and Glu, so the resulting isoelectric point (pI), where the **net** charge of the protein is **zero** (pI = pH) lies in the acidic range. In an electric field, the protein will migrate and stop at the pH where the net charge is zero. In this case, that is pH 4.3.

3–E. Southern blot analysis involves DNA (Northern blots involve RNA, and Western blots involve protein). The technique relies on the reversible denaturation of DNA immobilized on a membrane and "probed," with radioactive DNA annealing (binding) to its complementary sequence. Determining nonsense mutations requires DNA sequencing.

4–D. Northern blots are specific for RNA determination. Nonsense mutations in a gene or restriction fragment length polymorphisms (RFLPs) involve DNA (Southern blots), whereas an RNA binding protein might involve Western blots (protein). Transcription rate measurements involve "run-on" assays, not Northern blotting.

5–E. PCR **amplifies** specific double-stranded DNA sequences by heating (**denaturation**) to separate the strands and **renaturation** to two primers that will be extended in opposite directions by a heat-stable polymerase. The polymerases extend DNA into a polymer **but** are not critical to PCR since there is no amplification without denaturation/renaturation of DNA. An RNA primer is not required.

6–B. A precise difference in mass of even a few Daltons can be detected by mass spectrometry. PCR is for measuring DNA, and the number of nucleotides is the same. All the other choices can only differentiate larger mass differences of at least 30 amino acids.

7–B. Once coated with negatively charged sodium dodecyl sulfate (SDS), the isoelectric point (pI) becomes irrelevant, and proteins are run according to their mass. Therefore, based on size, smaller proteins are electrophoresed through the pores on the gel faster than larger proteins.

8–A. A 5′ "overhang" is a DNA sequence that extends as a single strand at the 5′ end. 5′ overhangs anneal to compatible 3′ overhangs. Annealing two "sticky" complimentary ends (5′ and 3′ ends) will cause the DNA to be readily "joined."

9–D. Two original DNA strands are templates. Each cycle doubles the amount of DNA present. After 30 cycles, the amplification in total DNA molecules is 2^{30}. Since $2^{10} = \sim 1000$, $2^{30} = \sim 1000 \times 1000 \times 1000 = 1,000,000,000 = 10^9$, an approximate billion-fold amplification in total DNA molecules.

10–C. There is a single amino acid replacement in HbS of a Val for Glu:

HbS: Val-His-Leu-Thr-Pro-**Val**-Glu
HbA: Val-His-Leu-Thr-Pro-**Glu**-Glu
beta 1 2 3 4 5 6 7

None of the other choices separate by electrophoretic mobility other than charge.

11–B. Size exclusion (gel) chromatography separates proteins by mass. Ion exchange chromatography involves anion exchange for separating proteins with a net positive charge. Nuclear magnetic resonance (NMR) spectra and x-ray crystallographic diffraction techniques require laborious effort and are not relevant to clinical use. SDS-PAGE does **not** yield the mass of a **native** (but denatured) protein.

12–D. The key is **isolation** as well as detection. The change of Arg to Leu alters the **1 charge** properties of the protein (+1 → 0 neutral). This can be separated via ion exchange chromatography. Mass spectrometry can differentiate the masses but cannot obtain material for analyses. Likewise, NMR and crystallography might detect a difference. A polyclonal antibody would not differentiate the two forms, although a monoclonal antibody, if designed properly, might separate the forms.

13–C. Since RFLP analyses involve DNA, a Southern blot would be performed. A Western blot is performed on protein, and a Northern blot is performed on RNA. Mass spectrometry could be used on the isolated protein, as could x-ray crystallography, but it is DNA that is being probed.

14–C. Because the mutation is known, probes that are specifically labeled with fluorescence or radioactivity can be synthesized to differentiate between normal and disease genotypes. DNA is spotted on nitrocellulose and probed. All of the other techniques involve electrophoresis on a gel based material. This takes longer and is more costly.

15–B. Net charge will differentiate between the isozymes, which are a combination of different M and H forms of the enzyme. We are interested in the proteins, so DNA is irrelevant. Affinity for effectors will not help either, and binding SDS is uniform among all proteins.

16–A. Since it is the 6th amino acid of the Hb β-chain that is different, only charge will separate the forms because the difference in mass is miniscule. Native gel electrophoresis will do this. SDS-PAGE blankets the protein with a uniform negative charge that will mask the inherent difference. Gel filtration and ultracentrifugation are not sensitive enough, and a C-terminal antibody will detect both forms.

17–C. A carboxymethyl cellulose column has a negative charge, and if a substance binds **less,** it must have a greater negative charge to repel binding. The protein deficiencies listed would make the protein more positive and bind better, not worse. A silent mutation would not change binding at all.

18–E. For the development of a PCR assay, one requires primers against the specific human immunodeficiency virus (HIV) target (choice A is incorrect) that are complementary and antiparallel (choices B and C are excluded) and require deoxy (not dideoxy;

primers that require dideoxy are used for sequencing because they terminate the reaction, thus choice D is excluded).

19–D. Since a chromosomal microdeletion and subsequent RFLP analyses is based on DNA, the optimal detection is by a Southern blot probe after digestion with a restriction enzyme whose site has been altered. SDS-PAGE or antibodies will not detect the disorder. Gene sequencing is not required for the Southern blot used to detect the polymorphism. An oligonucleotide cannot be amplified by PCR.

20–D. In an enzyme-linked immunosorbent assay (ELISA), antibody from patient serum is made in response to HIV proteins that binds to antigen. These tests **do not** identify the virus, only *antibodies* to the virus. Western blot also detects antibodies in response to HIV proteins that bind to antigens immobilized on strips. HIV antigens are coated on the ELISA plate, and serum antibody is detected, not circulating virus. Anti-human leukocyte antigen (HLA) antibodies may be present, but the test is not designed to measure them.

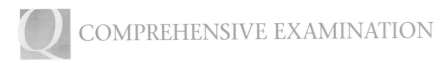

1. A 40-year-old male presents with a "burning" feeling in his upper central abdomen. This feeling occurs after eating spicy foods. He is prescribed a proton pump inhibitor medication, which prevents hydrochloric acid (HCl) production by the stomach. HCl:

(A) Is a strong acid
(B) Is a weak acid
(C) Dissociates to a limited extent
(D) Has a pH of 7
(E) Accepts protons

2. A 30-year-old female presents with fever, a severe infection, and low blood pressure. She is found to have an elevated level of lactic acid in her serum, causing a metabolic acidosis. Her body attempts to counteract this metabolic acidosis using one of the major buffers of the blood, which is:

(A) Bicarbonate
(B) Water
(C) Sulfuric acid
(D) Phosphoric acid
(E) Hydrochloric acid

3. A 12-year-old boy with asthma presents with wheezing and difficulty breathing. He is administered an asthma medication that has both R- and S-enantiomers present in it. Enantiomers are compounds that:

(A) Differ in the position of the hydroxyl group on only one asymmetric carbon
(B) Differ in the position of the hydroxyl group on one or more asymmetric carbons
(C) Are mirror images
(D) Are epimers
(E) Have different chemical formulas

4. A 20-year-old female presents with a tingling sensation on her upper lip. Her physician diagnoses herpes simplex virus-1 infection in a cold sore. To promote growth, this virus requires a positively charged amino acid for proper function, such as:

(A) Glycine
(B) Proline
(C) Arginine
(D) Aspartate
(E) Glutamate

5. A 5-year-old boy presents with cough and copious sputum production. He has had frequent bacterial infections in his lungs causing the same symptoms and is diagnosed with cystic fibrosis. This disease is passed on from the previous generation through:

(A) DNA
(B) RNA
(C) Protein
(D) Phenylalanine
(E) Carbohydrates

6. A 75-year-old male presents with progressive memory loss and dementia. He is diagnosed with Alzheimer disease, a condition in which multiple amyloid plaques form in the brain. These amyloid plaques are protein deposits that are composed of β-pleated sheets. Which of the following describes β-pleated sheets?

(A) Primary structure
(B) Secondary structure
(C) Supersecondary structure
(D) Tertiary structure
(E) Quaternary structure

7. A 50-year-old male presents with "dancing-like" movements of his arms and progressive dementia. He cannot control the movements in his arms. He states that he knows he has Huntington's disease because his mother has the same disease. This disease is caused by abnormal protein folding. Which of the following helps to mediate proper protein folding?

(A) ATP
(B) Leucine zippers
(C) Zinc fingers
(D) Transcription factors
(E) Chaperones

8. An 81-year-old male presents with weight loss, fatigue, and a relentless cough.

He has been smoking for the past 50 years. A radiologic scan performed on his chest shows a lung nodule. Biopsy of the nodule shows cancerous cells. He is placed on a cancer medication that inhibits post-translational modification of proteins. Which of the following is a post-translational modification?

(A) Denaturation
(B) Renaturation
(C) Folding
(D) Phosphorylation
(E) Binding to DNA

9. A 70-year-old male presents with back pain, fatigue, and frequent urinary tract infections. He is diagnosed with multiple myeloma, a cancer of blood cells, and is administered a drug that inhibits the proteasome. The proteasome:

(A) Mediates binding of ubiquitin to proteins
(B) Mediates misfolding of proteins
(C) Degrades intracellular proteins into peptides
(D) Digests extracellular proteins
(E) Inhibits proteases

10. An 80-year-old female presents with bleeding gums and pinpoint bleeding on her ankles. She is found to have severe vitamin C deficiency due to lack of intake in her diet. In vitamin C deficiency, patients have bleeding problems because the connective tissue around blood vessels is composed of collagen, which is improperly formed. In the synthesis of collagen, O_2 and vitamin C are required for:

(A) Adding glycine residues
(B) Hydroxylating proline and lysine residues
(C) Cleaving the signal sequence of pre-procollagen
(D) Forming the triple helix of procollagen
(E) Adding glucose and galactose

11. A 55-year-old male presents with difficulty breathing and swollen ankles. He is found to have a failing heart, resulting in blood backing up into his lungs and making it difficult for him to breathe. He is administered a drug that inhibits angiotensin-converting enzyme (ACE). By inhibiting this enzyme, which of the following will change about the reaction it catalyzes?

(A) Energy of activation
(B) Net free energy change
(C) Equilibrium concentration of substrate
(D) Equilibrium concentration of product
(E) Thermodynamics

12. A 37-year-old female presents with difficulty opening her eyelids, as well as an inability to raise herself up from a sitting position. She is diagnosed with myasthenia gravis, a disease that does not allow proper acetylcholine neurotransmission in her muscles. She is prescribed physostigmine, a competitive inhibitor of acetylcholinesterase, which increases the amount of available acetylcholine. Which of the following statements is true of competitive inhibitors?

(A) They inactivate the enzyme.
(B) V_{max} remains the same.
(C) The apparent K_m is decreased.
(D) They are dissimilar to substrate.
(E) They bind covalently to enzyme.

13. A 50-year-old male has had multiple bouts of a painful, red, swollen big toe. He is diagnosed with gout, a disease in which uric acid crystal deposits in joints cause severe pain. Xanthine oxidase converts hypoxanthine to uric acid. To decrease the serum uric acid level, the patient is prescribed allopurinol, a competitive inhibitor, which:

(A) Has a very similar structure to xanthine oxidase
(B) Binds to hypoxanthine and prevents it from binding to xanthine oxidase
(C) Binds to a site on xanthine oxidase that is distinct from the active site
(D) Inactivates xanthine oxidase
(E) Has activity that can be reversed by increasing levels of hypoxanthine

14. A 30-year-old male is depressed and commits suicide by ingesting cyanide salts. Cyanide is a noncompetitive inhibitor of cytochrome c oxidase. Noncompetitive inhibitors decrease V_{max} because:

(A) The substrate undergoes a conformational change
(B) The activity of the enzyme decreases
(C) The enzyme is inactivated
(D) The active site of the enzyme is occupied by inhibitor
(E) The amount of substrate decreases

15. A 35-year-old female presents with chronic fatigue. She is found to be anemic, with an abnormally low level of hemoglobin in her blood. In hemoglobin, the binding of O_2 to one subunit facilitates O_2 binding to the adjacent subunits. This is an example of:

(A) Enzyme cascade
(B) Allosteric activation
(C) Feedback inhibition
(D) Allosteric inhibition
(E) Michaelis-Menten kinetics

16. A 19-year-old female is running on a treadmill. Exercise increases her respiratory quotient. Respiratory quotient is:

(A) Higher for fat than carbohydrate
(B) Higher for protein than carbohydrate
(C) The ratio of CO_2 produced to O_2 utilized
(D) Increased in exercise toward fat metabolism
(E) Higher for a muscle at rest than at exercise

17. A 25-year-old male is intubated in the intensive care unit. He is being treated for an overwhelming infection. Through a gastric tube, he is being fed proteins that are broken down to amino acids. When his dietary nitrogen intake exceeds his excreted nitrogen, this is most accurately called:

(A) Negative nitrogen balance
(B) Positive nitrogen balance
(C) Nitrogen balance
(D) Biosynthesis
(E) An anabolic state

18. A 20-year-old male presents with a headache. He takes a headache medication that is metabolized to two products. For this biochemical reaction, the ΔG has a large positive value, which means the reaction:

(A) Will not proceed spontaneously
(B) Will release energy
(C) Is at equilibrium
(D) Occurs with a rapid rate
(E) Results in no net change in substrate concentration

19. A 30-year-old male presents with ankle swelling and weight gain. He is diagnosed with kidney failure. He is administered a drug that is reduced in a reaction that requires a large amount of ATP. Thus, this drug:

(A) Donates electrons
(B) Has a positive ΔE value
(C) Is an oxidant
(D) Has a negative ΔG value
(E) Is reduced in an energetically favorable process

20. A 45-year-old female presents with palpitations and dizziness. She is diagnosed with an abnormally fast heart rhythm. She is administered adenosine, a substance that can block electrical impulses in the heart. Adenosine:

(A) Is a nucleotide
(B) Contains adenine and ribose
(C) Can transfer phosphate groups
(D) Hydrolysis has a ΔG of -7.3 kcal/mole
(E) Contains a phosphate group esterified to the 5'-hydroxyl of its sugar

21. A 30-year-old Asian male presents with bloating, abdominal cramps, and diarrhea. He states that he develops these symptoms whenever he drinks milk or eats dairy products. He is diagnosed with lactose intolerance, a common condition in which lactose is not digested normally and accumulates in the gut. Lactase converts lactose into:

(A) Two glucose residues
(B) Glucose and fructose
(C) Glucose and galactose
(D) Fructose and galactose
(E) Sucrose and maltose

22. A 50-year-old female presents with severe upper abdominal pain. Her serum amylase and lipase levels are abnormally elevated, and she is diagnosed with pancreatitis. Which linkage between glucose residues does amylase cleave?

(A) α-1,4
(B) α-1,6
(C) β-1,4
(D) α-1 to β-2
(E) α-4,6

23. A 40-year-old female presents with bloating, abdominal discomfort, and diarrhea. She states that her stool floats in the toilet. She is found to have steatorrhea, which is excess lipids in the feces due to lipid malabsorption. In digestion of lipids, which of the following digests triacylglycerols to 2-monoacylglycerols and free fatty acids?

(A) Bile salts
(B) Pancreatic amylase
(C) Pancreatic lipase
(D) Micelles
(E) Bicarbonate

24. A 35-year-old male has been on the Atkins diet and has been taking in a large protein load. In the small intestine, which of the following enzymes is responsible for cleaving proteins at peptide bonds in which the carboxyl group is contributed by arginine or lysine?

(A) Trypsin
(B) Chymotrypsin
(C) Carboxypeptidase A
(D) Carboxypeptidase B
(E) Aminopeptidases

25. A 45-year-old female presents with a burning sensation in her upper abdomen and chest. She is diagnosed with gastroesophageal reflux disease (GERD), a condition in which stomach contents cause damage to the esophagus. Which of the following is responsible for this patient's symptoms?

(A) Hydrochloric acid
(B) Pepsinogen
(C) Endopeptidases
(D) Exopeptidases
(E) Enteropeptidase

26. A 50-year-old male presents with severe muscle pain and dark urine. He is found to have rhabdomyolysis (destruction of muscle cells) due to aldolase deficiency. Aldolase is an enzyme in glycolysis that cleaves 1,6-bisphosphate to the triose phosphates, and deficiency of this enzyme inhibits glycolysis in muscle cells. In glycolysis, what is the starting substrate and end product?

(A) Glucose to pyruvate
(B) Pyruvate to lactate
(C) Glucose to acetyl CoA
(D) Pyruvate to acetyl CoA
(E) Pyruvate to glucose

27. A 40-year-old male presents to the emergency room after being hit by a car. He has severe internal bleeding and is transfused with multiple units of red blood cells to replace his lost blood. In order for hemoglobin to release oxygen to his tissues, which of the following compounds is formed in red blood cells?

(A) 1,3-Bisphosphoglycerate
(B) 2,3-Bisphosphoglycerate
(C) Dihydroxyacetone phosphate
(D) Glyceraldehyde 3-phosphate
(E) Phosphoenolpyruvate

28. A 65-year-old male is brought to the intensive care unit presenting with fever, confusion, hypotension, and decreased urine output. He is found to be in sepsis (a state of severe systemic infection), and his serum is acidemic, with a very high lactate level of 6.0 mmol/L. When pyruvate is converted to lactate, which of the following is produced?

(A) NADH
(B) NAD$^+$
(C) CO_2
(D) H_2O
(E) Acetyl CoA

29. A 55-year-old mentally ill female refuses to eat for 2 weeks for fear that her food is poisoned. She is brought to the hospital to be given a glucose solution intravenously. When glucose enters glycolysis, it is converted to glucose 6-phosphate by

hexokinase. Hexokinase has a low K_m for glucose (about 0.1 mM). Which of the following is a characteristic of hexokinase?

(A) It is induced only when insulin levels are high.
(B) It is inhibited by high levels of glucose.
(C) Its rate is accelerated by high levels of glucose 6-phosphate.
(D) It works at a rapid rate, even at fasting blood glucose levels.
(E) It is only found in the liver.

30. An infant is rushed to the emergency room after aspirating a small toy. Upon arrival, the infant is limp, has blue-tinged skin, and is not breathing. Even in the absence of oxygen, glycolysis provides ATP for tissues. What is the net yield of ATP from one cycle of glycolysis?

(A) 2 ATP
(B) 4 ATP
(C) 6 ATP
(D) 24 ATP
(E) 36 ATP

31. A 35-year-old female presents with fatigue, shortness of breath, and decreased energy. She has been eating a balanced diet and sleeping well. A blood test shows that she is anemic (low red blood cell count). In red blood cells, ATP is generated using glycolysis but not using the tricarboxylic cycle because the latter occurs in:

(A) Lysosomes
(B) Cytosol
(C) Plasma membrane
(D) Golgi apparatus
(E) Mitochondria

32. An infant presents with severe lethargy, poor feeding, and tachypnea (rapid breathing). He is found to have pyruvate dehydrogenase deficiency. The pyruvate dehydrogenase complex is inhibited by increased levels of its product, which induces phosphorylation of the enzyme complex. Which of the following would be most likely to induce phosphorylation?

(A) Acetyl CoA
(B) CoASH
(C) NAD+
(D) Pyruvate
(E) Glucose

33. A 40-year-old male presents with excruciating pain in his right flank that radiates down to his right testicle. He is found to have a kidney stone and is prescribed citrate to help prevent future stones from forming. In the TCA cycle, citrate is isomerized to isocitrate. Isocitrate is subsequently oxidized to α-ketoglutarate by isocitrate dehydrogenase, a key regulatory enzyme of the TCA cycle. Which of the following would be most likely to inhibit isocitrate dehydrogenase?

(A) ADP
(B) Acetyl CoA
(C) CoASH
(D) NADH
(E) FAD+

34. A 45-year-old homeless male is brought to the emergency room after being found unconscious. He has a high serum level of ketone bodies, indicating that he has been starving. In starvation, oxaloacetate is used to synthesize glucose and is thus not available to condense with acetyl CoA to form citrate to begin the TCA cycle. Therefore, acetyl CoA is diverted from the TCA cycle to form ketone bodies. If 1 mole of oxaloacetate were available to condense with 1 mole of acetyl CoA for the TCA cycle, how many moles of ATP would be produced?

(A) 2
(B) 12
(C) 24
(D) 36
(E) 38

35. A 50-year-old alcoholic male presents with pain, numbness, tingling, and weakness in his feet. He is diagnosed with thiamine deficiency, and with repletion of this vitamin, his symptoms resolve. Thiamine and ATP form thiamine pyrophosphate, a cofactor important for enzymes that

catalyze oxidative decarboxylations (decarboxylation of α-ketoacids) in the TCA cycle, such as:

(A) α-Ketoglutarate dehydrogenase
(B) Citrate synthase
(C) Isocitrate dehydrogenase
(D) Fumarase
(E) Malate dehydrogenase

36. An 18-year-old college student is brought to the emergency room unconscious, with a very high serum alcohol level. Alcohol metabolism can result in high NADH levels. When NADH enters the electron transport chain, which of the following is the correct order in which electron transfer occurs?

(A) NADH, coenzyme Q, cytochrome c, FMN, O_2
(B) NADH, cytochrome c, coenzyme Q, FMN, O_2
(C) NADH, FMN, coenzyme Q, cytochrome c, O_2
(D) NADH, FMN, cytochrome c, coenzyme Q, O_2
(E) NADH, coenzyme Q, FMN, cytochrome c, O_2

37. A 40-year-old female presents with severe hypertension, with a blood pressure of 250/150 mm Hg (normal, 120/80 mm Hg). She is started on a nitroprusside drip to decrease her blood pressure. By mistake, the nitroprusside infusion rate is set too fast, and the patient becomes agitated and dizzy and starts having convulsions. Nitroprusside is metabolized to various substances, including cyanide. Cyanide inhibits cellular respiration by combining with:

(A) The NADH dehydrogenase complex
(B) O_2
(C) Cytochrome oxidase
(D) F_0–F_1 ATPase
(E) ATP-ADP antiport

38. A 25-year-old male is administered an anesthetic for routine surgery. His temperature rises to 105°F, he is drenched in sweat, and a cooling blanket is placed under him in an effort to bring his temperature down.

He is diagnosed with malignant hyperthermia, which is a reaction that some individuals may have to some anesthetics. Which of the following is the most likely etiology of the excessive heat generation?

(A) Excessive activity of the F_0–F_1 ATPase
(B) Uncoupling of oxidative phosphorylation from electron transport
(C) Oxidation of NADH with phosphorylation of ADP to form ATP
(D) Shutdown of the ATP-ADP antiport
(E) Uncontrolled reactive oxygen species generation

39. A 70-year-old smoker presents with weight loss, blood in his sputum, and fatigue. Imaging shows a nodule in his lung that is diagnosed as cancer by biopsy. It has been proposed that reactive oxygen species may induce mutagenesis and contribute to the initiation of cancer. Which of the following is the major source of superoxide within cells?

(A) NADH dehydrogenase complex
(B) FMN
(C) Coenzyme Q
(D) Cytochrome b
(E) Cytochrome c

40. A 3-year-old girl presents with fatigue and yellowing of her skin and eyes. She is found to be anemic (abnormally low red blood cell count) and is diagnosed with pyruvate kinase deficiency. This disease is the most common enzymopathy of glycolysis, resulting in deficient NADH production. For every NADH that does enter the electron transport chain and is oxidized, how many ATP are produced?

(A) 1
(B) 2
(C) 3
(D) 4
(E) 5

41. Shortly after birth, an infant presents with tremors, irritability, and seizures. His blood glucose is profoundly low, and he is fed glucose through a nasogastric tube. He is diagnosed with glycogen storage disease type 1, a disease that causes excessive buildup of liver glycogen, with an inability to release glucose, resulting in an abnormally low blood glucose level. In glycogen, the linkage at branch points is α-1,6, and linkage between glucose residues is:

(A) α-1,3
(B) α-2,3
(C) α-1,4
(D) β-1,3
(E) β-2,3

42. An infant presents with an enlarged heart, muscle weakness, and hypoventilation. She is diagnosed with glycogen storage disease type 2, a disease causing abnormal glycogen storage in the heart, skeletal muscle, and respiratory muscles. Glycogen synthase is the regulatory enzyme for glycogen synthesis. It adds glucose residues to the nonreducing ends of a glycogen primer from:

(A) Glucose 1-phosphate
(B) Glucose 6-phosphate
(C) UDP-glucose
(D) UTP
(E) ATP

43. A 30-year-old male presents with severe muscle cramps and pain while exercising. He is found to have muscle glycogen phosphorylase deficiency (McArdle disease, glycogen storage disease type 5). Glycogen phosphorylase degrades glycogen to produce:

(A) Glucose
(B) Glucose 1-phosphate
(C) Glucose 6-phosphate
(D) UDP-glucose
(E) Glycogen primer

44. A 15-year-old type 1 diabetic faints after injecting himself with insulin. He is administered glucagon and rapidly recovers consciousness. Glucagon induces activity of:

(A) Glycogen synthase
(B) Glycogen phosphorylase
(C) Glucokinase
(D) Hexokinase
(E) UDP-glucose pyrophosphorylase

45. A 30-year-old male presents with intractable vomiting and inability to eat or drink for the past 3 days. His blood glucose level is normal. Which of the following is most important for maintenance of blood glucose?

(A) Liver
(B) Heart
(C) Skeletal muscle
(D) Lysosome
(E) Spleen

46. A 5-year-old girl presents with muscle weakness, an enlarged liver, and intractable hypoglycemia. She is diagnosed with phosphoenolpyruvate carboxykinase (PEPCK) deficiency, a rare metabolic disorder. Which of the following is the reaction that phosphoenolpyruvate carboxykinase (PEPCK) catalyzes?

(A) Pyruvate to phosphoenolpyruvate
(B) Pyruvate to oxaloacetate
(C) Oxaloacetate to phosphoenolpyruvate
(D) Phosphoenolpyruvate to oxaloacetate
(E) Phosphoenolpyruvate to fructose 1,6-bisphosphate

47. A 10-year-old male presents with muscle cramping and dark urine after rigorous exercise. He is found to have a deficiency of lactate dehydrogenase. This enzyme converts lactate to form pyruvate, which can be converted to glucose during gluconeogenesis. Which is another important precursor for gluconeogenesis?

(A) Urea
(B) Amino acids
(C) Even-chain fatty acids
(D) ADP
(E) Acetyl CoA

48. An infant presents with growth retardation, weak muscle tone, and lethargy. He is diagnosed with pyruvate carboxylase deficiency. Which of the following cannot be produced by this infant?

(A) Pyruvate
(B) Ketone bodies
(C) Oxaloacetate

(D) Lactate
(E) Acetyl CoA

49. A 15-year-old male presents with increased thirst, hunger, urination, and weight loss. His fasting blood glucose level is 400 mg/dL (normal < 110 mg/dL), and he is diagnosed with type 1 diabetes mellitus. What is the reason for this patient's inability to maintain a normal blood glucose level?

(A) Decreased uptake of glucose by cells
(B) Abnormal response to glucagon
(C) Decreased glucagon:insulin ratio
(D) Decreased glucose output by the liver
(E) Increased ketone body production

50. A 45-year-old obese male presents for a routine physical. He has a sedentary lifestyle and eats a high-fat diet. His triglyceride (triacylglycerol) level is abnormally elevated. When glycerol (which is derived from adipose triacylglycerols) is converted to glucose, how many moles of high-energy phosphate are required?

(A) 1
(B) 2
(C) 3
(D) 4
(E) 6

51. A 5-year-old boy presents with rapid breathing, mild jaundice (yellowing of the skin), and an enlarged liver. His mother states that he seems to get like this every time he eats fruit or table sugar. After several tests, the patient is diagnosed with aldolase B deficiency. Which of the following is the reaction that this enzyme catalyzes?

(A) Fructose to fructose 1-phosphate
(B) Fructose 1-phosphate to DHAP and glyceraldehyde
(C) Sorbitol to fructose
(D) Glucose to sorbitol
(E) Galactose to galactose 1-phosphate

52. A 30-year-old male presents with fatigue and shortness of breath with minimal exertion. He recently started taking antimalarial drugs in preparation for a trip to Africa. His red blood cell count is abnormally low. He is diagnosed with glucose 6-phosphate dehydrogenase (G6PD) deficiency. This enzyme is important in producing:

(A) NAD^+
(B) NADH
(C) NADPH
(D) FAD^+
(E) FADH

53. A 20-year-old male presents with knee pain. The pain started after he was tackled playing football. Imaging reveals a tear in the cartilage, a substance rich in glycosaminoglycans. Which of the following is a characteristic of glycosaminoglycans?

(A) Positively charged
(B) Located intracellularly
(C) Degraded by lysosomal enzymes
(D) Noncompressible
(E) Dehydrated compounds

54. A 30-year-old female presents with profuse vomiting of bright red blood. Her blood is crossmatched (blood cell typing) and found to have blood group antigen (A) In blood group antigens, carbohydrates are linked to a serine or threonine residue in the protein, which is characteristic of:

(A) N-linked glycoproteins
(B) O-linked glycoproteins
(C) Dolichol phosphate
(D) UDP-sugars
(E) GDP-mannose

55. A 30-year-old pregnant female presents to her obstetrician for a prenatal visit. She has been conscious of her weight gain and has not been taking a multivitamin. Her red blood cells are found to have decreased transketolase function. Transketolase transfers 2-carbon units from the substrates of the pentose-phosphate pathway. Transketolase requires:

(A) Pyridoxine
(B) Cobalamin
(C) Thiamine
(D) Riboflavin
(E) Folate

56. A 35-year-old chef experiments with various cooking oils to give just the right taste to his new entree. Cooking oils contain fatty acids, such as palmitate, stearate, oleate, and linoleate. Which of the following reacts with fatty acid synthase to supply carbons for fatty acid synthesis?

(A) Glucose
(B) Pyruvate
(C) Acetyl CoA
(D) Oxaloacetate
(E) Malate

57. A 45-year-old chemist is trying to create a new medication that interferes with fatty acid synthesis. To try to figure out the best approach, he writes out the steps of fatty acid synthesis, which include:

(A) Elongation by 3-carbon units
(B) Oxidation of the β-keto group to a β-hydroxy group
(C) Hydration of the β-hydroxy group produces an enoyl group.
(D) Linoleate is released by the fatty acid synthase complex.
(E) Malonyl CoA provides carbon units that add to a fatty acyl CoA.

58. A 45-year-old male who has acquired immunodeficiency syndrome (AIDS) presents with profuse watery diarrhea and weight loss for the past month. Although he is being treated with proper medication, his diarrhea is continuing. Since he cannot take in proper nutrition by mouth, he is started on intravenous total parenteral nutrition, which supplies essential fatty acids required in the diet. In the liver, when two fatty acyl CoAs react with a glycerol moiety, which of the following is formed?

(A) Phosphatidic acid
(B) Diacylglycerol
(C) Triacylglycerol
(D) Arachidonic acid
(E) Glycerol 3-phosphate

59. A 40-year-old female presents with pain in her legs that is elicited upon walking and relieved by rest. Imaging reveals that diffuse atherosclerosis is causing her leg

pain. She is found to have no functional apoprotein C_{II}. Which of the following will be elevated in this patient's blood?

(A) Triglycerides
(B) Chylomicrons
(C) LDL
(D) HDL
(E) Cholesterol

60. A 45-year-old female presents with severe abdominal pain and vomiting. She is diagnosed with pancreatitis, and in the workup, it is found that the likely cause is an abnormally elevated triglyceride (triacylglycerol) level. Out of the blood lipoproteins, the highest component of triacylglycerols is found in:

(A) Chylomicrons and LDL
(B) Chylomicrons and VLDL
(C) LDL and VLDL
(D) LDL and HDL
(E) HDL and VLDL

61. A 20-year-old male presents with intermittent ataxia (abnormal gait), paralysis of eye muscles, and confusion. After an extensive workup, he is diagnosed with carnitine acyltransferase I (CATI) deficiency. The reaction catalyzed by CATI forms:

(A) Fatty acyl CoA
(B) Fatty acyl carnitine
(C) Fatty acid
(D) Malonyl CoA
(E) Carnitine

62. A 40-year-old obese male attends a nutrition course to revise his diet regimen. The nutritionist teaches about breakdown of long-chain fatty acids. When the 18-carbon oleate is oxidized, which of the following is released as the end product?

(A) Acetyl CoA
(B) Propionyl CoA
(C) Malonyl CoA
(D) Enoyl CoA
(E) β-Hydroxyacyl CoA

63. An infant presents with difficulty moving his limbs, facial abnormalities, and seizures. His blood level of very long–chain fatty acids is abnormally elevated, and he is diagnosed with Zellweger syndrome. Which of the following is true of oxidation of very long–chain fatty acids?

(A) Occurs in mitochondria
(B) Oxidized at the β-carbon
(C) Produces acetyl CoA
(D) Generates no ATP
(E) Degraded 2 carbons at a time

64. A 25-year-old female has a Malaysian meal rich in palm oil, which has a high content of palmitate. What is the approximate net ATP generation from the oxidation of palmitate to CO_2 and H_2O?

(A) 2
(B) 5
(C) 10
(D) 30
(E) 130

65. An infant presents with lethargy, sweating, and irritability. He is admitted to the pediatrics unit, where the nurses note that, when the time between feedings is prolonged, his symptoms are pronounced. After multiple tests, he is diagnosed with an enzyme deficiency that catalyzes the first step in the fatty acid β-oxidation spiral, which is:

(A) Fatty acid synthase
(B) Acyl CoA dehydrogenase
(C) Enoyl CoA hydratase
(D) L-3-hydroxyacyl CoA dehydrogenase
(E) β-Ketothiolase

66. A 35-year-old male presents with chest pain with exertion (angina). His cholesterol level is 500 mg/dL (normal, < 200 mg/dL), and he is diagnosed with familial hypercholesterolemia. In the liver, from which of the following is cholesterol synthesized?

(A) Acetyl CoA
(B) Triacylglycerol
(C) Fatty acids
(D) LDL
(E) HDL

67. A 45-year-old male presents with crushing substernal chest pain that radiates to his arm and jaw. He is diagnosed with a myocardial infarct (heart attack). He is placed on a statin medication, which inhibits HMG-CoA reductase. This enzyme reduces cytosolic HMG-CoA to:

(A) Acetyl CoA
(B) Mevalonic acid
(C) Squalene
(D) Lanosterol
(E) Cholesterol

68. A 50-year-old male presents with weakness in his leg. Imaging of his brain shows that he has had a stroke. If his blood cholesterol level is abnormally elevated, which of the following would also be expected to be abnormally elevated?

(A) Chylomicrons
(B) VLDL
(C) IDL
(D) LDL
(E) HDL

69. A 6-month-old infant presents with stools that are pale colored, bulky, and foul smelling. Deep tendon reflexes are absent, his vision is poor, and he has difficulty walking. He is diagnosed with abetalipoproteinemia, causing an inability to make and transport an apolipoprotein. His serum level of LDL and VLDL are found to be abnormally low. Which of the following apolipoproteins is most likely to be deficient?

(A) Apo A
(B) Apo B
(C) Apo C_{II}
(D) Apo E

70. An 8-year-old boy presents with severe abdominal pain and vomiting. Blood tests show that he is experiencing pancreatitis at a remarkably young age. Further testing shows that he has lipoprotein lipase deficiency. The level of chylomicrons in his blood is severely elevated. Which of the following would also be expected to be elevated?

(A) Fatty acids
(B) Cholesterol
(C) Triacylglycerols

(D) Glycerol

(E) LDL

71. A 17-year-old female with type 1 diabetes mellitus presents with lethargy, vomiting, and an odor of acetone on her breath. Blood tests show a severely elevated glucose level and an increased level of ketone bodies. These ketone bodies in her serum are synthesized from:

(A) Acetyl CoA

(B) Triacylglycerol

(C) Fatty acids

(D) Glycerol

(E) Cholesterol

72. A 50-year-old alcoholic male presents with persistent vomiting after binge drinking. He has not eaten any food in 2 weeks. He is found to have an abnormally elevated level of ketone bodies in his serum and urine, which is indicative of prolonged starvation and glycogen depletion. Which of the following is an example of a ketone body?

(A) Acetoacetate

(B) Phosphatidic acid

(C) Lecithin

(D) Ceramide

(E) Diacylglycerol

73. Immediately after birth, a premature infant has difficulty breathing, takes rapid breaths, and has blue-colored skin due to lack of oxygenation. He is diagnosed with respiratory distress syndrome of the newborn, which occurs due to surfactant deficiency. He is admitted to the neonatal unit, where he is administered exogenous surfactant. Surfactant is primarily composed of:

(A) Phosphatidic acid

(B) Phosphatidylinositol

(C) Phosphatidylethanolamine

(D) Phosphatidylcholine

(E) Phosphatidylserine

74. A 5-month-old infant presents with spasticity and seizures. On exam, the infant is found to be hypertonic (excessive muscle tone) and hyper-reflexic (excessive reflex response). β-Galactosidase levels are found to be abnormally low, and he is diagnosed with Krabbe disease. This disease causes accumulation of sphingolipids in cells. The backbone of sphingolipids is composed of:

(A) Serine

(B) Glycerol

(C) Ceramide

(D) Acetyl CoA

(E) Propionyl CoA

75. A 13-year-old boy presents with painful burning in his hands and feet, as well as lipid globules in his urine. He has an abnormally low level of the α-galactosidase A enzyme, and he is diagnosed with Fabry disease. Which of the following accumulates in this patient's cells?

(A) Phosphatidic acid

(B) Phospholipases

(C) Palmitoyl CoA

(D) Sphingosine

(E) Glycosphingolipids

76. In the nursery, an infant with blond hair and blue eyes is noted to have a mousy odor to his urine upon diaper changes. As is mandated by the state, all infants are screened for multiple inborn errors of metabolism, and he is found to have phenylketonuria (PKU), a disease resulting from a defect in phenylalanine hydroxylase. This enzyme converts phenylalanine to:

(A) Tyrosine

(B) Serine

(C) Glycine

(D) Cysteine

(E) Alanine

77. A 60-year-old male with liver failure presents with confusion and disorientation. He is diagnosed with hepatic encephalopathy and is placed on a low-protein diet. This is because a consistently high-protein diet will:

(A) Decrease urea production

(B) Increase ammonia production

(C) Reduce deamination of nitrogenous compounds

(D) Inhibit urea cycle enzymes
(E) Transfer amino groups from one amino acid to an α-ketoacid

78. A 60-year-old female undergoes major reconstructive surgery for third-degree burns. Branched-chain amino acid nutritional support has been hypothesized to improve nitrogen balance and decrease skeletal muscle catabolism in patients who undergo major surgical stress. Which of the following is an example of a branched-chain amino acid?

(A) Valine
(B) Aspartate
(C) Citrulline
(D) Arginine
(E) Glutamate

79. A 45-year-old female presents with severe dehydration and decreased urine output. Her blood urea nitrogen level is abnormally elevated because her kidneys are not able to properly excrete urea in the urine. In the production of urea, which is an important intermediate?

(A) Serine
(B) Glutamate
(C) Proline
(D) Ornithine
(E) Leucine

80. A 55-year-old male presents with pain in his hips. Physical examination reveals a blue-black tinge to his fingernails. His urine sample turns black upon sitting. He is diagnosed with alkaptonuria, a deficiency of homogentisic oxidase, resulting in accumulation of homogentisic acid, which is derived from:

(A) Tyrosine
(B) Lysine
(C) Threonine
(D) Isoleucine
(E) Tryptophan

81. A 40-year-old female is in a locked psychiatric unit, presenting with hallucinations and delusions. She hears voices and sees insects crawling on her skin. She is diagnosed with a disease called schizophrenia and is prescribed a dopamine antagonist. Dopamine is a neurotransmitter derived from:

(A) Creatine
(B) Nitric oxide
(C) Tyrosine
(D) Serotonin
(E) GABA

82. A 60-year-old male presents with fatigue, weakness, and shortness of breath. His red blood cells are abnormally enlarged. He is found to have a deficiency in a compound that transfers 1-carbon groups to purine precursors and is required for DNA and RNA synthesis. This compound is:

(A) Thyroid hormone
(B) Melanin
(C) Catecholamine
(D) Tetrahydrofolate
(E) *S*-adenosylmethionine

83. A 50-year-old male is brought to the emergency room with chest pain and shortness of breath. He is given a medication that activates cGMP, resulting in relaxation of vascular smooth muscle. This medication is most likely a derivative of:

(A) Creatine phosphate
(B) *S*-adenosylmethionine
(C) Glutathione
(D) Melatonin
(E) Nitric oxide

84. A 40-year-old female presents with sweating, diarrhea, tremors, and nervousness. Blood tests reveal she has excessive production of a compound derived from iodine and tyrosine, which is:

(A) Dopamine
(B) Thyroid hormone
(C) Melanin
(D) Epinephrine
(E) Norepinephrine

85. A 5-year-old boy presents with runny nose, itchy eyes, and sneezing. His symptoms are exacerbated in the summertime. He is prescribed a medication that blocks the bronchoconstriction, vasodilation, and allergic reactions caused by:

(A) Catecholamines
(B) *S*-adenosylmethionine
(C) Creatine phosphate
(D) Serotonin
(E) Histamine

86. A 5-year-old boy presents with mental retardation and self-mutilation. Blood tests show an elevated uric acid level. He is diagnosed with Lesch-Nyhan syndrome, a disease caused by a defect in hypoxanthine-guanine phosphoribosyl transferase (HGPRT). HGPRT is most significant in:

(A) Purine synthesis
(B) Purine salvage
(C) Purine degradation
(D) Pyrimidine synthesis
(E) Pyrimidine degradation

87. An infant presents with recurrent infections and a markedly decreased lymphocyte count. He is diagnosed with severe combined immunodeficiency due to adenosine deaminase (ADA) deficiency. Intracellular accumulation of dATP and dGTP is toxic and results in immune cell destruction. In purine degradation, adenosine deaminase catalyzes the conversion of:

(A) AMP to adenosine
(B) Adenosine to inosine
(C) Guanosine to guanine and ribose 1-phosphate
(D) Inosine to hypoxanthine and ribose 1-phosphate
(E) Hypoxanthine to xanthine

88. An infant presents with developmental delay, muscle weakness, and anemia. Urine analysis reveals a high level of excreted orotic acid. This patient has hereditary orotic aciduria due to a defect in UMP synthase. In which pathway is orotic acid and UMP synthase most directly involved?

(A) Purine synthesis
(B) Purine degradation
(C) Purine salvage
(D) Pyrimidine synthesis
(E) Pyrimidine degradation

89. A 10-year-old boy is hit on the leg by a baseball pitch, leaving a bruise. Over the next few weeks, the bruise starts to change color from dark red to green and yellow. Which of the following is responsible for this color change?

(A) Fe is converted to the ferrous (Fe^{2+}) state
(B) Heme production by δ-amino-levulinic acid (δ-ALA) synthase
(C) Conversion of heme to biliverdin and bilirubin
(D) Oxidation of iron by ceruloplasmin
(E) Increased erythropoietin production

90. An infant presents with neonatal jaundice. After several weeks, the jaundice becomes more exaggerated. The patient has an enzyme deficiency that inhibits conjugation of bilirubin. Which of the following reacts with bilirubin to conjugate it?

(A) Vitamin C
(B) Iron
(C) Ceruloplasmin
(D) Porphyrin ring
(E) UDP-glucuronate

91. An infant is born with a congenital brain malformation and dies shortly after birth. An enzyme screen shows that the patient was deficient in pyruvate carboxylase, the enzyme that converts pyruvate to oxaloacetate. Which of the following is the cofactor required for function of pyruvate carboxylase?

(A) Thiamine pyrophosphate
(B) Biotin
(C) Pyridoxal phosphate
(D) Acetyl CoA
(E) Vitamin B_{12} (cobalamin)

92. A 60-year-old female presents with burning on urination, fever, and chills. She is admitted for treatment of a severe urinary tract infection and is placed on an antibiotic. After a few weeks of taking this antibiotic, she develops bleeding gums and oozing of blood from her intravenous line site. Depletion of which of the following vitamins is most likely to be responsible for her symptoms?

(A) Vitamin A
(B) Vitamin B
(C) Vitamin C
(D) Vitamin D
(E) Vitamin K

93. An intern is scrubbing into a complicated surgery that is anticipated to last for 15 hours. In preparation, the intern has not eaten or drunken anything for the past 15 hours so that he will not have to go to the bathroom in the middle of the surgery. After 30 hours of fasting, which of the following is most important for maintenance of normal blood glucose?

(A) Glycogenolysis
(B) Gluconeogenesis
(C) Triacylglycerol synthesis
(D) Increased insulin release
(E) Decreased muscle protein breakdown

94. A 70-year-old female with Alzheimer dementia wanders away from her home into the woods. She gets lost in the woods for 5 days without food or water. After 5 days of starvation, which of the following is the primary source of energy for the body?

(A) Carbohydrate
(B) Lipid
(C) Protein
(D) Vitamins
(E) Minerals

95. A 70-year-old male presents with a fever, productive cough, and rust-colored sputum. He is diagnosed with bacterial pneumonia, and his antibiotic dose is adjusted according to his creatinine clearance rate. The creatinine clearance rate measures function for which of the following tissues?

(A) Heart
(B) Skeletal muscle
(C) Brain
(D) Liver
(E) Kidney

96. A 16-year-old type 1 diabetic female checks her fingerstick blood glucose before a meal. She injects herself subcutaneously with exogenous insulin and then starts to eat. As insulin is absorbed into her blood, it binds to insulin receptors that activate:

(A) Tyrosine kinase
(B) Adenylate cyclase
(C) Cyclic AMP (cAMP)
(D) Protein kinase C
(E) Phospholipase C

97. A 30-year-old female presents with headaches and blurry vision. Her blood pressure is 200/100 mm Hg (normal, 120/80 mm Hg). Imaging reveals that she has a tumor that is overproducing the hormone most responsible for regulating salt and water balance for blood pressure control, which is:

(A) Growth hormone
(B) Thyroid-stimulating hormone
(C) Glucocorticoid
(D) Aldosterone
(E) Epinephrine

98. A 30-year-old female presents to an infertility clinic with a wish to become pregnant. She states that she and her husband have been unsuccessfully trying to have a baby for 2 years. Over the next few months, her physician runs some tests, which show that she may not be ovulating. Which of the following is responsible for ovulation?

(A) Increased FSH
(B) Increased estradiol
(C) LH surge
(D) Increased progesterone
(E) Increased progesterone and estradiol

99. A 65-year-old male presents with difficulty starting urination, difficulty emptying his bladder, and frequent urination at night. He is diagnosed with benign prostatic hyperplasia, a common condition that causes enlargement of the prostate with resultant compression of the urethra, which inhibits urine from passing out of the bladder. He is prescribed a 5-α reductase inhibitor called finasteride. Which of the following hormones is most likely inhibited by finasteride?

(A) Leydig cell secretion of testosterone
(B) Sertoli cell production of androgen-binding protein (ABP)
(C) Dihydrotestosterone
(D) Progesterone
(E) Estradiol

100. A 60-year-old female presents with severe back pain for the past week. Imaging reveals a compression fracture of one of the vertebrae and diffuse osteopenia. She is diagnosed with osteoporosis, which is a common condition resulting from calcium depletion in bones. As treatment, she is prescribed:

(A) Oxytocin
(B) Prolactin
(C) Estradiol
(D) Calcitonin
(E) Parathyroid hormone

101. A 25-year-old female who is 10 weeks pregnant presents with intractable vomiting from morning sickness. She is admitted for intravenous glucose administration and hydration. Glucose enters pancreatic β cells and activates the insulin gene. The insulin gene is transcribed into insulin messenger RNA. Which of the following best describes the structure of messenger RNA?

(A) B form with 10 base pairs per turn
(B) Double-stranded circular
(C) Cap structure and poly(A) tail
(D) Contains many loops and extensive base pairing
(E) Cloverleaf structure

102. A 60-year-old female presents with burning on urination and blood in her urine. She is diagnosed with a urinary tract infection. She is prescribed an antibiotic that inhibits an enzyme that prevents extreme supercoiling of DNA. Supercoiling of DNA would result from unwinding at a replication fork, but this enzyme breaks and rejoins DNA chains. Which of the following is most characteristic of this enzyme?

(A) Helicase
(B) Single-stranded binding protein
(C) Topoisomerase

(D) DNA polymerase I
(E) DNA polymerase III

103. A 40-year-old male presents with an enlarged nose, ears, and jaw, sausage-like fingers, and excessive sweating. He is diagnosed with acromegaly, a disease of excessive growth hormone production. The gene for growth hormone is transcribed by RNA polymerase in the pituitary. At what part of the gene does RNA polymerase bind?

(A) Promoter
(B) TATA box
(C) CAAT box
(D) Consensus sequence
(E) Enhancer

104. An infant presents with pale skin, an enlarged liver, and a severe anemia. The hemoglobin in his red blood cells is deficient in β-globin chains. He is diagnosed with β-thalassemia, in which the β-globin gene possesses mutations that affect RNA splicing. Regarding cleavage and splicing from hnRNA to mRNA, which of the following statements is true?

(A) The poly(A) tail is removed.
(B) Small nuclear RNAs (snRNPs) are involved.
(C) mRNA contains introns and exons.
(D) It occurs in the cytoplasm.
(E) mRNA is always the same size or larger than hnRNA.

105. A 30-year-old female presents with a feeling of fullness in her lower abdomen. Her physician notes an abnormally enlarged ovary and ascites (fluid) in her abdomen. The ascites fluid is sampled, and the cytology report returns as ovarian cancer. Radiation is discussed as a possible treatment, but the patient is concerned about DNA damage because she still wishes to become pregnant. When insults such as radiation cause DNA mutagenesis, which of the following is involved in DNA repair?

(A) Leading and lagging strands
(B) Exonuclease
(C) Okazaki fragments

(D) Reverse transcriptase
(E) Transposon

106. A 14-year-old African female presents with extreme pain in her chest and legs. A peripheral smear shows sickling of her red blood cells. She is diagnosed with sickle cell anemia, a disease in which red blood cells lyse and, due to an abnormal sickle shape, can occlude the lumens of blood vessels. Sickle cell anemia is caused by a mutation that results in one amino acid being replaced by another, which is also called a:

(A) Missense mutation
(B) Nonsense mutation
(C) Insertion
(D) Deletion
(E) Frameshift mutation

107. A 50-year-old male presents with fever and hypotension, and his blood cultures are positive for bacteria. He is prescribed an antibiotic called an aminoglycoside. Aminoglycosides bind to the 30S subunit of bacterial ribosomes. Since mammalian ribosomes do not have a 30S subunit, translation of the patient's proteins can proceed normally. Which of the following is a step in the initiation of translation?

(A) Binding of methionyl-tRNA$_i^{Met}$ to the small ribosomal subunit
(B) Binding of aminoacyl-tRNA to the A site
(C) Formation of a peptide bond
(D) Translocation of peptidyl-tRNA to the P site
(E) Termination codon in the A site

108. A 20-year-old male presents with severe anemia. After extensive testing, he is diagnosed with a rare disease called Diamond-Blackfan anemia. In this disease, most cases are caused by a mutation in the ribosomal protein S19. Secreted proteins are synthesized on ribosomes attached to the rough endoplasmic reticulum. Which of the following is unique to the synthesis of secreted proteins?

(A) Initiation factor
(B) Elongation factor

(C) Peptidyl transferase
(D) Signal sequence
(E) Polysome

109. A 65-year-old female presents to the emergency room with fever, chills, and a kidney infection caused by *Escherichia coli*. *E. coli* use the *lac* operon, a set of genes that are coordinately controlled, to adjust for their environment. Which of the following statements is true of *lac* operon?

(A) Binding of a repressor protein to the operator activates transcription.
(B) Allolactose inhibits the lac operon.
(C) It is induced only in the absence of glucose.
(D) Proteins produced inhibit the utilization of lactose.
(E) RNA polymerase binds to the inducer to transcribe the operon.

110. A 75-year-old male is brought to the emergency room after being hit by a car. His leg bone is broken in half, and the bone is protruding through the skin. After orthopedic surgery, he is recovering well. After several days, the wound starts to turn red, warm, and painful. The wound culture reveals a new bacterial organism that is resistant to all antibiotics currently available. The effort toward creating new antibiotics requires targeting of characteristics exclusive to bacteria and not to humans. Which of the following statements is exclusively true of prokaryotes but not eukaryotes?

(A) Transcription and translation occur at the same time.
(B) Most cells are diploid.
(C) Each gene has its own promoter.
(D) DNA is complexed with histones.
(E) Genes contain introns.

111. A 5-year-old boy presents with a large mass on his jaw. Biopsy reveals Burkitt lymphoma, a cancer of lymph nodes. In Burkitt lymphoma, the myc gene, which is normally found on chromosome 8, is translocated to chromosome 14. Myc is an example of the group of proteins that contain amino acid sequences with motifs, such as helix-loop-helix, leucine zipper, and zinc finger domains. This group is called:

(A) Growth factors
(B) Signal transducing proteins
(C) Nuclear transcription factors
(D) Cell cycle regulators
(E) Tumor-suppressor genes

112. A 65-year-old female presents with enlarged lymph nodes in her neck. She noticed them a month ago but they subsided, so she did not seek medical attention. Now the lymph nodes have enlarged again. Lymph node biopsy reveals follicular lymphoma, which is a tumor of B cells that overexpresses bcl-2, which is a product from a:

(A) Tumor-suppressor gene
(B) Growth factor gene
(C) Anti-apoptotic gene
(D) Philadelphia chromosome
(E) Oncogene

113. A 65-year-old male presents with weight loss, fever, and night sweats. Imaging of his abdomen shows a large liver nodule that is diagnosed as primary liver cancer. Major liver resection is not an option because of the location of the cancer. He is given tumor necrosis factor (TNF), which kills cancer cells, but has severe side effects. TNF stimulates the activation of:

(A) Caspases
(B) Bax
(C) bcl-2
(D) Fas ligand
(E) p53

114. A 65-year-old female presents with a hard lump in her breast. She has never undergone a routine mammogram. Core biopsy reveals cancerous cells that express the HER2/neu oncogene, which portends a poor prognosis. Targeting of this oncogene is currently treated with:

(A) Ionizing radiation
(B) Tyrosine kinase inhibitor
(C) Retroviruses
(D) Monoclonal antibody
(E) BRCA-1 inhibition

115. A 40-year-old male presents with café-au-lait spots, a peripheral nerve sheath tumor (schwannomas), and a tumor of the 7th cranial nerve (acoustic neuroma). This disease is caused by a mutation in a gene product that has intrinsic GTPase activity, which is:

(A) WT-1
(B) Cyclin D
(C) NF-1
(D) Rb
(E) p53

116. A 25-year-old female is sexually active with a new partner and would like to have an HIV test. The current standard for HIV testing is to start with an enzyme-linked immunosorbent assay (ELISA). HIV antigens are coated on a plate, and the patient's serum is added. If the patient has HIV antibodies, binding of these antibodies to the antigens on the plate will be detected. If the ELISA test is positive, a confirmatory test is done. In this confirmatory test, the patient's serum is added to HIV antigens, which are on a nitrocellulose membrane. This confirmatory test is a:

(A) Northern blot
(B) Southern blot
(C) Western blot
(D) Gel electrophoresis
(E) Restriction endonuclease

117. A 50-year-old male presents with weight loss, fever, and night sweats. Imaging shows that he has a lung nodule suspicious for cancer. The patient does not wish to undergo surgical resection of a lobe of his lung. Biopsy is taken of the nodule, and pathology reveals cancerous cells. mRNA is isolated from the biopsy, is reverse transcribed into complementary DNA (cDNA), and is labeled with a blue probe. mRNA from normal lung tissue is reverse transcribed to cDNA and is labeled with a red probe. These cDNAs are mixed and are applied to a chip. The chip has 20,000 genes that are often implicated in cancer adherent to it. Which of the following best defines this assay?

(A) Reverse transcriptase
(B) DNA microarray
(C) DNA fingerprinting
(D) DNA sequencing
(E) DNA cloning

118. An 18-year-old girl is found dead in her apartment. A forensics pathologist takes a hair found at the crime scene. He isolates DNA from the hair and replicates it in an exponential fashion to generate a much larger amount of DNA. This method is called:

(A) Expression
(B) Genotyping
(C) Polymerase chain reaction
(D) Single nucleotide polymorphism
(E) Mapping

119. Much controversy has surrounded stem cell research. Which of the following best defines stem cells?

(A) Differentiated
(B) Pluripotent
(C) Only found in the embryo

(D) Only found in the bone marrow
(E) Mature

120. A 26-year-old pregnant female has sickle cell trait (heterozygous hemoglobin S). She states that the baby's father also has sickle cell trait, and she is concerned that her baby may have sickle cell disease (homozygous hemoglobin S). A test is performed that detects a mutation that occurs in a site that is within or tightly linked to a gene. An enzyme can cleave normal DNA at this site but not the mutant. Thus, normal DNA will appear as two fragments, while the mutant DNA will appear as one fragment. This assay is called:

(A) Variable number of tandem repeats (VNTR)
(B) Restriction fragment length polymorphism (RFLP)
(C) Amplification
(D) Polymerization
(E) Labeling

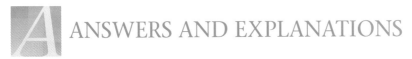

A ANSWERS AND EXPLANATIONS

1–A. HCl is a strong acid that dissociates completely. Weak acids include acetic acid and dissociate only to a limited extent. The pH of pure water is 7, and the pH of an HCl solution is acidic and lower than 7. Acids donate protons, and bases accept protons.

2–A. Bicarbonate and carbonic acid act as one of the major buffers of the blood. Water does not dissociate to form the acid-base conjugate pairs required in a buffer. Sulfuric acid, phosphoric acid, and hydrochloric acid are major acids produced in the body and do not serve as buffers.

3–C. Enantiomers are stereoisomers that are mirror images of each other. Stereoisomers have the same chemical formula but differ in the position of the hydroxyl groups on one or more of their asymmetric carbons. Epimers are stereoisomers that differ in the position of only one asymmetric carbon.

4–A. Arginine is a positively charged amino acid that is present on the side chains of basic amino acids. Glycine does not have a side chain and is not positively or negatively charged. Proline is an imino acid, in which nitrogen is part of a ring. Aspartate and glutamate are negatively charged amino acids that are present on the side chain of acidic amino acids.

5–A. Genetic diseases, such as cystic fibrosis, are passed from the previous generation through the DNA. DNA is transcribed into RNA, which is then translated into protein. The mutated protein in cystic fibrosis has a loss of a phenylalanine residue at position 508. RNA, protein, and carbohydrates are not passed down from the previous generation.

6–B. The primary structure is defined as the amino acid sequence of a polypeptide chain. In secondary structure, α-helices or β-sheets are created. The tertiary structure refers to the overall three-dimensional conformation of a protein. Quaternary structure refers to the spatial arrangement of the subunits in a protein containing more than one polypeptide chain.

7–E. Chaperones are proteins that interact with a polypeptide to mediate proper folding into the correct tertiary structure. ATP is a nucleotide that is required for many energy-requiring activities of cells. Leucine zippers and zinc fingers are motifs that are often found in transcription factors, which help to mediate binding of proteins to DNA.

8–D. Phosphorylation is an example of a post-translational modification of a protein. Denaturation of proteins occurs due to heat or urea treatment and results in unfolding of polypeptide chains without causing hydrolysis of peptide bonds. Renaturation is the process of a denatured protein returning to its native state. Folding of a polypeptide results in tertiary structure. Binding to DNA is not a post-translational modification.

9–C. The proteasome degrades intracellular proteins into peptides. Ubiquitin is a protein that covalently attaches to proteins targeted for degradation by the proteasome, in a process called ubiquitination. Extracellular proteins are degraded within lysosomes. The proteasome is a multi-protein complex composed of proteases.

10–B. In the synthesis of collagen, O_2 and vitamin C are required for hydroxylating proline and lysine residues. Approximately one third of collagen is made of glycine residues.

The cleaving of the "pre-" signal sequence of preprocollagen, the forming of the triple helix, and the addition of galactose and glucose to hydroxylysine residues do not require vitamin C.

11–A. Enzymes decrease the energy of activation for a reaction and thus speed up a reaction. The thermodynamics of a reaction, such as the net free energy change and the equilibrium concentrations of substrate and product, remain unchanged.

12–B. Competitive inhibitors compete with substrate for binding at the active site of the enzyme, and thus they are similar to substrate in structure. V_{max} remains the same, and the apparent K_m is increased. Irreversible inhibitors bind covalently to the enzyme and inactivate it.

13–E. Allopurinol is a competitive inhibitor, and thus, its activity can be reversed by increasing substrate. Competitive inhibitors have a similar structure to substrate (not enzyme), and they bind to enzyme (not to substrate). Noncompetitive inhibitors bind to the enzyme at a site distinct from the active site. Irreversible inhibitors inactivate the enzyme they covalently bind to.

14–B. V_{max} is the maximum velocity of an enzyme, or how fast an enzyme can go at "full speed." V_{max} is reached when all of the enzyme is bound to substrate (without inhibition). The V_{max} decreases when noncompetitive inhibitors bind to enzyme because the activity of the enzyme decreases. Binding of noncompetitive inhibitor to enzyme at a site distinct from the active site does not change the substrate or inactivate the enzyme. Noncompetitive inhibitors do not affect the amount of substrate.

15–B. Allosteric activators (such as O_2 binding to hemoglobin) cause the enzyme to bind substrate more readily. Allosteric inhibitors cause the enzyme to bind substrate less readily. Allosteric enzymes do not obey Michaelis-Menten kinetics. Enzyme cascades are enzymes arranged such that they exponentially amplify the availability or activity of products in the path. Feedback inhibition is where the concentration of the end product of a pathway shuts off the first enzyme of that pathway.

16–C. Respiratory quotient (R.Q.) is the ratio of CO_2 produced to O_2 used (CO_2/O_2) by a tissue in oxidation of a foodstuff. The R.Q. for fat is 0.7, 0.8 for protein, and 1.0 for carbohydrate. R.Q. is increased in exercise toward carbohydrate metabolism and is thus higher for a muscle at exercise than at rest.

17–B. Positive nitrogen balance describes the state when dietary nitrogen exceeds excreted nitrogen. Negative nitrogen balance occurs when dietary nitrogen is less than excreted nitrogen. Nitrogen balance occurs when dietary nitrogen equals excreted nitrogen. Anabolism describes biosynthetic pathways, which require energy. Catabolism describes degradative pathways, some of which yield energy.

18–A. ΔG is the change in free energy, or the energy available to do useful work at a constant pressure and temperature. If ΔG is negative, the reaction will proceed spontaneously with the release of energy. If ΔG is positive, the reaction will not proceed spontaneously. If ΔG is at zero, the reaction is at equilibrium and results in no net change in substrate or product concentrations. ΔG is not related to the rate of a reaction; the rate of a reaction depends on the enzyme that catalyzes the reaction.

19–C. An oxidant accepts electrons. An oxidant is reduced by a reductant, which donates electrons. ΔE is the change in reduction potential. The larger the positive value for ΔE, the larger the negative value for ΔG ($\Delta G = -nF\Delta E$). Thus, a positive ΔE indicates an energetically favorable process.

20–B. Adenosine is a nucleoside that contains adenine linked to ribose. AMP is a nucleotide that contains adenosine with a phosphate group esterified to the 5′-hydroxyl of its sugar. ATP can transfer phosphate groups to compounds such as glucose, with ADP as a product. Hydrolysis of ATP to ADP and P_i has a ΔG of −7.3 kcal/mole.

21–C. Lactase converts lactose into glucose and galactose. Maltose is cleaved by maltase to two glucose residues. Sucrase converts sucrose to glucose and fructose. Sucrose, maltose, and lactose are disaccharides.

22–A. Amylase cleaves α-1,4 linkages between glucose residues. The α-1,6 linkage creates the unbranched component of glycogen. The enzyme β-1,4 endoglucosidase is required to digest the polysaccharides found in cellulose, which is the carbohydrate storage found in plants. The α-1 to β-2 bond is found in sucrose. α-4,6 linkages are found in the branches of glycogen.

23–C. Pancreatic lipase digests triacylglycerols to 2-monoacylglycerols and free fatty acids, which are then packaged into micelles. The micelles are absorbed by intestinal epithelial cells. Bile salts emulsify dietary lipids in the small intestine. Pancreatic amylase cleaves α-1,4 linkages in carbohydrates. Bicarbonate is released with pancreatic enzymes and neutralizes stomach acid, raising the pH into the optimal range for these digestive enzymes.

24–A. Trypsin cleaves peptide bonds in which the carboxyl group is contributed by arginine or lysine. Chymotrypsin cleaves peptide bonds at the carboxyl group of aromatic amino acids or by leucine. Carboxypeptidase A cleaves aromatic amino acids from the C-terminus. Carboxypeptidase B cleaves the basic amino acids, lysine and arginine, from the C-terminus. Aminopeptidases are produced by intestinal cells and cleave one amino acid from the N-terminus.

25–A. GERD is caused by the reflux of HCl from the stomach to the esophagus. Pepsinogen is the inactive zymogen that autocatalyzes to form active pepsin. Endopeptidases (such as trypsin, chymotrypsin, and elastase) and exopeptidases (such as carboxypeptidase A and B) are produced by the pancreas. Enteropeptidase (enterokinase) cleaves trypsinogen to form trypsin and is produced by intestinal cells.

26–A. In glycolysis, 1 mole of glucose is converted to 2 moles of pyruvate. Pyruvate can be converted to lactate by lactate dehydrogenase to regenerate NAD^+. Pyruvate can also enter mitochondria and be converted by pyruvate dehydrogenase to acetyl CoA.

27–B. 2,3-Bisphosphoglycerate is a compound that decreases the affinity of hemoglobin for oxygen, so that oxygen can be released from hemoglobin in red blood cells to tissues. 2,3-Bisphosphoglycerate is formed from 1,3-bisphosphoglycerate, and this latter compound is formed from glyceraldehyde 3-phosphate (which is formed in glycolysis). Dihydroxyacetone phosphate and phosphoenolpyruvate are formed in the process of glycolysis.

28–B. Pyruvate can be reduced in the cytosol by NADH to form lactate, thus regenerating NAD$^+$, which is needed so that glucose can keep flowing through glycolysis. Acetyl CoA enters the TCA cycle to form CO_2, H_2O, and energy.

29–D. Hexokinase is one of the regulatory enzymes of glycolysis and converts glucose to glucose 6-phosphate. Hexokinase has a low K_m for glucose, which means that it works near its maximum rate (V_{max}), even when blood glucose is low. It is inhibited by its product, glucose 6-phosphate. Hexokinase is present in most tissues.

30–A. Glycolysis produces only 2 moles of ATP (2 moles of ATP are used, and 4 moles of ATP are produced) from 1 mole of glucose. Two moles of pyruvate that undergo oxidative phosphorylation generate approximately 6 moles of ATP. Two moles of acetyl CoA that are oxidized in the TCA cycle generate approximately 24 moles of ATP. Overall, when 1 mole of glucose is oxidized to CO_2 and H_2O, approximately 36 or 38 moles of ATP are produced (depending on which shuttle is used).

31–E. The tricarboxylic acid cycle occurs in mitochondria, and red blood cells do not have mitochondria. Glycolysis occurs in the cytosol. Lysosomes are vesicles that contain enzymes that degrade proteins at an acidic pH. The Golgi apparatus is important in intracellular membrane trafficking.

32–A. Pyruvate dehydrogenase converts pyruvate to acetyl CoA, which can then enter the TCA cycle. This enzyme complex is present in an active (dephosphorylated) form and an inactive (phosphorylated) form. When the concentration of the substrates, CoASH and NAD$^+$, is high, the enzyme is active. When the concentration of the products, acetyl CoA and NADH, is high, the enzyme is inactive.

33–D. NADH and FADH$_2$, produced from the TCA cycle, donate electrons to the electron transport chain for generation of ATP. Inhibition of isocitrate dehydrogenase occurs when there are high levels of products from the TCA cycle. Therefore, high levels of NADH and high levels of ATP (a low ADP:ATP ratio) will allosterically inhibit isocitrate dehydrogenase. Acetyl CoA is produced from pyruvate by pyruvate dehydrogenase, with CoASH as a substrate.

34–B. One mole of glucose produces 2 moles of ATP (2 moles of ATP are used, and 4 moles of ATP are produced) and 2 moles of pyruvate in glycolysis. One mole of pyruvate is converted to acetyl CoA, which is oxidized in the TCA cycle to generate approximately 12 moles of ATP. Thus, 2 moles of pyruvate would generate 24 moles of ATP. Overall, when 1 mole of glucose is oxidized to CO_2 and H_2O, approximately 36 or 38 moles of ATP are produced (depending on which shuttle is used).

35–A. α-Ketoglutarate dehydrogenase and pyruvate dehydrogenase are the major α-ketoacid dehydrogenases, which catalyze oxidative decarboxylations in a sequence of reactions that involve the cofactors of thiamine pyrophosphate, lipoic acid, coenzyme A, FAD, and NAD$^+$. Citrate synthase, isocitrate dehydrogenase, fumarase, and malate dehydrogenase are other enzymes in the TCA cycle.

36–C. Electron transfer occurs from NADH to FMN to coenzyme Q to cytochromes to O_2, which is reduced to H_2O. Electrons from FADH$_2$ enter the electron transport chain at the coenzyme Q level.

37–C. Cyanide combines with cytochrome oxidase and blocks the transfer of electrons to O_2. NADH passes electrons via the NADH dehydrogenase complex to FMN. As electrons are passed from complexes I–IV, an electrochemical potential or proton-motive force is generated. Protons can re-enter the matrix only through the ATP synthase complex, complex V (the F_0–F_1 ATPase), causing ATP to be generated. ATP is exchanged for ADP by the ATP-ADP antiport in the inner mitochondrial membrane.

38–B. Malignant hyperthermia is a reaction that genetically prone individuals may have to some inhaled anesthetics. Uncoupling of oxidative phosphorylation from electron transport results in excessive heat generation and decreased ATP production. Excessive activity of the F_0–F_1 ATPase would result in increased ATP generation. Oxidation of NADH with phosphorylation of ADP to form ATP simply defines oxidative phosphorylation. Shutdown of the ATP-ADP antiport would inhibit transfer of ATP (in exchange for ADP) to the cytosol. Reactive oxygen species are byproducts of pathways of oxidative metabolism.

39–C. Coenzyme Q is the major source of superoxide within cells. Coenzyme Q occasionally loses an electron in the transfer of reducing equivalents through the electron chain, and this electron is transferred to dissolved oxygen to produce superoxide. The NADH dehydrogenase complex, FMN, cytochrome b, and cytochrome c are other key components in the electron transport chain.

40–C. For every NADH that is oxidized, one-half O_2 is reduced to H_2O, and approximately 3 ATP are produced. For every $FADH_2$ that is oxidized, approximately 2 ATP are generated because electrons from $FADH_2$ enter the chain via coenzyme Q, bypassing the NADH dehydrogenase step.

41–C. In glycogen, the linkages between glucose residues are α-1,4, except at branch points, where the linkage is α-1,6. There are no β linkages in glycogen.

42–C. Glycogen synthase adds glucose residues from UDP-glucose to the nonreducing ends of a glycogen primer. Glucose is phosphorylated to glucose 6-phosphate, which is converted to glucose 1-phosphate, which reacts with UTP, forming UDP-glucose.

43–B. Glycogen phosphorylase uses inorganic phosphate (P_i) to cleave α-1,4 bonds, producing glucose 1-phosphate. Glucose 1-phosphate is converted to glucose 6-phosphate, which releases inorganic phosphate, and free glucose enters the blood. UDP-glucose and glycogen primer are used in glycogen synthesis, not degradation.

44–B. Glucagon, a peptide hormone, acts on liver cells to stimulate glycogen degradation. Glycogen phosphorylase is activated to cleave glucose residues from the nonreducing ends of glycogen chains, producing glucose 1-phosphate, which is eventually converted to free glucose. Glucagon decreases glycogen synthase activity. Glucokinase, hexokinase, and UDP-glucose pyrophosphorylase are not induced by glucagon.

45–A. Liver glycogenolysis and gluconeogenesis are most important in maintaining blood glucose during fasting or exercise. Skeletal muscle does not contain glucose 6-phosphatase and, therefore, does not contribute to the maintenance of blood glucose. Lysosomal glycogen is degraded by an α-glucosidase and is not necessary for maintaining normal blood glucose levels. The heart and spleen are other organs that can store glycogen.

46–C. Oxaloacetate is decarboxylated by PEPCK to form phosphoenolpyruvate (and not the reverse). Pyruvate is not directly converted to phosphoenolpyruvate. Pyruvate carboxylase converts pyruvate to oxaloacetate. Phosphoenolpyruvate is converted to fructose 1,6-bisphosphate by reversal of the glycolytic reactions.

47–B. The primary precursors for gluconeogenesis are lactate, amino acids, and glycerol. Amino acid nitrogen is converted to urea. Even-chain fatty acids are oxidized to acetyl CoA, which enters the TCA cycle. For every 2 carbons of acetyl CoA that enter the TCA cycle, 2 carbons are released as CO_2, thus there is no net synthesis of glucose from acetyl CoA. ATP (or GTP) is required for gluconeogenesis.

48–C. Pyruvate carboxylase converts pyruvate to oxaloacetate for gluconeogenesis. Since oxaloacetate cannot be produced, citrate cannot be produced for the TCA cycle. Pyruvate is shunted to alternate pathways to produce lactate, alanine, and acetyl CoA. Acetyl CoA cannot produce citrate without oxaloacetate and is thus shunted to produce ketone bodies.

49–A. Type 1 diabetes mellitus causes autoimmune destruction of pancreatic β cells, which produce insulin. Due to insulin deficiency and a high glucagon level, these patients manifest with hyperglycemia because of decreased uptake of glucose by cells and increased glucose output by the liver. The glucagon:insulin ratio is abnormally increased. Ketone body production is also increased. Since patients have a normal response to insulin (and glucagon), they are treated with exogenous insulin.

50–B. Since 2 moles of glycerol are required to form 1 mole of glucose during gluconeogenesis, 2 moles of high-energy phosphate are required for synthesis of 1 mole of glucose. Glycerol enters gluconeogenesis at the DHAP level. In contrast, two moles of pyruvate are required to form 1 mole of glucose, so 6 moles of high-energy phosphate are required for synthesis of 1 mole of glucose.

51–B. Fructose 1-phosphate aldolase cleaves fructose 1-phosphate to form DHAP and glyceraldehyde. Patients who are deficient in this enzyme are asymptomatic until they ingest fructose. The major dietary sources of fructose are table sugar and fruit. Fructokinase converts fructose to fructose 1-phosphate. Sorbitol dehydrogenase converts sorbitol to fructose. Aldose reductase converts glucose to sorbitol. Galactokinase converts galactose to galactose 1-phosphate.

52–C. G6PD is the first enzyme of the pentose phosphate pathway. G6PD deficiency results in insufficient amounts of NADPH to be produced under certain conditions of oxidative stress (such as taking some antimalarial drugs). As a result, glutathione in red blood cells is not adequately reduced and, in turn, is not available to reduce antimalarial drug metabolites. This results in a hemolytic anemia (red blood cell lysis).

53–C. Glycosaminoglycans are degraded by lysosomal enzymes. Glycosaminoglycans are negatively charged, located extracellularly, highly compressible, and heavily hydrated.

54–B. O-linked glycoproteins are carbohydrates linked to a serine or threonine residue in the protein. UDP-sugars and GDP-mannose are some of the precursors. N-linked glycoproteins are carbohydrates linked to an asparagine residue in the protein. Dolichol phosphate is involved in the synthesis of N-linked glycoproteins.

55–C. Transketolase requires thiamine pyrophosphate. Pyridoxine, cobalamin, riboflavin, and folate are other important B vitamins.

56–C. Acetyl CoA reacts with the phosphopantetheinyl residue of fatty acid synthase. Pyruvate, oxaloacetate, and malate are involved in the conversion of glucose to acetyl CoA.

57–E. Malonyl CoA provides the 2-carbon units that add to palmitoyl CoA or longer chain fatty acyl CoAs. Fatty acids are elongated by 2-carbon units. The β-keto group is reduced by NADPH to a β-hydroxy group. Dehydration occurs, producing an enoyl group with the double bond between carbons 2 and 3. Palmitate is released by the fatty acid synthase complex.

58–A. Glycerol 3-phosphate provides the glycerol moiety that reacts with two fatty acyl CoAs to form phosphatidic acid. The phosphate group is cleaved to form a diacylglycerol, which reacts with another fatty acyl CoA to form a triacylglycerol. Arachidonic acid is a polyunsaturated fatty acid that is present in the phospholipids of cell membranes.

59–B. Apoprotein C_{II} is transferred from HDL to chylomicrons and VLDL. Apoprotein C_{II} activates lipoprotein lipase, which hydrolyzes the triacylglycerols of chylomicrons and VLDL to fatty acids and glycerol. LDL contains the highest content of cholesterol and its esters.

60–B. Triacylglycerols synthesized by intestinal epithelial cells become a component of chylomicrons. In the liver, triacylglycerol is incorporated into VLDL. LDL has the highest content of cholesterol but less triacylglycerol. HDL has the lowest triacylglycerol content.

61–B. In fatty acid oxidation, CATI catalyzes the transfer of acyl groups from fatty acyl CoA to carnitine to form fatty acyl carnitine. CATI is inhibited by malonyl CoA. Fatty acids are activated by ATP and CoA to form a fatty acyl CoA.

62–A. Acetyl CoA is the end product in the oxidation of even-chain fatty acids. Oxidation of odd-chain fatty acids produces acetyl CoA and propionyl CoA. Malonyl CoA is an intermediate in fatty acid synthesis. Enoyl CoA and β-hydroxyacyl CoA are intermediates in fatty acid oxidation.

63–D. Oxidation of very long–chain fatty acids occurs in peroxisomes and generates no ATP. Oxidation occurs at the α-carbon, so the fatty acid is degraded one carbon at a time, producing CO_2.

64–E. Oxidation of fatty acids provides a rich source of ATP. The net ATP produced from palmitate is 129. Two ATP are used to activate palmitate to palmitoyl CoA, and oxidation of palmitoyl CoA to CO_2 and H_2O generates 131 ATP ($131 - 2 = 129$).

65–B. Acyl CoA dehydrogenase is the enzyme that catalyzes the first step in the fatty acid β-oxidation spiral. Fatty acid synthase is the first enzyme involved in fatty acid synthesis. Enoyl CoA hydratase, L-3-hydroxyacyl CoA dehydrogenase, and β-ketothiolase are the other enzymes involved in the β-oxidation spiral.

66–A. Cholesterol is synthesized from cytosolic acetyl CoA. Triacylglycerols are produced from fatty acids. LDL and HDL are examples of lipoproteins, which are composed of triacylglycerols, cholesterol, cholesterol esters, phospholipids, and proteins.

67–B. HMG-CoA is reduced to mevalonic acid by HMG-CoA reductase. Acetyl CoA, squalene, and lanosterol are other intermediates involved in cholesterol synthesis.

68–D. LDL has the highest content of cholesterol and its esters and is known as the "bad" lipoprotein. Chylomicrons and VLDL have a high content of triacylglycerols. IDL, which is derived from VLDL, has less than one half the amount of triacylglycerol. HDL is known as the "good" lipoprotein because it can transport cholesterol from the periphery back to the liver for excretion or re-utilization.

69–B. Apo B is the major apolipoprotein of LDL and VLDL. Apo A is the major apolipoprotein of HDL. Apo C_{II}, which is transferred by HDL to chylomicrons and VLDL, is an activator of lipoprotein lipase. Apo E is transferred by HDL to nascent chylomicrons to form mature chylomicrons.

70–C. Chylomicrons and VLDL have a high content of triacylglycerols. Lipoprotein lipase hydrolyzes the triacylglycerols of chylomicrons and VLDL to fatty acids and glycerol. Blood cholesterol or LDL level is not usually elevated.

71–A. Ketone bodies are synthesized from acetyl CoA. Triacylglycerols are synthesized from fatty acids and glycerol. Cholesterol is used as the backbone for components such as bile salts and steroids.

72–A. Ketone bodies include acetoacetate and 3-hydroxybutyrate. Phosphatidic acid releases inorganic phosphate to form diacylglycerol, which is involved in the synthesis of phosphoglycerides, such as lecithin. Ceramide forms the backbone of sphingolipids.

73–D. The primary component of surfactant is dipalmitoyl phosphatidylcholine (DPPC), also called lecithin. Phosphatidic acid is involved in the synthesis of phosphoglycerides, such as phosphatidylinositol, phosphatidylethanolamine, and phosphatidylserine.

74–C. The backbone of sphingolipids is composed of ceramide. β-Galactosidase is important for degradation of β-galactose–containing sphingolipids. Sphingolipids are formed from serine, not glycerol. Odd-chain fatty acids are oxidized to acetyl CoA and propionyl CoA.

75–E. Patients with Fabry disease have a deficiency of α-galactosidase A, resulting in accumulation of glycosphingolipids in cells. Phosphatidic acid is an intermediate in phosphoglyceride synthesis. Phospholipases hydrolyze phosphoglycerides. Palmitoyl CoA is involved in forming a derivative of sphingosine, which combines with other compounds to form sphingolipids.

76–A. Phenylalanine hydroxylase converts phenylalanine to tyrosine. A defect in this enzyme results in accumulation of phenylketones in the urine, which gives it a characteristic odor. PKU is treated by restriction of phenylalanine in the diet. Serine, glycine, cysteine, and alanine are similar in being derived from intermediates of glycolysis.

77–B. Amino acids release their nitrogen in the form of ammonia or ammonium ion, which is toxic to the central nervous system. Ammonium ion (and aspartate) provides the nitrogen that is used to produce urea. A consistently high-protein diet will increase urea production and excretion by inducing urea cycle enzymes and by making more nitrogenous compounds available for deamination. Transamination is defined as the transfer of amino groups from one amino acid to an α-ketoacid.

78–A. The three branched-chain amino acids are valine, leucine, and isoleucine. Aspartate, citrulline, and arginine are involved in the urea cycle. Glutamate is an important amino acid for transamination reactions.

79–D. Ornithine serves as a carrier that is regenerated in the urea cycle. Serine, glutamate, proline, and leucine are not involved in the urea cycle.

80–A. Homogentisic acid is a product of tyrosine or phenylalanine metabolism. Lysine, threonine, isoleucine, and tryptophan are similar in that they all can form acetyl CoA.

81–C. Phenylalanine forms tyrosine, which forms dopa. Decarboxylation of dopa forms dopamine. Creatine is converted to creatine phosphate by creatine kinase. Nitric oxide induces relaxation of smooth muscle. Serotonin is a neurotransmitter derived from tryptophan. GABA is an inhibitory neurotransmitter produced by decarboxylation of glutamate.

82–D. Folate is reduced in two subsequent reactions, which require NADPH and dihydrofolate reductase, to tetrahydrofolate. The 1-carbon groups that tetrahydrofolate receives are transferred to purine precursors. Thyroid hormone, melanin, catecholamine, and S-adenosylmethionine do not transfer 1-carbon groups to purine precursors and are not required for DNA and RNA synthesis.

83–E. When medications called nitrates enter the blood, they release nitric oxide, which relaxes vascular smooth muscle. Sublingual nitroglycerin is used to dilate coronary arteries if a patient may be having a myocardial infarct. Creatine phosphate is made in the heart, brain, and skeletal muscle. S-adenosylmethionine donates methyl groups to various compounds. Glutathione reduces oxidized proteins. Melatonin is most important in the light-dark cycle and is derived from serotonin (which is derived from tryptophan).

84–B. Thyroid hormones (T_3 and T_4) are produced upon iodination of tyrosine residues and subsequent coupling reactions. Melanin forms pigments in skin and hair and is derived from dopa. Dopamine, norepinephrine, and epinephrine are catecholamines.

85–E. Histamine causes bronchoconstriction, vasodilation, allergic reactions, and stomach acid production. Histamine blockers inhibit this response. Catecholamines are inhibited by monoamine oxidase. S-adenosylmethionine, creatine phosphate, and serotonin are not involved in any of these processes.

86–B. Hypoxanthine-guanine phosphoribosyl transferase (HGPRT) and adenine phosphoribosyl transferase (APRT) are the purine-salvage enzymes. Purine bases can be salvaged by reacting with PRPP to re-form nucleotides. If purine bases cannot be salvaged due to a defect in one of these enzymes, purines will instead be converted to uric acid, which will rise in the blood.

87–B. ADA converts adenosine to inosine. AMP is degraded to adenosine by removal of a phosphate by 5′ nucleotidase. There are two reactions catalyzed by purine nucleoside phosphorylase (PNP): (1) guanosine is converted to guanine and ribose 1-phosphate, and (2) inosine is converted to hypoxanthine and ribose 1-phosphate. Like ADA deficiency, PNP deficiency also results in SCID. Hypoxanthine is converted to xanthine by xanthine oxidase.

88–D. In pyrimidine synthesis, orotate reacts with PRPP, producing orotidine 5′-phosphate, which is decarboxylated to form uridine monophosphate (UMP). Both of these reactions are catalyzed by UMP synthase, which acts as orotate phosphoribosyltransferase and as OMP decarboxylase.

89–C. When it is combined with oxygen, heme gives red blood cells its red color. In heme breakdown, heme is oxidized and cleaved to produce CO and biliverdin, a green pigment. Biliverdin is reduced to produce bilirubin, which has a yellow color. The iron in heme combines with oxygen when it is in the ferrous (Fe^{2+}) state. Heme is produced using the enzyme δ-ALA. Ceruloplasmin is involved in the oxidation of iron. Erythropoietin induces heme synthesis in the bone marrow.

90–E. UDP-glucuronate reacts with bilirubin to form bilirubin monoglucuronide. This reaction is catalyzed by bilirubin uridine diphosphate gluconyl transferase (UDP-GT). Vitamin C increases uptake of iron in the intestinal tract. Iron is in the center of the porphyrin ring in heme. Ceruloplasmin is involved in the oxidation of iron.

91–B. Biotin is an important cofactor in the carboxylation of pyruvate (to oxaloacetate), acetyl CoA (to malonyl CoA), and propionyl CoA (to methylmalonyl CoA). Thiamine pyrophosphate, pyridoxal phosphate, and vitamin B_{12} are B vitamins that also serve as cofactors for other enzymes.

92–E. Vitamin K is involved in the activation of precursors of prothrombin and carboxylation of clotting factors. Deficiency results in bleeding problems. Vitamin A is necessary for light reactions of vision. The B vitamins act as cofactors for enzymes. Vitamin C is important for hydroxylation of prolyl residues in collagen, in the absorption of iron, and as an antioxidant. Vitamin D is involved in calcium metabolism.

93–B. Approximately 2–3 hours after a meal, the liver maintains normal blood glucose by glycogenolysis. Within 30 hours, liver glycogen stores are depleted, leaving gluconeogenesis as the primary process for maintaining normal blood glucose. Ketone bodies are generated, triacylglycerols are broken down, and muscle protein breakdown increases. In the fed state, insulin increases; in the fasting state, glucagon increases.

94–B. In the starvation state (3–5 days of fasting), the body uses its fat stores as its primary source of energy, conserving functional protein. Liver gluconeogenesis decreases, muscle protein is spared, and the brain uses ketone bodies to derive energy.

95–E. Creatinine is derived from creatine phosphate, which is derived from creatine from skeletal and heart muscle. Daily creatinine excretion by the kidney is constant and depends on body muscle mass. Thus, the creatinine clearance rate is used to measure kidney function. The heart, skeletal muscle, brain, and liver are not involved in creatinine excretion.

96–A. Insulin binds to a cell surface receptor that acts as a tyrosine kinase. Hormones such as epinephrine and glucagon activate adenylate cyclase, which converts ATP to cAMP. Hormones such as thyrotropin-releasing hormone (TRH) and oxytocin activate protein kinase C. Subsequent complexes then activate phospholipase C, which cleaves PIP_2 into diacylglycerol (DAG) and inositol bisphosphate (IP_3).

97–D. Aldosterone increases Na^+ absorption in the kidney, and water is resorbed, resulting in an increase in blood volume and blood pressure. Growth hormone stimulates release of insulin-like growth factors and is responsible for proper growth and development. Thyroid-stimulating hormone stimulates release of T_3 and T_4 from the thyroid, which increase basal metabolic rate. Glucocorticoids are important in the response to stress. Epinephrine is the "fight or flight" hormone that stimulates glycogenolysis and lipolysis.

98–C. A surge of LH at the midpoint of the menstrual cycle stimulates the egg to leave the follicle. Initially, FSH acts on immature follicles to promote maturation. Estradiol causes the endometrium to thicken and vascularize in preparation for implantation. After ovulation, the residual follicle secretes both progesterone and estradiol. Progesterone also causes the endometrium to thicken and vascularize.

99–C. 5-α reductase converts testosterone into the more potent androgen dihydrotestosterone (DHT). DHT is responsible for masculinization and growth of the prostate. LH stimulates Leydig cells to produce and secrete testosterone. FSH acts on Sertoli cells to promote synthesis of ABP. Progesterone and estradiol are not affected by finasteride.

100–D. Calcitonin inhibits release of calcium from bone and also decreases calcium levels by stimulating its excretion in urine. For this reason, calcitonin, calcium, and vitamin D may be prescribed to help treat osteoporosis. In contrast, parathyroid hormone promotes calcium and phosphate mobilization from bone, increasing calcium levels. Oxytocin, prolactin, and estradiol are not significant for calcium level regulation.

101–C. Messenger RNA has a cap structure with a poly(A) tail. Nuclear DNA is the B form and contains 10 base pairs per turn. Mitochondrial DNA is double stranded and circular. Ribosomal RNA contains many loops and extensive base pairing. Transfer RNA has a cloverleaf structure and is relatively small.

102–C. Quinolone antibiotics inhibit DNA gyrase, which is a topoisomerase that is only present in prokaryotes. Humans have different topoisomerases than prokaryotes. During DNA replication, helicase unwinds the helix, and single-stranded binding proteins hold it in a single-stranded conformation. DNA polymerase I is involved in repair during DNA synthesis. DNA polymerase III is the replicative enzyme.

103–A. RNA polymerase binds at the promoter region for RNA synthesis. The TATA box is located about 25 base pairs upstream from the transcription start site. The CAAT box is located about 70 base pairs upstream from the transcription start site. A consensus sequence consists of the most commonly found sequence of bases in a given region of all DNAs tested. An enhancer is a DNA sequence that stimulates the transcription rate.

104–B. Small nuclear RNAs (snRNPs) are involved in RNA splicing. A poly(A) tail is added to the 3′ end of the transcript. hnRNA contains introns, which are spliced out in a lariat structure, and only the remaining exons are combined to form mRNA. RNA splicing occurs in the nucleus, and when complete, the mRNA exits the nucleus to the cytoplasm. hnRNA is always the same size or larger than mRNA.

105–B. Endonucleases, exonucleases, a DNA polymerase, and a ligase are involved in DNA repair. Leading and lagging strands and Okazaki fragments are involved in DNA synthesis. Reverse transcriptase converts RNA into DNA. A transposon is a "jumping gene," or mobile DNA element that facilitates movement of genes.

106–A. A missense mutation results when one amino acid is replaced by another. In sickle cell anemia, T replaces A in the β-globin gene, changing the codon GAG (glutamate) to GTG (valine). A nonsense mutation results in premature termination of the growing polypeptide chain (the correct amino acid is replaced by a stop codon). Insertions occur when one or more bases are added to DNA. Deletions occur when one or more bases are removed from DNA. Frameshift mutations occur when the number of bases added or deleted is not in a multiple of three.

107–A. Translation is initiated when methionyl-tRNA$_i$^{Met} binds to the small ribosomal subunit. Elongation occurs with binding of aminoacyl-tRNA to the A site, formation of a peptide bond, and translocation of peptidyl-tRNA to the P site. Translation is terminated when a termination codon occupies the A site.

108–D. A hydrophobic signal sequence at the N-terminus of a secretory protein causes the nascent protein to pass into the lumen of the RER. The signal sequence is cleaved, such that the protein may be glycosylated within the RER. Initiation factor, elongation factor, and peptidyl transferase is involved in protein synthesis. A polysome is a complex of mRNA with multiple ribosomes.

109–C. The *lac* operon is inducible but only in the absence of glucose. If glucose is not present but another sugar is available, *E. coli* produces the proteins that allow the cell to derive energy from that sugar. Binding of the repressor to the operator inhibits transcription. Allolactose activates the *lac* operon. RNA polymerase binds to the promoter to transcribe the operon.

110–A. In prokaryotes, transcription and translation occur at the same time. Eukaryotes contain nuclei, so transcription is separated from translation. In eukaryotes, most cells are diploid, each gene has its own promoter, DNA is complexed with histones, and genes contain introns. These characteristics are not true of prokaryotes.

111–C. Nuclear transcription factors contain amino acid motifs that allow them to bind to DNA. Growth factors, signal transducing proteins, cell cycle regulators, and tumor-suppressor genes do not contain these motifs.

112–C. bcl-2 is an anti-apoptotic gene. Rb is a tumor-suppressor gene that is associated with retinoblastoma. EGF is a growth factor. The Philadelphia chromosome is bcr-abl and is associated with chronic myelogenous leukemia. Ras is the most commonly mutated oncogene in cancer.

113–A. The pro-apoptotic cytokines, TNF and Fas ligand, each activate pro-apoptotic enzymes called caspases. Caspases are proteins that contain cysteine and aspartic acid protease activity, resulting in DNA laddering (fragmentation). Bax is a pro-apoptotic gene activated by p53.

114–D. The HER2/neu oncogene is currently targeted using Herceptin, a monoclonal antibody. Ionizing radiation such as x-rays and γ-rays cause direct damage to DNA, resulting in radiation carcinogenesis. A tyrosine kinase inhibitor, such as Gleevec, has been shown to be effective in treating chronic myelogenous leukemia. Retroviruses have carcinogenic potential by inserting regulatory elements next to cellular proto-oncogenes or by expressing viral homologues (v-oncs) of cellular proto-oncogenes (c-oncs). BRCA-1 is a DNA repair gene implicated in familial breast and ovarian cancer. There is no direct known association between BRCA-1 and HER2/neu.

115–C. The neurofibromatosis (NF)-1 gene product has intrinsic GTPase activity, activating the GTPase function of Ras and converting GTP to GDP. This results in the suppression of the growth-promoting function of Ras. Wilms tumor (WT)-1 is mutated in the most common kidney tumor in children. Cyclin D is a regulator of the G_1 to S transition, and increased expression is commonly found in tumors. Rb, the retinoblastoma gene, is a tumor-suppressor gene that is an important negative regulator of cell growth. p53 functions as the gatekeeper of cellular proliferation. p53 assures adequate DNA repair before proceeding through the cell cycle, and if DNA cannot be repaired, p53 induces pro-apoptotic genes to induce cell death.

116–C. HIV testing starts with an ELISA. If the ELISA is positive, a Western blot is performed. If the Western blot is positive (if the patient's serum contains HIV antibodies that bind to the HIV antigens on the nitrocellulose membrane), then the patient is diagnosed as HIV positive. A Northern blot is when a DNA or RNA probe hybridizes with RNA on a nitrocellulose blot. A Southern blot is when a DNA probe hybridizes with DNA on a nitrocellulose blot. Gel electrophoresis separates DNA, RNA, or proteins based on molecular size. A gel is performed first, and the components are transferred to a nitrocellulose membrane. A restriction endonuclease cleaves DNA into fragments.

117–B. This describes a DNA microarray. mRNA is reverse transcribed into cDNA before being added to the DNA chip. DNA fingerprinting is the detection of variable number of tandem repeats (VNTRs), which differ from one individual to another. DNA sequencing by the Sanger dideoxynucleotide method determines the nucleotide sequence. DNA cloning is when foreign DNA is inserted into a DNA vector and inserted into bacteria. As the bacteria grow, the foreign DNA is replicated, or cloned.

118–C. Polymerase chain reaction (PCR) replicates a much larger amount of DNA from a very small amount of DNA. DNA expression results in generation of mRNA. Genotyping of genomic DNA can detect mutations or polymorphisms. Single nucleotide polymorphisms are single bases in DNA that are different between 99% of individuals. Mapping of the human genome is an attempt to sequence all 3 billion bases.

119–B. Stem cells are pluripotent, undifferentiated cells that can mature into different types of cells. Embryonic stem cells have the potential to become a variety of specialized cell types. Adult stem cells can only differentiate to specialized cell types of the tissue from which they originated.

120–B. RFLPs detect a mutation that occurs in a restriction enzyme cleavage site that is within or tightly linked to a gene. VNTRs are regions of human DNA that differ between individuals. DNA amplification and polymerization can be performed during PCR. DNA can be labeled with radioactivity or substrates that change color.

Index

Page numbers in *italic* designate figures; page numbers followed by the letter "t" designate tables; *(see also)* cross-references designate related topics or more detailed subtopic listings.